Sofa Dodger

Sam Taylor

Copyright © Sam Taylor 2016

Contents

Chapter 1 – The Challenge 8
The 100 List 9
Preparing for the Challenge 13
Chapter 2 - Challenge 1 – 10 15
Nordic Walking – Number 1 15
Bowls – Number 2 17
Boxing – Number 3 19
Cricket – Number 4 21
Body Combat – Number 5 24
Petanque – Number 6 26
Bums, Tums & Thighs – Number 7 28
Baseball – Number 8 31
Yoga – Number 9 34
Croquet – Number 10 36
The Challenge So Far - Number 1 to 10 39
Chapter 3 - Challenge 11 – 20 40
Pole Fitness – Number 11 40
Stand Up Paddleboarding – Number 12 43
Horse Riding – Number 13 46
Fencing – Number 14 48
Powerhooping – Number 15 50
Badminton – Number 16 52
Canoeing – Number 17 54
Trampolining – Number 18 57
Tai Chi – Number 19 60
Handball – Number 20 62
The Challenge So Far - Number 11 to 20 64
Chapter 4 - Challenge 21 – 30 67
Insanity – Number 21 67
Rowing – Number 22 69
Aikido – Number 23 72
Rounders – Number 24 75
Wild Swimming – Number 25 77
American Football – Number 26 80
Running, Number 27 83
Tang Soo Do – Number 28 85

Krav Maga – Number 29..87
Orienteering – Number 30 90
The Challenge So Far - Number 21 to 30 92

Chapter 5 - Challenge 31 – 40 94
Archery – Number 31..94
Coasteering – Number 32 96
Aqua Aerobics – Number 33..98
Ice Skating – Number 34 99
Angling – Number 35..101
Korfball – Number 36..104
Surf Life-Saving – Number 37 106
Pilates – Number 38 108
FitSteps – Number 39..111
Circuit Training – Number 40 113
The Challenge So Far - Number 31 to 40 116

Chapter 6 - Challenge 41 – 50 118
Segway – Number 41... 118
Special Olympics – Number 42.................................120
Judo – Number 43 122
Dodgeball – Number 44..124
Lacrosse – Number 45 126
BarreConcept – Number 46 128
Climbing – Number 47..130
Karting – Number 48..133
Football – Number 49...135
Roller Skating – Number 50 137

Chapter 7 - Challenge 51 – 60 139
Netball – Number 51...139
Karate – Number 52.. 141
Spinning – Number 53...144
Piloxing – Number 54 145
Cheerleading – Number 55 147
Golf – Number 56 150
Rugby – Number 57 153
TRX – Number 58...155
Cardio Tennis – Number 59..158
Snooker – Number 60.. 160
The Challenge So Far - Number 51 to 60 163

Chapter 8 - Challenge 61 – 70 165
Online Exercise Class – Number 61 165
Clubbercise – Number 62 167
Kettlercise – Number 63 169
Table Tennis – Number 64 171

CrossFit – Number 65...173
Gymnastics – Number 66 176
Volleyball – Number 67 179
Kickboxing – Number 68..182
Squash – Number 69 184
Kickboxing Aerobics – Number 70............................186
The Challenge So Far - Number 61 to 70 188
Chapter 9 - Challenge 71 – 80 192
Zumba – Number 71 192
Walk Football – Number 72......................................194
Wrestling – Number 73..196
Wheelchair Rugby – Number 74...............................199
Basketball – Number 75...202
Hockey – Number 76 204
Skiing and Snowboarding – Number 77 & 78...........206
TyreFit – Number 79..209
Dance – Number 80...212
The Challenge So Far - Number 71 to 80 214
Chapter 10 - Challenge 81 – 90 216
Personal Training – Number 81................................216
Parkour – Number 82..218
Buggyfit – Number 83...221
PoolBiking – Number 84 224
Athletics – Number 85..226
Surfing – Number 86 229
Capoeira – Number 87..233
Gaelic Football – Number 88...................................236
Water Polo – Number 89 238
Tennis – Number 90 240
The Challenge So Far - Number 81 to 90 242
Chapter 11 - Challenge 91 – 100 244
New Age Kurling – Number 91 244
Sailing – Number 92 246
Ultimate Frisbee – Number 93 248
Underwater Hockey – Number 94............................251
Shooting – Number 95.. 253
Gig Rowing – Number 96 256
Floorball – Number 97.. 259
Cycling – Number 98 261
Bootcamp – Number 99...263
Wakeboarding – Number 100 266
Chapter 12 - My Five Minutes Of Fame 270
Chapter 13 - My Favourites................................274

Martial Arts 274
Extreme Sports... 276
Individual Sports.. 279
Team Sports 281
Water Sports.. 283
Dance Inspired Fitness Classes 284
Fitness Classes.. 285
Chapter 14 - What Next?.. 288
Chapter 15 - The People Who Inspired Me................ 292
Chapter 16 - Get Involved 341
Chapter 17 - Thanks.. 345

Introduction

This book is a story of my adventures over the course of the year, as I tried 100 different sports and fitness classes in a year, from the highs and lows and everything in between. As well as my own view, some of the coaches, instructors and people I have met along the way have been kind enough to tell me their story about the passion they have for their own activity. I hope you enjoy reading my experiences; it was certainly a unique year for me and one I will treasure forever.

Thanks to everybody who helped me, encouraged me and motivated me throughout, especially my long-suffering family.

Chapter 1 – The Challenge

I am one of those people who have loads of ideas. They germinate, I get excited about them. I convince myself they are world changing ideas and then I dawdle, talk myself out of them and move on to the next hair-brained idea, which will keep me up at night. My last great idea was conceived out of the frustration of not knowing what was going on locally to me. Why did I have to trawl through google to find out what fitness classes were going on, whilst trying to work out what free time I had between dropping kids at their clubs? My big idea was to try and get every fitness class provider, gym and sports club to list on one place and like a TV listing; I could actually find what suited me.

That was a year ago and instead of chucking out the idea, I actually only went and bloody launched the website – I gave birth to it at Easter and I named it SofaDodger.co.uk.

I am very proud of my new bouncy website but it turns out you can't just have a great idea and release it to the world; you have to tell people about it. As I had no money left in the pot, I thought about doing something which would get a bit of publicity. I discussed this with my partner Paul, and he said: "Well, if you are going to do something, go mad and do something big." I gave it some thought, whilst ironically dwelling on my sofa and egged on by a glass of wine, the lightbulb went off and I thought, how about 100 sports and fitness classes in a year?

100 activities are viable – that's only 2 a week for a year. Logistically, it is doable but a quick glance of the mirror suggested other obstacles: I am 35 now, a mother of three kids and the most out of shape I have ever been, due to my love of chocolate and wine! On top of the visual clues as to why this is a bad idea is that I know that I am really unfit, I have no flexibility, no rhythm and I

have never done well in the few experiences of instructor-led classes.

The last time I went to a fitness class was four years ago, when my friend Sarah convinced me to give PUMP ago. I had no idea what it was but thought I would give it a try anyway. Turns out PUMP is hard but made harder when I kept doing it continually wrong. My poor instructor sounded patient but struggled to stifle the irritation in her voice, repeating: "Like this Sam...No, like this." Halfway through she told me I could "Do want I want." The pain in my bingo wings and my embarrassment meant that I didn't go back the week after.

I am more comfortable in a team sports environment. I have played hockey since I was 13 for Bodmin Hockey Club, then Southgate Hockey Club and back to Bodmin, once Paul and I started a family. The benefit for me of playing a team sport is that with my limited willpower, I am expected at training, or I let other people down - letting myself down is far easier than 10 other people down. I am now the oldest and most unfit in the team. Debs, who retired last season at 42, was by far the fittest and would run up and down the wing with relative ease. My excuse of "being too old" never held sway until now, but am I ready to just accept that at 35 it is all downhill from here?

So sat here on my sofa on a Sunday morning, with bleak pouring rain outside and yet another cold, I have decided to start on a daunting journey and take on the challenge of 100 different sports and classes in a year and see what happens.

The 100 List

OK, the decision is made now and I am going to try doing "100 different sports and fitness classes in a year." My general outlook on life since coming up with the idea of SofaDodger is just to carry on until someone tells me that whatever I am doing is a very bad idea and I must stop. I keep waiting for the intervention and still nothing, so I carry on.

First things first: I need to work out which 100 I am going to do. This should be a fairly simple process of elimination, based on the things I am not prepared to do on account of fear of death/heights and excreting in public. People, don't be fooled here; I am a wuss (I have never typed that word before). Anyway, first on the NO list are:

1. Caving
2. Flying
3. Jet Ski
4. Mountain Boarding
5. Paragliding
6. Powerkiting
7. Sand & Land Yachting
8. Skydiving

I have spent a good half an hour on my YES list and reached 91:

1. AeroBiking
2. Aikido
3. Angling
4. Aquafit
5. Archery
6. Athletics
7. Badminton
8. Baseball
9. Basketball
10. Bokwa
11. Bootcamp
12. Bowls
13. Boxercise
14. Boxing
15. Buggyfit
16. Bums, Tums & Thighs
17. Canoeing
18. Capoeira
19. Cardio Tennis
20. Cardio Bike
21. Chair Exercise
22. Cheerleading
23. Circuit Training
24. Clay Pigeon Shooting
25. Cricket
26. Croquet
27. Curling
28. Cycling
29. Dance
30. Darts

31. Dodgeball
32. Fencing
33. Floorball
34. Football
35. Freestyle Martial Arts
36. Futsal
37. Gig Rowing
38. Golf
39. Gymnastics
40. Handball
41. Hockey
42. Ice Skating
43. Insanity
44. Judo
45. Jujitsu
46. Karate
47. Kettlercise
48. Kickboxing
49. Kitesurfing
50. Kung Fu
51. Korfball
52. Krav Maga
53. Lacrosse
54. Netball
55. Nordic Walking
56. Orienteering
57. Personal Training
58. Petanque
59. Pilates
60. Qigong
61. Rallying
62. Rambling
63. Roller Derby
64. Rounders
65. Rugby League
66. Running
67. Sailing
68. Self-Defence
69. Skiing
70. Snooker
71. Spin Class
72. Squash
73. Step N'Tone

74. Street Hockey
75. Surf Life-Saving
76. Surfing
77. Swimming
78. Table Tennis
79. Taekwondo-do
80. Tai Chi
81. Tang Soo Do
82. Tennis
83. Trampolining
84. Triathlon
85. Tug of War
86. Ultimate Frisbee
87. Volleyball
88. Water Polo
89. Windsurfing
90. Yoga
91. Zumba

I am really apprehensive of a high percentage of these activities and the only reason I'm not scared of the others is because I don't know what they are. So now I have to delve into the NO list. I cannot believe that I am committing this to paper/screen but based on the process of elimination by what I am least terrified of, I have gone with:

1. American Football - fits firmly into my fear of death
2. Coasteering – See above and add fear of heights
3. Horse Riding – never been on a horse
4. Ice Hockey – I like hockey but not a fan of ice – 50/50 on this
5. Karting – this could be OK if the kart is a peddle kart
6. Octopush – I think this is underwater and I'm claustrophobic
7. Snowboarding – very un-coordinated, this will end in tears
8. Wakeboarding – already covered most of the phobias around this
9. Wrestling – really? What the hell am I doing!

So there we have it: The List!

Preparing for the Challenge

Since taking this public, I've had a number of adjectives thrown at me but mostly positive ones. My mother is now the only person to convince, as she winces every time I mention the subject. I'm not sure if she thinks I am too unfit, incapable or like me, she has major reservations about me jumping off a cliff when I get to Coasteering!

Maybe she'll come around when she sees the snazzy new t-shirt and hoody that arrived earlier. Obviously, I need to dress the part and when people ask me what I am doing, I can just point to my back. I also thought that anyone behind me in the fitness classes would be distracted from my lack of coordination by reading about my plans. But, in retrospect, I may have ordered them just a couple of sizes too big.

Like a lot of ladies thinking about going to the gym, I'm concerned about what to wear and if my wobbly bits are fully covered as I jump about. Operation "cover the bum" is in full swing. I still need to worry about shorts - or leggings. What do people wear when they exercise indoors now?

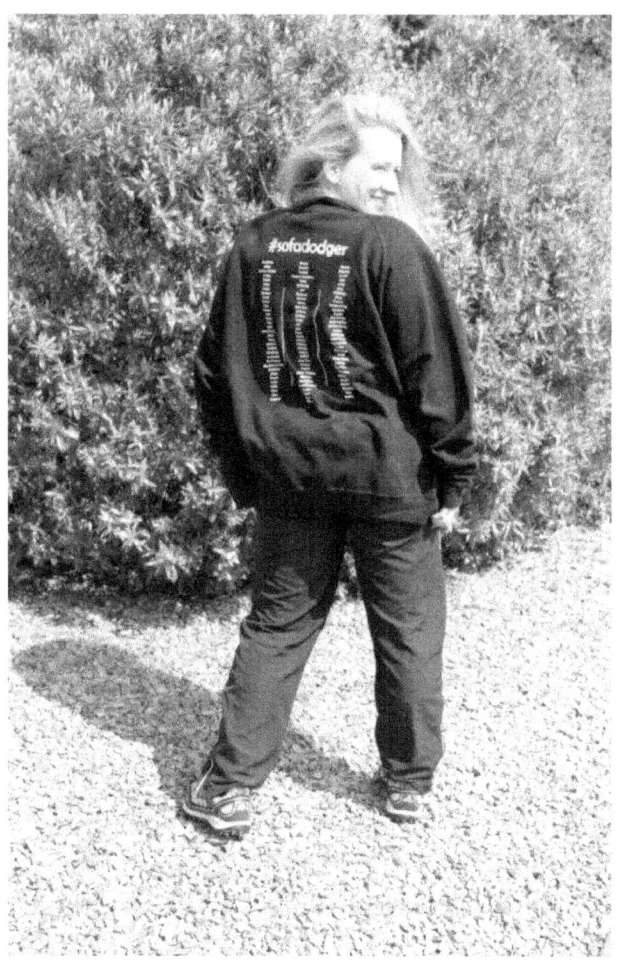

Now that I am togged up, I need to decide what to do first. Luckily, the social media is paying off and I've had a number of clubs/instructors come forward to offer me a taster session or class. One of them was Kelly at Walk Kernow. Now my knowledge of Nordic Walking is pretty limited - it seems to be just walking with sticks. The Nordic part I am sure I will get acquainted with but the walking side of it is still within my comfort zone.

So there is officially no turning back now, as tomorrow I wake up to the start of what I am sure will be the most interesting, challenging and varied years of my life.

Chapter 2 - Challenge 1 - 10

Nordic Walking – Number 1

So finally the day has come; when the talking and typing must stop and I have to actually get off my sofa and start my challenge. After a few ill-advised glasses of wine the night before, I sacrifice an hour of my sacred Saturday morning lie in and drive 45 minutes down to Tresillick Gardens.

I have experience of the benefits of walking - not for myself but my partner Paul, who gets up at 6am and walks with his mate Mat for an hour every morning. He has never been particularly big, as he is one of those irritating people who can eat mostly what they like without putting on weight. If I ate what he ate, I would be 10 times the size. Anyway, after 18 months of walking, he has lost loads of weight and has never been in better shape. He scoffed at the idea of using "sticks" while walking and it does seem fairly alien to use an aid for doing something which is natural to most people. Hopefully, I'll soon find out why they're needed.

I arrive on time and introduce myself to the group of people taking a Beginners Workshop with Walk Kernow. Having the list of my sports on my back really helps explain my challenge, but I start thinking I should have printed it on my front, as I end up having conversations with people reading behind me.

We start with a short introduction of the benefits of Nordic walking, a warm-up and a quick introduction to each other and why we were looking to take up Nordic Walking. A number of people cited the need "to be able to eat cake" whilst not piling on the pounds but generally it was for the health benefits and the motivational aspect of exercising with a group.

Walking in a certain way is easy; adding poles and thinking about walking in another way is tricky. We practise up and down a few times. My main concerns are not tripping over my pole or stabbing any of the curious dogs who were bounding over. Turns out walking up a hill is much easier with poles, as it helps with your posture and is particularly good if you suffer from a sore lower back. Kelly tells us that Nordic walking burns 46% more calories than walking itself. The cake eaters among us lap that bit of information up as we look around smugly at the dog walkers, who are poleless and obviously not in the know.

Having mastered our basic techniques, we set off for a woodland walk. The scenery around this National Trust estate is absolutely stunning and as I walk through the bluebells, with the coast on the other side, I wonder if I would find my 99 other activities as enjoyable. Walking is great for allowing chatting as well, and I met some really interesting people. The chats were interspersed with further instruction and techniques to conquer pesky obstacles such as stairs and hills. We got the techniques really quickly - until Kelly came over to check on us. Somehow, you'd then immediately forget what you'd been doing for the past hour and completely mess it up!

By the finish of the walk, we had covered 4 miles with several stops. I could feel my arms aching. Kelly assured us we would wake up and "gently ache" all over. Although this is only my first activity and I'm planning to try all types of activities, I can definitely see me taking up Nordic Walking after my challenge. It is lower intensity than running but apparently, mile for mile; you can burn as many calories as a runner. Yes, it will take longer to get somewhere but it's gentler on the joints. It's also very social, as you get to walk a couple of times a week with a group of people.

After a warm down, I wave goodbye to everybody, who all wish me luck with my challenge, and head for a slice of guilt-free cake in the cafe. So, one down and 99 to go.

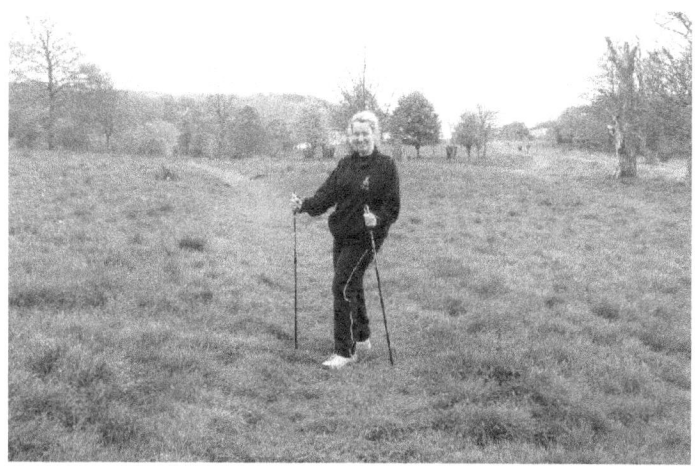

Check out my poles!

Bowls – Number 2

I am not silly; I know that with my current level of fitness, I will probably break if I try and join a running club or cycling club this early into my challenge. Bowls, therefore, seems like a good second sport to progress with. In fact, it is not just bowls; it is short mat bowls – not to be confused with Bowling Crown, Bowling Flat Green, Bowling Indoor, Lawn Bowls or Outdoor Bowls.

I'm enthusiastically welcomed into the Village Hall by Blisland Short Mat Bowls Club. Given the time of day (Tuesday afternoon) it's no surprise that most of the players looked retirement age but don't be fooled: this is a competitive and skilful game. Betty was also "new" and she told me not to worry. However, Betty didn't tell me that she was only new to the club and was actually a county player!

There are two green mats laid over the hall floor and this is where the action happens – clever really, as unlike their outdoor sibling sport, they are not interrupted by the English weather. I like watching most sports, but I've never watched a game of bowls in my life and am a bit perturbed to see a long wooden obstacle in the middle of the floor. This is definitely going to cramp my style. After smacking my first attempt into the floor, as if I'm going to score a strike in the ten-pin variety, and knocking down the wooden slab, it soon becomes clear that I might need to change tactics. Steady and smooth, not fast and furious, is the order of the day.

Everybody's very encouraging and clap whenever my ball doesn't go off the mat. However, I must have a latent competitive streak because there's no way I'm leaving until I hit the jack. After an hour and a half, I hit the damned thing, which is met with riotous applause and "she's a natural...sign her up!"

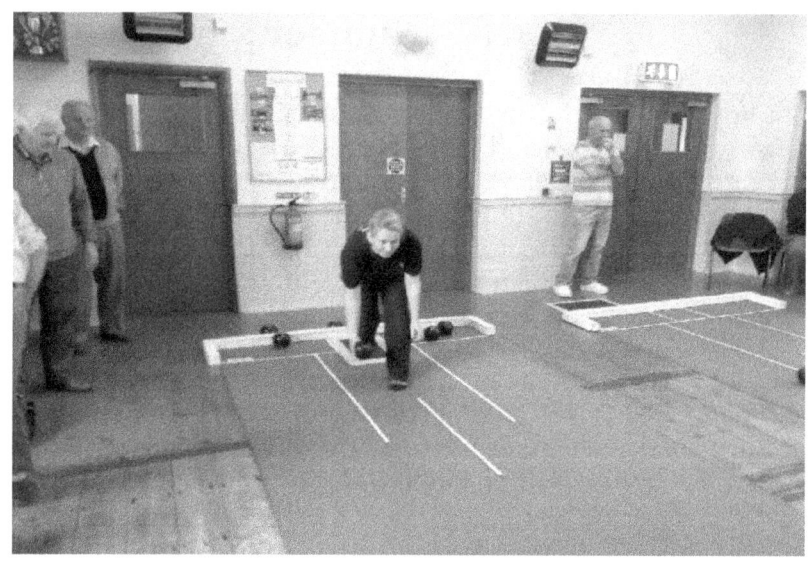

Getting the hang of it

I worked out that I must have a 5% hit rate, but I decided to retire at that point. I helped score 2 points for my side and I left on a high.

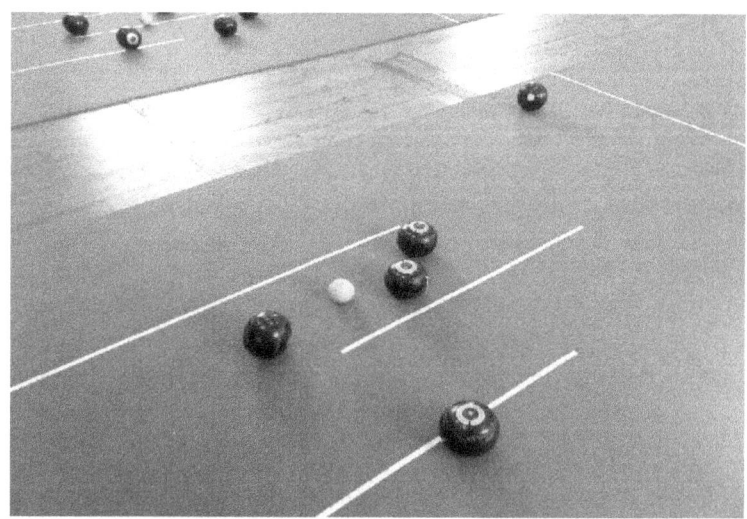

Mine are the two at the top

I know I've only done 2 of my challenges and I don't want to get too far ahead of myself but I have a feeling there is a sport for everybody. Although bowls is no way just a sport for older people, approximately 775,000 older people (that's 7% of those aged 65 or over in the UK) say they are always or often feel lonely. That's a tragic situation when there are so many clubs and activities up and down the country. At Blisland, the members can play competitively or just enjoy playing the game on the afternoons they meet up, so is an ideal activity for anybody who's interested in meeting new people and taking up a new challenge. There was a lot of banter and a cuppa in the interval. I was also offered the chance to do bell ringing, but that isn't on the list!

Boxing – Number 3

Yesterday, I was at Bodmin Boxing Club, run by Denis. Immediately, the list of sports on my back was scrutinised and boxercise was roundly scoffed at...I sensed a certain sneering at its gym counterpart and I can't wait to see what boxercise say about boxing.

And so to the warm-up, where I was sent to run after a young, fit guy: maybe this boxing malarkey wouldn't be so bad! The young, fit guy had lapped me within a few minutes and I went my usual, attractive, beetroot colour.

Next was skipping. So far, so Rocky. The guys faced the floor-to-ceiling mirror on one of the walls. I generally have a policy of avoiding full-length mirrors and went to one side, facing the non-judgemental wall. These boys could skip! They were like galloping steeds, changing speed and putting in bursts of effort, while I looked like a My Little Pony....a chubby little My Little Pony, cantering along as though I was looking for a 4-leaf clover in a field of rainbows! Skipping went on for three bursts over 10 minutes and was an absolute killer on the bingo wings.

Then it was sprints, or for me, jogging and then walking fast. I must say, I was really admiring the effort those guys were putting in. Once warmed up and dripping with sweat, it was on to shadow boxing. Denis told me I had to learn in front of the damned mirror. Left foot forward, right leg back, left for jabbing, right for something else. The lads next to me were making swooshing noises with their fists and dancing backwards and forwards – I looked like I was fencing and when I threw a punch, I resembled a beetroot, which wouldn't pose a threat in a salad bowl!

Then, it was onto the serious stuff and on with the gloves and onto the bags. Denis's daughter Rachel gave me some tips on technique. To counteract my bouncing, she told me to imagine there was a piece of paper under my feet and I had to slide the paper. That helped. Then work on my left jab, punch high and control the bag. The interval bell rang and Denis beckoned me into the ring for some "light sparring." Light sparring for me is not doing a full shop at the local convenience store; I was unprepared to actually go in the ring.

Denis bounced about with gloves on, whilst giving punch instructions – left jab, right hook, left upper cut, etc. It was absolutely knackering. I have a new respect for the boxers who stand up for 12 rounds. At my current fitness level, I'd struggle with one. Denis told me that the club supports all levels – they could accommodate unfit novices like me, to juniors, right through to national contenders. I am definitely going to suggest to the hockey team that we come for a pre-season fitness session!

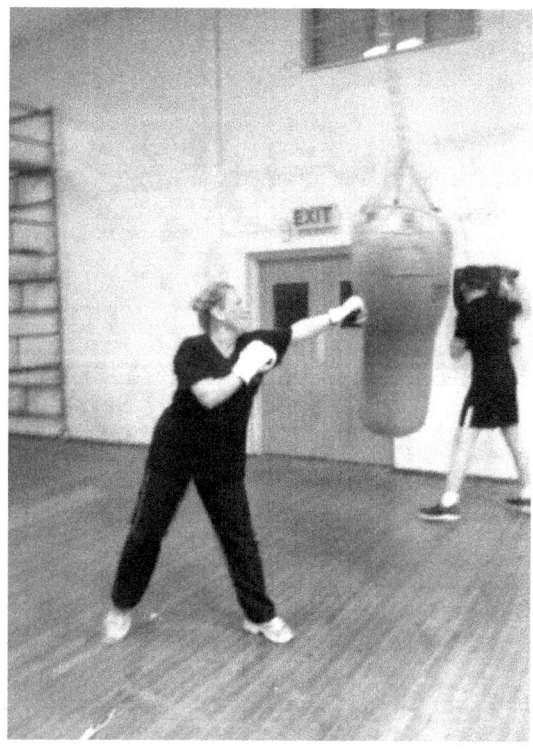

Take that bag!

We were then instructed to get into the ring to "ab crunch" and got given a medicine ball and some more exercises to do. The guys were putting it in: I sat back in awe and used my medicine ball as a back rest. After some warm down stretches (which I was really good at) it was time to go.

I didn't expect to like boxing but it was really exhilarating, not just to push my body but to try something I'd never done before. It wasn't in any way elitist and I was welcomed and encouraged. Certainly, if I kept this up after my challenge, I wouldn't ever become a champion boxer, nor would I want to, but I would be really fit.

With Nordic Walking, I was told I would "gently ache" the next day. With boxing, I was told I would "ache like hell" the day after tomorrow. And as for getting my 6 pack, I think I'll just stop and pick some up at the local Spar.

Cricket – Number 4

Last night was sport number 4: cricket at Wadebridge Cricket Club. This session was going to be a bit different, as 3 of the hockey girls (Tamar, Sugar and Tara) came along to give it a go. I was a little unsure as to whether they would cramp my style, but thought it would be different to go along with friends.

At this point, I will fess up that I am or was a complete cricket nerd. I don't like cricket, no, no, I love it and this sentence will only make sense if you know the song! So much of a nerd that when I was a teenager I watched every ball of the 1994-1995 Ashes series, played in Australia. I was never into bands or popstars; my pin-up was Darren Gough. I followed England in the 90s when they were rubbish. I even have a 2005 Ashes injury from when I jumped up at Hoggard's match-winning eighth-wicket partnership with Ashley Giles and I took a painful lump out of my knee. People, I love cricket - but I have never played.

Sure, I have knocked about on a beach with a tennis ball but never have I used a proper cricket ball. So when picking it up for the first time, I was surprised how light it was. Immediately, I set about polishing the knackered old ball nicely around the seam, just to help with my turn. My hockey friends asked what the hell I was doing. I ignored them.

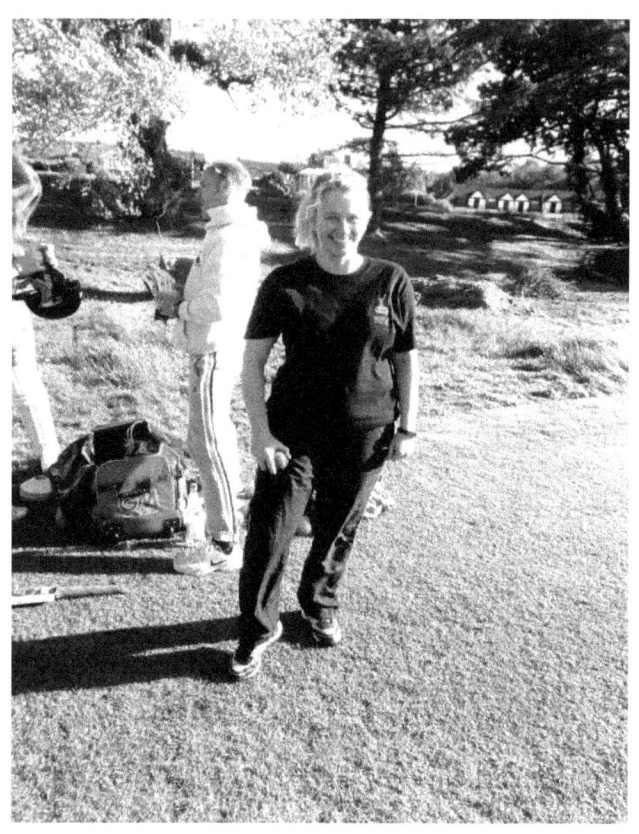

Pro Shining

First things first. Before I could unleash my pent-up yorker, we had to warm-up, which was led by Coach Mark. The hockey girls are a competitive lot, so took this on with vigour. After we had thrown, rolled and caught, we moved on to the nets. This was my time. I largely ignored the coaching instructions provided - I knew how to bowl. I took a couple of steps run up, gripping the ball and aiming for middle stump. I released the ball and it went flying over the nets into the grass to my left. This was the first of many bowling disappointments of the evening.

Thankfully the hockey girls were equally rubbish at bowling. We regrouped and decided that batting was definitely our thing, given that we hit hockey balls around on a Saturday. Two by two, we went into the nets to give it a go. Tara was no Lara, which I chortled at her. She looked blankly at me. I was in next. Again, I channelled my inner Pietersen, whilst putting on the pads and getting ready to face my first ball in anger. Unfortunately, as my friends were equally useless at bowling, it took about 3-4 balls before I could face anything I could actually hit. The first ball I went for, I smacked the bat into the wickets...dammit! Wickets back and a step forward then I was away. I absolutely loved it. I am sure if the nets weren't in the way, I would have been consistently scoring boundaries. Probably...possibly.

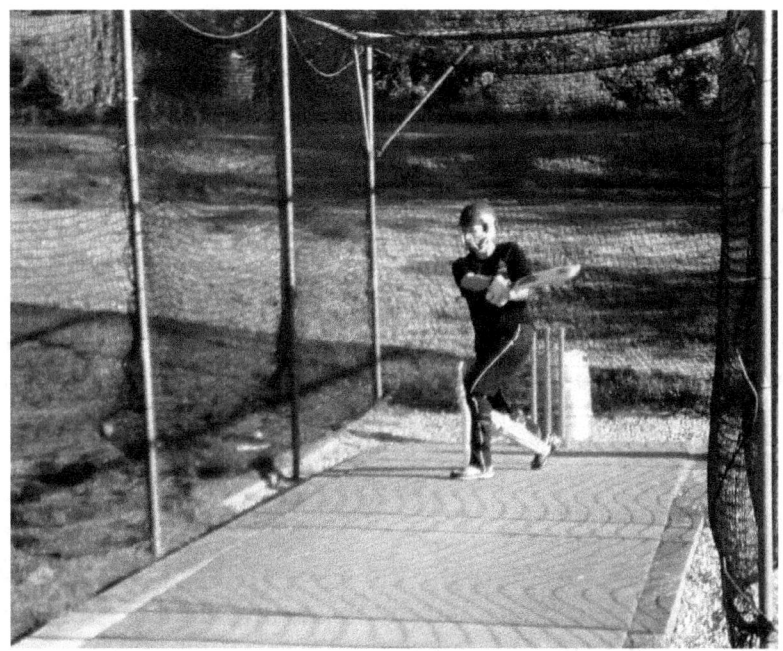

Take that ball

The session was a really chilled out one, with passers-by wandering past and watching family members of those playing encouraged to have a bowl. After reluctantly giving up the bat, we moved onto catching and throwing. I liked throwing. As a bit of a tomboy at school, I had worked hard not to have a "girly" throw. I was also good at catching but that was with a tennis ball. This ball is hard and I really wasn't keen on trying to catch this one.

So batting - tick, throwing - tick, bowling - fail, catching - fail. Never mind, there are some cricketers who have had successful careers focusing on only one of them!

The hockey girls enjoyed themselves and hopefully we can get the cricket ladies to come and give hockey a go when our season starts again. Maybe there is something in "sport-swapping" when you are out of season?

As for me, I'm delighted to have given something a go which I have always wanted to do. It's never too late. If you have always wanted to ride a horse or jump on a trampoline, go do it! You may only do it once but definitely, do it. Life is short. You have to make your own opportunities and memories.

Body Combat – Number 5

The sun is finally out and that usually in my book, means one thing at the end of the day, sitting in the garden with a glass of something chilled.

However, this is a different day to my usual day, as I am attending a gym class down at The Core in Falmouth to try Body Combat. I love wine in the sun. I hate Lycra. I hate me in Lycra, so I was already sulking before I had to leave. One hour previous, I had emptied the drawer where I keep my old sports clothes, onto my bed and rifled through, deciding what to wear. I don't even know what people wear in the gym these days. I have been to one gym class in the past 6 years. Me in Lycra running shorts is not a good look – thankfully I have the world's biggest T-Shirt to cover the lumps, bumps and camel toe!

Apart from my relationship with wine, I have a new and recent friend, which I am embracing and this is my FitBit. A FitBit is an activity tracker, worn around your wrist that tells you how many calories you burn, steps you take, etc. I gave one to Dad last Christmas, which he neglected to do anything with, so I've repossessed it for the purposes of my challenge. Although weight loss isn't the point of this challenge, it would be a welcome by-product.

After an unplanned 25 minutes stuck in rush hour traffic, I was in full flapping mode, as I rushed to find the gym, find somewhere to park and actually find the door to get inside the building. Ironically, the building was set in between a pub and an Italian restaurant, two places that I would much rather be just then. But I was welcomed in by a very friendly guy, who pointed me in the direction of the changing area and then into the class itself.

Immediately, I recoiled at the 360-degree mirrors. I don't need to see my Lycra-clad arse in 3D. Then the first thing I had to do was figure out where the back was, so I could tuck myself away and make my mistakes out of the full glare of the instructor. Body Combat is a martial arts based aerobics class, set to high energy music, where you punch, jab and karate kick throughout. I wondered what Denis from my boxing challenge would feel about this bastardised version of boxing.

As a class, it was something I could follow...for maybe 75% of the time. I was mostly out of time and had to apologise to the token man next to me for nearly kicking him. It was intense but to give me extra encouragement my FitBit buzzed in approval, which meant I must be actually working out (equally it could have meant the battery was low). My FitBit has never buzzed before. I am working out, people!

Body Combat was enjoyable and it certainly worked arms and legs but I am pretty gym-phobic, so it's going to take more than one class to make me feel at ease in this environment. 15% of my challenge will be in a gym class, so it will be interesting to see if I get over my phobia at all. It was a good start – they seemed a friendly lot and the instructor didn't point out my mistakes and try to "help" me, which I have found mortifying in the past. I certainly drove back feeling more energetic and my mood had lifted. When I got back, I looked momentarily at the wine in the fridge, but then poured myself a glass of water instead.

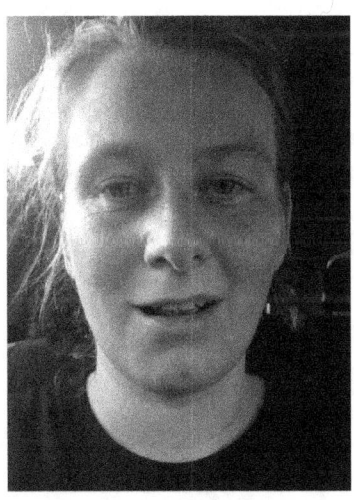

How knackered do I look after?

Petanque – Number 6

I've spoken to about a dozen people so far about this challenge and only one person had heard of petanque, so I was intrigued to join the guys at Tregony Petanque Club yesterday evening to find out more about it. From my research on YouTube, I felt my Fitbit and sports bra were not required for this particular sport.

I arrived on a beautifully sunny evening at the Village Sports Club, where I met Graeme and his wife Susan. As I was early, I was given a run through of the history and basics of the sport. My first question was how you pronounced it: I don't want to be regaling some hapless listener with my story of trying it out and getting it wrong. Apparently it is pronounced P-TONK and it hails from France, where it is widely played and very popular.

The game is played on a rectangular, gravel playing area. No line painting here, as a stick is sufficient to mark out playing circles. Graeme took me through the health and safety aspect of the sport, which basically comprised of not throwing a boule at somebody's head. You certainly wouldn't want a direct hit by one of these metallic balls as they are fairly heavy (apparently a jam jar and a half in weight.) I imagined hitting somebody with a king-sized jam jar. Maybe this was an extreme sport after all?

Unlike when I tried bowling, the idea isn't to bowl underarm but to grip the ball with your fingers and flick it out of your hand, aiming for the little jack. Now, I'm not foolish enough to think I could pick up tactics and gameplay in one session for any of my sports, so I try to focus on just one element of the game. In this case, it's to try and bowl the ball as near to the jack as possible and hope that my fellow contenders fail to disturb my attempt.

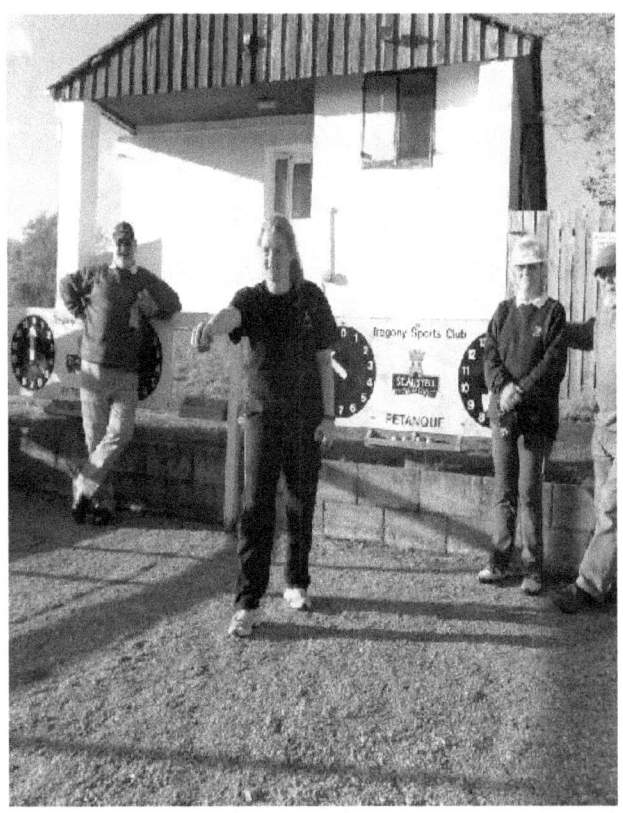

Pre-throwing stance

Technique is a tricky business, so before we were joined by the rest of the club, I managed to get my practise in and stay out of the limelight. A further 8 people arrived and after introductions and the obligatory inspection of the list of sports on the back of my back, the game commenced. At this point, I was asked if I wanted a drink and a couple of people then skipped off to the sports club bar, reappearing with several pints. The sport immediately jumped up in my rankings, as it was rapidly ticking off my favourite things:

1. being outside
2. being outside in company
3. being outside in company, in the sun
4. being outside in company, in the sun, drinking a pint of cider.

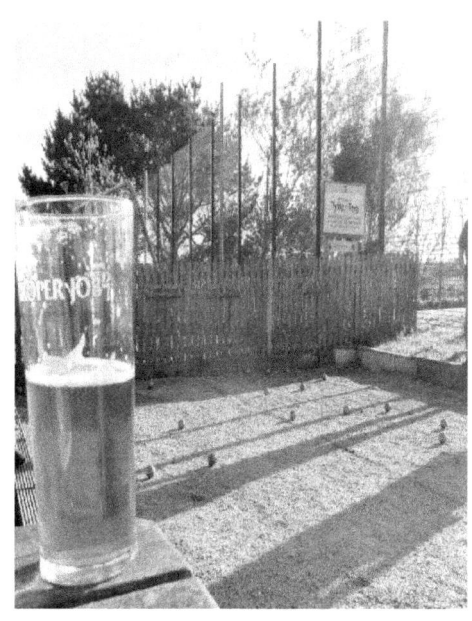

A Proper Job Sport

So far, so good. Now, I just had to prove myself in the game play situation. Getting close to the jack would be easier if we weren't playing on gravel, where one rogue stone would change the direction of the boule completely. I embraced this excuse until I actually got better at throwing and my attempts weren't so wild. I think at one point, I even scored a point for my team, which received much congratulation.

Again, petanque seems to be played at any level, from the players who played in the County championships to the more social and novice players. And I'm sensing a common theme here – the club were very friendly, very welcoming and very social. So much fun, in fact, I am just about to go online and get myself a beach version for the family to play!

Bums, Tums & Thighs – Number 7

You know when you've had a good old workout; you can't walk down stairs or bend down the next day! I am now in this very position. This is because I voluntarily went to what can only be described as low-level torture session, disguised as a Bums, Tums and Thighs class yesterday at Lakeview Country Club.

Due to my gym phobia and a dislike of the horrible pre-class hanging around, when you don't know anybody and you just look at your phone and wait for the instructor, I decided to invite my friend, Sarah along. Sarah is currently on a fitness drive and she is also great at photography, so could take some pictures.

Kai, the very lovely instructor, started with a "warm-up." Now, a warm-up in my book is a gentle stretching but no, this was Kai's warm-up, whereby we would run and sprint on the spot. The class progressed to all types of crunches, stretches and culminated in a "bear relay". This was a personal low for me as I frolicked ungracefully like a monkey, with my arse in the air and my knees slightly bent. There is no picture of this: there will never be a picture of this.

Once our dignity was fully spent, we got to take a field trip outside to take some of the class in the fresh air. We were promised that it wouldn't be in front of windows, as the thought of bear racing, in front of a holidaying family of four as they ate their dinner, made me queasy. We continued our punishing workout outside with the benefit of a slight breeze, which was more than welcome. At this point, I had mouthed "Sorry" to Sarah approximately half a dozen times.

Next, Kai ushered us in front of a steep bank and told us to sprint up and down it 5 times. Kai was relishing our reluctance and answered the groans by walking on his hands. We finished off with everybody's nightmare – burpees! After skipping back to the class, we had 12 minutes left. *Phew*, I thought, *a warm down*. Oh no, no warm down; that happened 30 seconds to the end. This was where the phrase "no pain, no gain" comes in.

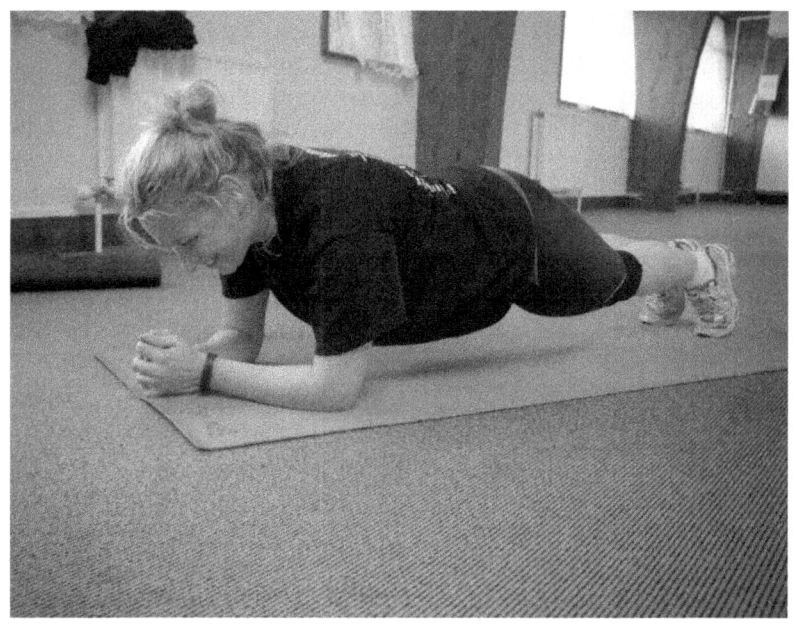

Do I look a plank?

We concentrated on the thighs, as we hoisted one leg in the air and rotated it to start and then did several kicks, whilst still not letting it go down. I felt the cramps and as soon as Kai went to address the music situation and his back was turned, I lay sprawled flat out. When he turned back, I immediately resumed the pose. We finished the class with some yoga positions and we were done. Everybody looked suitably knackered.

As soon as I dropped Sarah home, I went to check what FitBit thought of my evening. Surely it would be pleased with me? Apparently, FitBit doesn't measure pain and effort and told me patronisingly that I had moderately worked out. FitBit is now FitBitch!

The saving grace for my aches and pains is that I lost 2lbs – which is quite a triumph and would make me consider going back again. The first time must be the worst. It was also a good class for me, as it wasn't rhythmic. This is where I know I struggle, so roll on Zumba.

Sarah must be really cross with me, though, as she has just sent me over the pictures and she has photoshopped in a couple of chins in the pictures, which is very naughty!

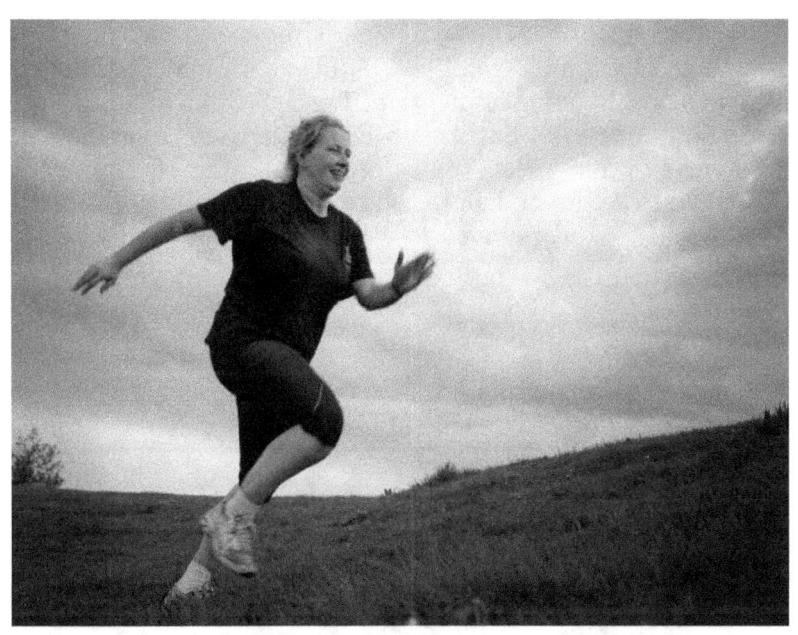

Sarah must have photoshopped in some chins on me!

Baseball – Number 8

With my list of 100 sports, I have categorised them in my mind in 3 sections: excited to try, sceptical and dreading it. Baseball fits into the first. It is the most popular game in the US, with 40 million people playing some form of the game and it is one of the fastest growing sports in the UK but, unfortunately, those facts are not reflected in my home county of Cornwall, as we don't have a team. So, off I go to my first "away" cross-border fixture in Torquay, home to the Torbay Barons.

In the films, you see flood lit, huge stadiums with thousands of roaring spectators. In Torquay, it happens on the playing field, behind the leisure centre, encircled by dog walkers. I am now getting used to randomly rocking up and interrupting a team's training session. Mid-introduction to Laurence (who runs the team) and the rest of the guys, I mentally kick myself for forgetting to pack my baseball cap to complete the look.

After introductions, Laurence hands me a baseball mitt to try on. This specially imported glove is heavy. In fact, it feels like I have half a cow hanging off my arm. The first thing to master is the catching. Sounds easy, but it does feel quite alien. Imagine a crab with a glove on its pincer; this is my initial attempts before I was encouraged to catch the ball in the centre of the mitt, which made far more sense. I also moved to a lighter glove, which was much better.

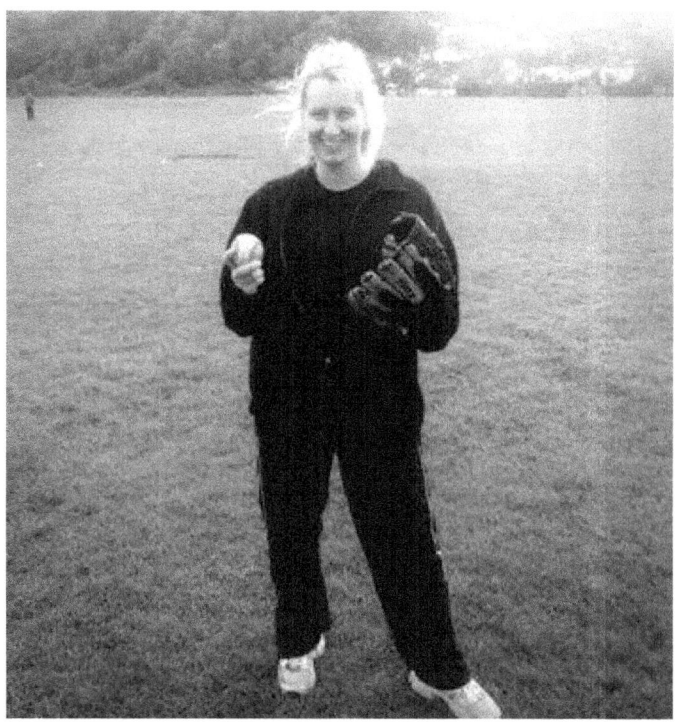

Smitten with my mitten

After a bit of catching, we went to a game situation and I tried to select the place in the pitch where I would cause the least damage to my team. The first time seeing a ball pitched is quite something to behold: this thing travels! So much so, that getting a connection with the ball doesn't happen that often. However, when it does, the ball is collected in the field and in most cases thrown to first base. My self-allocated job was to clap – a mitt muffled clap which produced no noise.

Unfortunately, my catching seems to be a massive weakness and as with cricket, this is what continually lets me down. When the ball is hit in the air and I have to get under it to catch it, I follow a 4 step process. Firstly, I emit a noise like a pterodactyl. Secondly, I swear – usually one word which I stretch out for at least three seconds. Thirdly, I duck and cover. Lastly, after the ball lands beside me, I apologise. I call it the old SH approach to catching: SHOUT, SH*T, SHELTER and SHAME – not to be found in any good coaching manual. The lads were very encouraging and pointed out that I "covered the space" well as the batter jogged triumphantly around the diamond for a home run.

Just as I was getting into the banter and my confidence was building, it was my turn to bat. Having seen the ball being pitched at somebody's thumb, somebody's thigh and lastly somebody's head, I wasn't relishing giving it a go. However, I didn't want to be pity pitched to (I have a bit of self-respect and pride) but at the same time, I didn't want to go home with a trophy bruise. I was given a quick tutorial on holding and swinging. The catcher behind reiterated that I had to keep hold of the bat, not let go of it and hit him on the head (he was the one who had just been hit in the head with the ball).

As I couldn't pitch and couldn't catch, I was determined to hit the thing and hit it I did. In fact, I managed to connect most of the time, which was really exhilarating. I have hand-eye-ball coordination, people. I have some sort of co-ordination! If only there were piñata style dances on a dance floor, I would no longer be ridiculed.

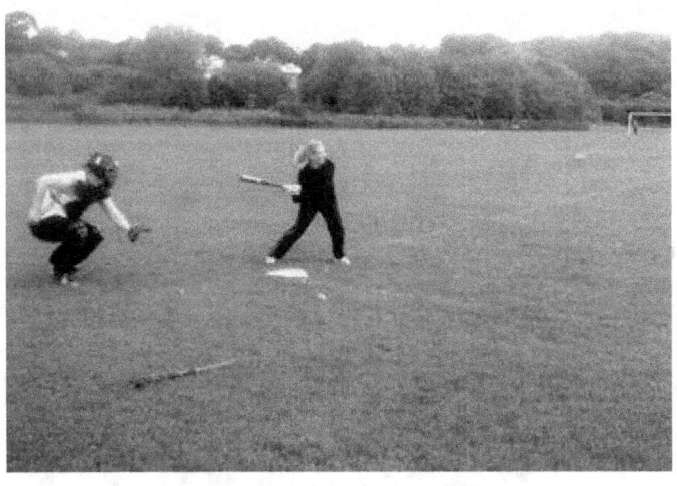

Bitchin' with the pitchin'

We finished up with a "whoever catches the ball can go home" activity. Obviously, given my previous attempts, I expected to be there until dusk. Being last, I did encourage a pity throw and on my first attempt, caught the damned thing without squawking! Progress!

Baseball didn't disappoint at all. I mockingly suggested to friends beforehand that it was just rounders with a hat but certainly there is a lot of skill involved and providing you can find a team near you, I would definitely encourage anybody, young or old, to give it a go. Don't forget the hat, though!

Yoga – Number 9

Since I started writing about my adventures I have found that my writing style leans toward the self-deprecating. I assumed, therefore that yoga, my number 9 challenge, would be rich pickings. I could talk about my fear of flatulence whilst in a pose, with either me being the emitter or the receiver. Or the fact, that I forgot that it was bare-foot and I hadn't re-painted my half chipped toe-nail paint or that I wore my Lycra shorts instead of loose fitting bottoms like everybody else. However, this bit will be different and dare I say it, a bit emosh (which is, I gather, a trendy word for emotional). I actually found something I truly connected with.

I tried yoga once before, and that was pregnancy yoga 12 years ago, when I was carrying my first child. We lived in North London then and I took myself off to Crouch End to give it a go. I must have found myself in an advanced class because I certainly couldn't follow the instructions, the group felt clique-y and I remember leaving feeling slightly humiliated. Until now, it has put me off going back again. But I'm doing a challenge and yoga is on the list.

I was invited by Aimee at the Cornwall Yoga Centre to try out two different styles of yoga; the first being Vinyasa, which is, I would say a fairly physically demanding form of yoga. Aimee took us through a built up sequence of poses, with a further link added after each repetition. Instead of clock-watching, which I invariably do in any type of class, I was surprised when the hour had finished.

To get a more balanced overview of yoga, Aimee invited me to the general class, which followed on. In contrast, this was a far less physically intense form, where we focused on movement and breathing. Aimee's gentle voice guided us through the steps and we concentrated on different parts of the body.

The session culminated in a meditative focus on breathing and mentally identifying parts of the body to be thoughtful of. At this point, laying on the mat, under a blanket, I stopped doing what I was told and my thoughts drifted away to what I was like when I entered the building. Getting through rush hour traffic, finding the building, finding a parking spot, checking my phone, checking that the battery was charged in the camera... I had been just a ball of frenzy and now lying there, it felt peaceful. It felt quiet. It felt quite alien.

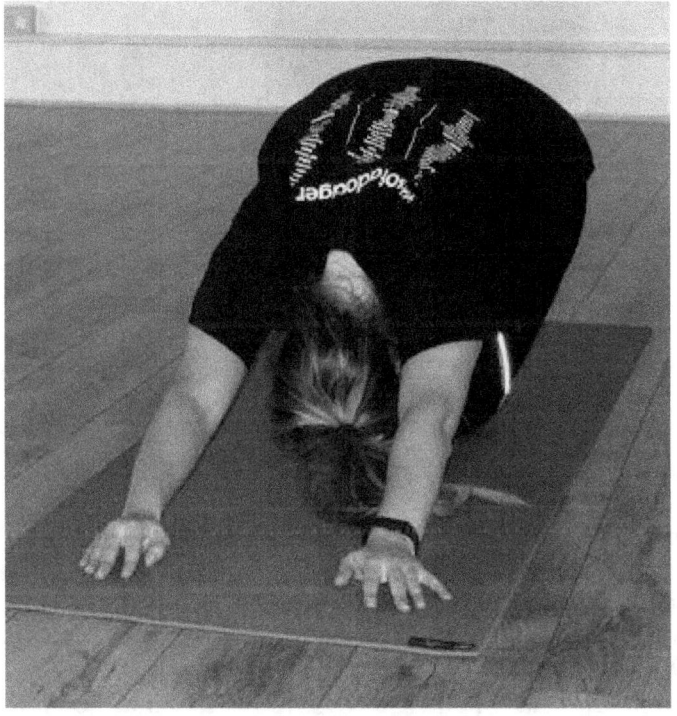

As I drove home, I thought about those alien feelings. As a busy mum of three primary aged children, my life is non-stop with afterschool clubs and play dates. I also run two businesses; I am the club secretary of the local hockey club and am taking on this mad challenge of trying this bewildering number of activities in a short period of time. Don't get me wrong, I have a very happy and fulfilled life and I count my blessings every day but sitting in the car on the journey home, I started to cry.

I seemed to have tapped into something, which maybe I didn't know I needed: quiet. Some time to stand still, to breath and reflect. The tears weren't from a place of self-pity. It reminded me a little of the scene in Pretty Woman when Vivian is taken to the Opera for the first time and cries. She cries out of wonder and discovery. Maybe she cried because it was like finding a new friend, who she didn't know was missing in her life. That was why I cried and when this crazy year is over, I know that I will come back looking for this new friend.

Croquet – Number 10

After my rather emotional yoga experience, I was glad that my next challenge gave me the chance to hit a ball; something I'm far more comfortable with. Off I went to the Cornwall Croquet Club in Porthpean and I couldn't have picked a more beautiful afternoon. I was introduced to a multitude of friendly -if not - perplexed faces. I did stand out slightly in my black tracky bottoms and black T-Shirt, contrasting with the Wimbledon whites everybody else was sporting. The initial confusion as to my attendance was replaced with warm enthusiasm and questions about why I was doing what I was doing. Good question and my answer tends to change on different days and how I progress. I decided to think on it later.

Croquet is played in two teams with two players on each side. The aim is to hit the ball through the hoops and unlike golf, you do not finish a hole and pick up the ball, you carry on the last shot to the next hoop. First to 7 hoops wins. This all seemed quite straightforward. After my baseball challenge and the discovery that I possess hand- eye- ball coordination, my confidence was running high. This was just hitting the ball. I had no catching or bowling to worry about, so bring it on and where was my Pimms?

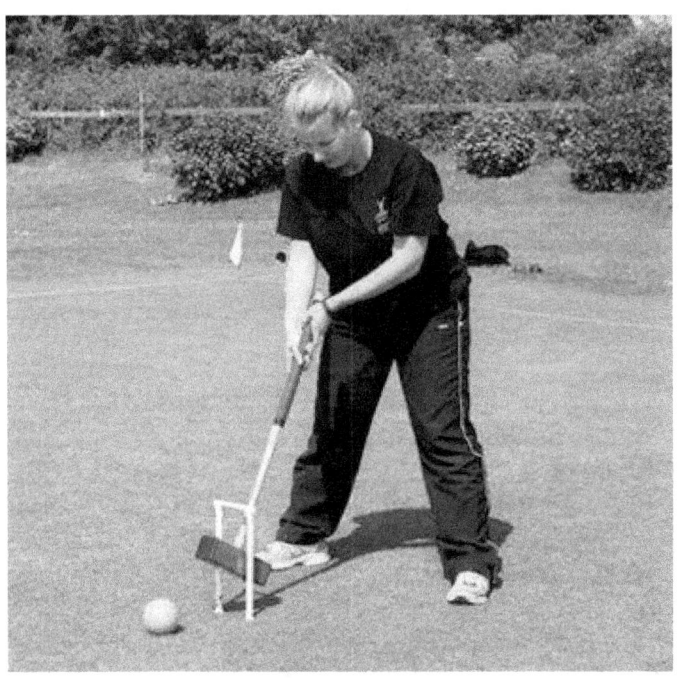

Ball through hoop

Preconceptions over, I was paired with Ron, the team coach. Poor Ron probably made the journey that day looking forward to improving his own game. Instead, he was paired with a complete novice. I was given my own mallet and the basic instruction of holding and hitting the ball. I took a few swings and on the third or fourth attempt, I worked out that you had to swing the mallet through your legs to get the required welly to move the ball more than a metre.

While the game continued, I carried on practicing my shots. For no particularly good reason and thankfully out of sight, I forgot the main principle of having your legs apart when taking the shot and proceeded to swing the heavy mallet into my own leg. You may not have swung a mallet into your own leg before, but let me tell you, it hurts! In order to maintain dignity, I covered my grimace with a smile and corrected the hobbling gait that my body wanted to adopt. In hockey, we have shin pads on, so I'm not used to shin ache.

I found the game very reminiscent of snooker, where you can almost snooker an opponent. It was chess-like in its strategy, with Ron obviously thinking 3 or 4 shots ahead, while I focused on not inflicting further damage on myself. When I started to get the hang of it, I played a few half decent shot, with the ball going roughly where I wanted it to go. Ron and I progressed to a 3 hoop lead, with the end clearly in sight. With this knowledge, my very rudimentary progress ground to a sudden halt when I essentially missed an open goal. With all of 20 centimetres between my ball and the unopposed hoop, I missed it. It was harder to miss than to put the damn thing through the hoop! I am the Torres of croquet.

I then effortlessly moved from one embarrassment to another. Ron coached me on where the ball should go. I then overshot it and usually in the wrong direction. I believe I have invented a new type of shot – the banana shot. At 6 all and with one hoop to get, Ron pretty much abandoned me and took matters into his hands. He would never get a cup of tea with me cocking it up the whole time. With a few deft swings, he single-handily won the last hoop and I unashamedly celebrated for being on the winning team.

I can see the game is one of skill and strategy and again very enjoyable on a beautiful day. It seems ironic to me that I have boxed and played baseball and I get an injury playing croquet. I went home to ice my injury and used half of the ice cubes in a tea towel for my swelling, and the other half for my glass of Pimms!

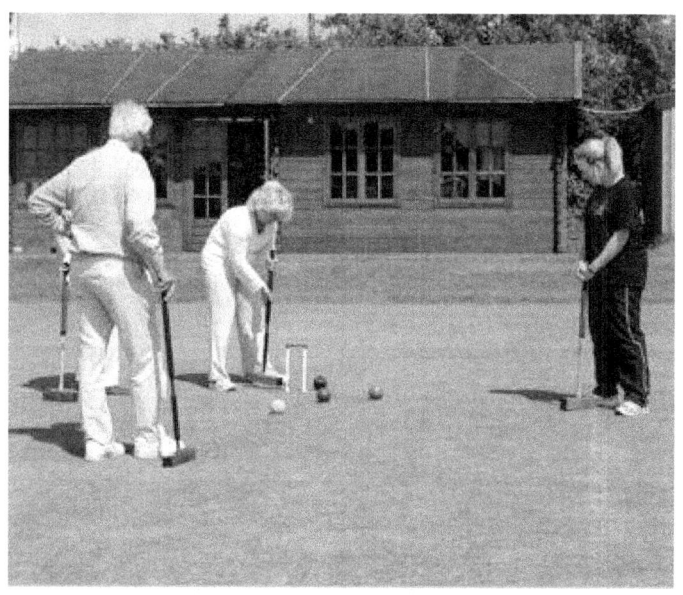

Close game

38

The Challenge So Far - Number 1 to 10

I thought as I have reached the 10 milestone of my 100 challenge, I would take stock and review the adventure so far. I am sure when I get to the middle of my challenge, I might find myself a bit grumpy or cantankerous but at the moment, like a new mum, I am excited by my and I am generally filled with the wonder and excitement of this new world.

So far, I have Nordic walked, short mat bowled, boxed, played cricket, taken part in a body combat and bums, tums and thighs class, played petanque, croquet and baseball and tried yoga. All of which have been completely new for me and a challenge in their own right. I have looked forward to some and not to others but so far, so good. Going to a fitness class is a big deal for me, as it isn't something I really enjoy, but there is such a variety of classes out there... surely I'll find one which will float my boat?

I'm a little worried about the winter months when it is dark and rainy. Will I want to get off my sofa then? It's all very well skipping off to play croquet on a beautiful day on the coast but what about a howling rainy day, where I will have to leave the warmth of my house, drive in the rain to a place I haven't been to before and spend an hour getting sodden playing a game I don't know? This is all to come I guess and the real challenge will be to keep focused and not give up.

I've met a range of different people, all of whom have been friendly and keen to show off their sport or help me in a gym class and, I must admit, I have enjoyed people's reactions when I explain the challenge. Everyone just says "good for you" or "why not, life is short" (the last phrase was said by an 85-yearold I met at one of the clubs!) I'm also enjoying writing up my experiences; something which I haven't previously done and I might not be a professional but the few people who have read it (my mum) have been very complimentary. I guess I'll learn along the way and regardless about the number of people, who read about my adventure, it'll always be a diary for me to look back on - maybe when I am 85.

Chapter 3 - Challenge 11 – 20

Pole Fitness – Number 11

Grace, poise, balance, upper body strength and a strong core: you can see where this is going! How better to prove that I have none of these elements by attending a Pole Fitness taster session, at the Atlantic Reach Hotel? My partner, Paul, spent the afternoon randomly showing me pole-dancing fails on YouTube, which started to foster a deep sense of dread that the pole would fall down that evening and I would be ridiculed. I shared these feelings with him and got told to make sure I got it on film so we could make £250 from You've Been Framed.

I wasn't sure what to wear, so went with the usual Lycra shorts, teamed with my fat pants, just to make sure everything stayed in place. I considered using gaffer tape for extra protection of lumps and bumps but thought it might chafe. So, I took my heavily corseted and un-moisturised body off to give it a go!

When I arrived, Vicky was erecting four poles in the middle of the floor. I took the chance to chat with some of the other girls. I was relieved to discover that not everyone was twenty-something and light looking. Most of them had come along with friends and had the same look of anticipation as me.

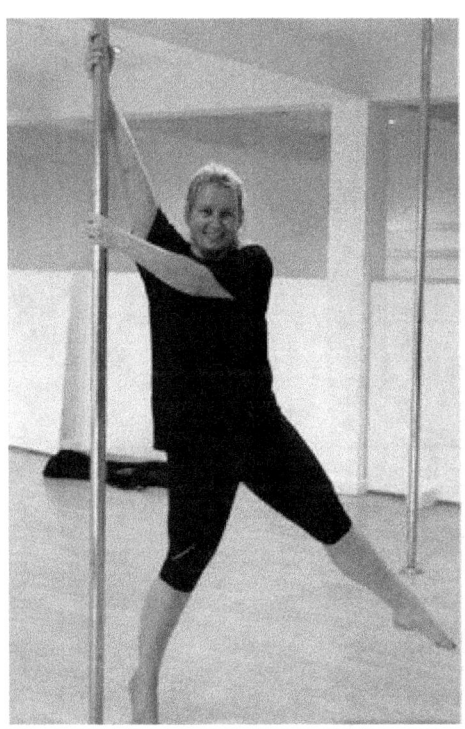

Grace and poise...

We started with a gentle warm-up to cheesy music and then over to the poles. I managed to land myself in the group with the only person in the room who had tried it before. She was immediately labelled "The Pro." Vicky instructed us to prance around the pole on the balls of our feet to get used to it. She said it would feel a bit strange at first. I placed myself last. The atmosphere in the room changed to laughter and giggles as we got over our initial reticence.

Before we moved on, Vicky told us that "there was no such word as can't" and praised us for already showing that we were encouraging each other. Next up was more of a swing around the pole, which graduated to swinging and crossing our legs around the pole as we got to the end of the spin. At this point, I started to blame the pole for my dismal efforts and felt that cleaning the pole with the cloth would indicate that the blame didn't lie with me.

Everybody was having a good old time and there was more Girl Power emanating from the room then a Spice Girls concert. There was clapping, cheering and encouragement for our sisters.

However, as with everything I do, as soon as I get the hang of something, it moves on.

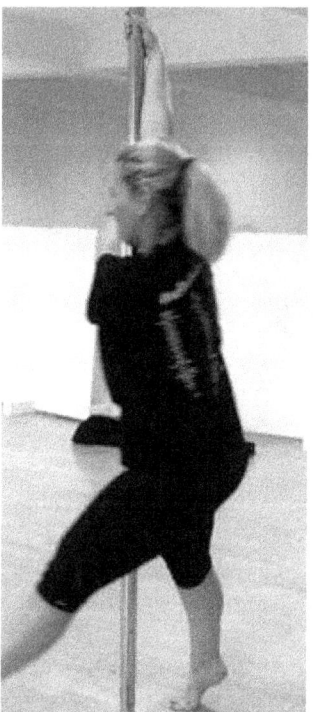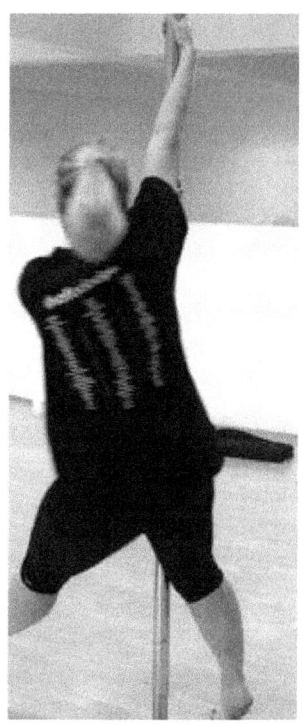

and around...

My own humiliation arrived when we had to climb the pole and squeeze various muscles to maintain the position. Again, I put myself last after The Pro and her two friends. The two friends hadn't got the other exercises immediately but this time, they scuttled up the pole with ease. My turn next. Inner thigh muscles are not something which I possess, so this was always going to be a challenge. However, after two failed attempts, which involved me lifting my arms up and clinging on for dear life as I slid down like a slug, the Pro decided to help me by hoisting my foot and telling me to squeeze. Squeeze what? I have nothing to squeeze! My Lycra shorts were achieving the same effect as rolling around in oil and no, I couldn't pull them up. Remember I am corseted in; I couldn't roll them up even by an inch!

Thankfully, after encouraging my team to have an extra-long go each, it was time to warm down. Overall, I really enjoyed myself and can see that going with a friend would be a great laugh. I'm sure it would give your body great tone and strength, but I think I would need to locate some of the essential muscles before I would benefit from it.

Stand Up Paddleboarding – Number 12

Watergate Bay is one of my special places. It was my childhood beach and I take my 3 kids there now. Memories are stored over the expanse of that beach; from hitting my hockey ball from one end to the other, as the 11-year-old me dreamed of making it to the Olympics one day, to having a birthday party there where Mum fell over a rock, but managed not to drop the cake. I didn't make it to the Olympics, but I did keep my relationship with cake going.

So, I turned up on a beautiful day to try Stand Up Paddle with The Extreme Academy, feeling quite at home in my surroundings. I should have remembered that my treasured memories were land based and not so much in the sea. I managed to prise myself into my wetsuit and stepped out ready to go: I looked like a fat Baywatch extra. Jan and Tony, a couple who had tried it the previous evening for half an hour, joined me and I felt a bit more encouraged about it all.

Carl took us down to the beach to give us a substantive run through of the equipment, technique and safety instructions. The board, at about 10ft long, was a big old beast and the sea looked fairly flat and calm - I felt confident that even I could stand up. Once we finished our land-based practises, I was feeling cocky. I didn't fall off and managed to mount and dismount with aplomb but, saying that, we were still on the sand.

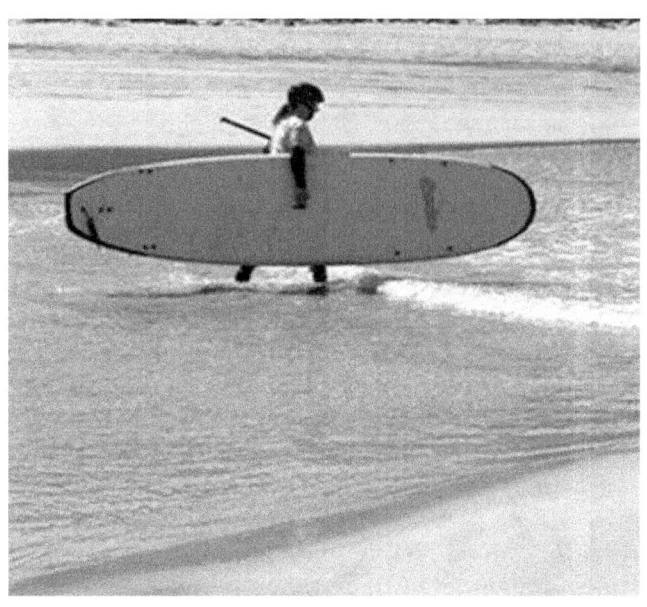

Highly confident at this point

We lifted the boards down to the waterfront and I forgot the whole previous half hour of instructions. As I flailed about, Carl repeated all the salient points and launched me into the wind, where I maintained a kneeling stance. I flapped my paddle around and gained no ground whatsoever. The calm, flat sea I saw from the beach, was actually turning out to be 6ft and choppy in my mind. Jan and Tony were already off standing up and paddling about.

I could no longer put it off. I had to attempt to stand up. Slowly, slowly was the key to this. After several aborted efforts, I rose to my feet, only to emit my pterodactyl scream as my legs wobbled and turned to jelly. The approaching ripple of a wave sent me flying off. Carl checked me and then urged me to remount and give it another go, which I did, resulting in the same outcome. I resorted to my knee-paddling and when I found that tiring, I sat on my bum and paddled about. This was great. Maybe I could lie down on it and use it as a lilo?

Then I tried to distract Carl with questions, but he got wise to it and suggested he launch me into a wave to get the feeling of catching one. He reassured me I didn't need to stand up "unless I felt like it." He pulled me into position, awaiting a wave I could be propelled into. My paddle was poised, head forward, and then whoosh, I got caught in the wave. I stayed with it momentarily but

44

I could feel my balance going. I tried desperately to right myself but could only stem the tide for a split second, before I was once more gobbled up by the white monster. As I lay washed up, like a beached whale, I looked up and I kid you not, I saw a dog...the dog was surfing. A surfing dog was better than me!

I was determined not to be outdone by a surfing Spaniel. Carl was determined that I was going to get the full experience. We resumed the previous position. This time, Carl would swim behind me, keeping the board upright. We caught the smallest wave possible to feasibly catch and coupled with Carl's dogged babysitting of me and my dogged determination not to be outdone by a dog, I caught the elusive wave and I surfed it, on my knees, all the way to the shallows. Victory and exhilaration! I might actually be an adrenaline junkie...

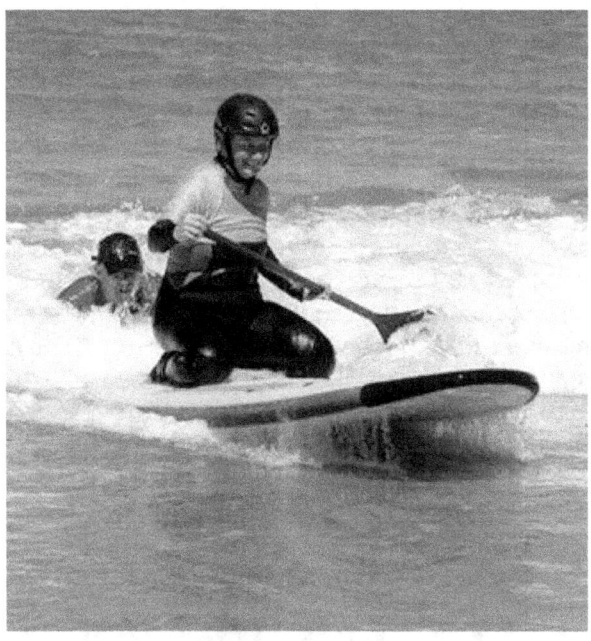

Take that Spaniel!

Horse Riding – Number 13

Now, otters - I love a good otter. A horse not so much, which is odd for most people to understand, as I live in the country and am surrounded by them. I have never been on a horse and am suspicious of them as a species. I'm not good with heights and as I've remembered on my challenge so far, I have very little to no balance. This is my 13th challenge and I'm hoping it isn't an omen of doom.

With my activities so far, I've gone to publically available classes or clubs where I try things out, then write about how I get on and maybe inspire a few people to give it a go. In this particular situation, I'm so nervous about getting on a horse that I wanted a friendly face to help me along, so I went to see my friend, Nina. I often see Nina clopping along past my window, chatting to other riders and seemingly having a good old time, so she seems perfectly qualified to take on my equine issues.

When I arrived at Nina's stable, she introduced me to her horse Spot. Spot is a big, 18-year-old, white horse, who adopts a long-suffering, disinterested look when I speak to him. It soon becomes apparent why Spot looks like this: his neighbour Gem farts...a lot! I have seen enough programmes, films and cartoons to know that horses like apples, so I brought one along to help with the bonding process. I only brought one, so I halved it, meaning Spot and Gem could both have a piece. I held my hand out for them to indulge. Spot chewed it monotonously. Gem gobbled it up and then farted.

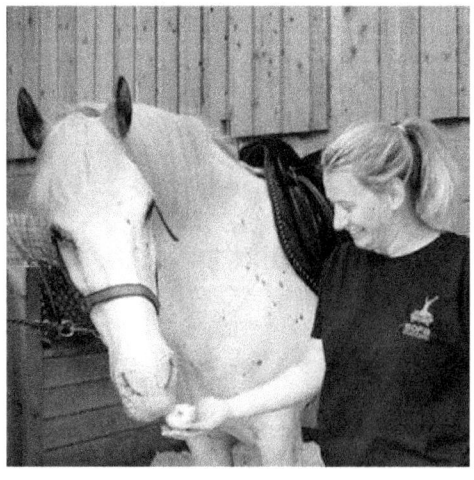

Nice Horsey....

Nina put the saddle on Spot and a hat on me and led out Spot to a step, where I was to get ready to mount him. I put my foot in the stirrup but didn't feel brave enough to swing my leg over, so I grasped the fence and once I felt my leg was over, I removed my hands. Nina told me to breathe. Apparently, it was important to Spot that he felt I was breathing. I adopted a pre-childbirth fast panting and I gripped the reins with my white knuckles glowing.

When I visit adventure parks with the family, I refuse to go on the high, adrenaline pumping rides and encourage the kids to come with me on the teacups. So, there I was on top of a horse for the first time and I could feel my heart racing and the irrational fear of falling entering my head. As Nina led us out and turned to shut the gates, all I could do was cling on for dear life, breathe/pant and try not to scream. I didn't like it. I didn't like it all. Nina coaxed me to relax, maintain a good posture and try and sit back into the saddle. At this point, Spot started getting annoyed with the flies and was swishing his tail and giving his head a bit of a shake. I felt a bit sick.

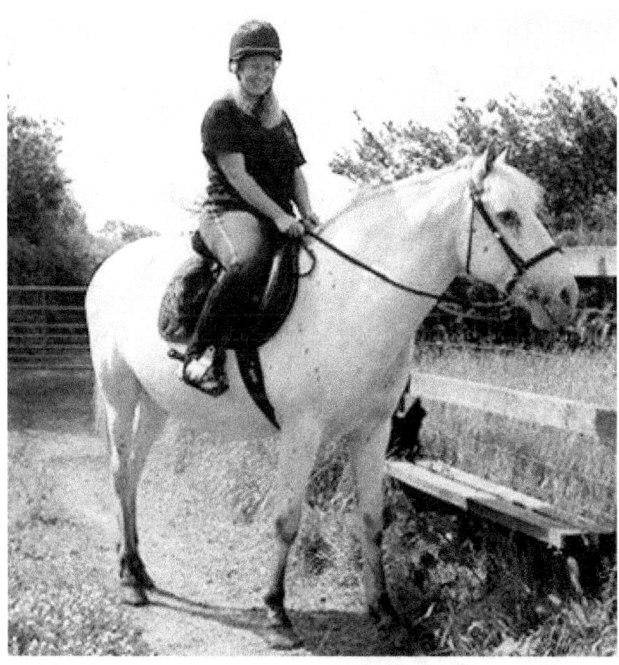

Yeah, I'm on a horse....

Nina led us out onto the country road. She reassured me Spot was fine in traffic and there was nothing to worry about. Spot trotted on and seemed wholly disinterested in what was going on and didn't react as I apologised to him for having such a fat arse. I loosened my grip on the reins slightly and could see the blood returning to my hands. My heart rate slowed as I started to overcome my initial panic. We went on further and although I was relaxing more, I was keen to turn back. We'd all had a good time, I'd been on a horse and had a picture to prove it, plus we'd done enough to write about it. However, Nina suggested we do the loop, which meant we had only done a third of the way.

I mutely nodded my assent to the idea and we continued. The more I rode, the more comfortable I became. Spot was a right old character. Like me going for a run, he slowed to a standstill when there was any kind of incline and I felt confident enough to tap him with both legs to go forward. Apart from a small wobble towards the end, we got back to the stable safely. I resumed the clinging onto the fence to dismount and then spent a couple of minutes walking like John Wayne as my muscles relaxed. I said goodbye to Spot, but I am not sure he heard me as he looked like he had gone to sleep.

It feels kind of good to face your fears a little bit – not sure if I would do it again but at least I can say that I have done it. As it turns out, I didn't have a fear of horses; it is my fear of heights which made me not want to go on a horse. I thanked Nina for my adventure and quickly exited as Gem looked like he was brewing one again!

Fencing – Number 14

As an avid reader of history, especially The War of the Roses and Tudor times, the thought of doing something derived from sword fighting is right up my street. Along with my last challenge of horse riding and if you throw in a bit of archery as well, I reckon I could navigate my way around the Middle Ages quite happily - as long as I managed to avoid the plague, being persecuted as a witch or requiring any kind of medical assistance.

I arrived on a boiling hot day at Truro Fencing Club and was introduced to Jon, my instructor. As I usually do, I asked about the club and prepared to empathise with the trials and tribulations of trying to run an amateur sports club, struggling along season by season, but it was very different here. Jon had represented GB. Linda, who managed the office was a double Olympian, and training at the same time as me were Rio 2016 hopefuls representing other countries. The club has a burgeoning number of members and I was very impressed. In fact, I was pretty gobsmacked that Cornwall could boast such an internationally renowned club for an Olympic sport. The only sport I thought we were world-renowned for was Cornish Wrestling.

Jon took me through the equipment and clothing I had to wear and the safety message of not waggling around a pointy object, for fear of injury. I donned an under-protector over my shoulder, what can only be described as a Madonna-esque boob protector, a protective jacket, a glove, and then finally and to my disgruntlement, a mask. Claustrophobia and I are not the best of friends, which is one of the multitudes of reasons why I haven't taken up bee-keeping or tried being a firewoman. It took a few minutes to adjust and then I was ready to go.

First off, Jon told me how to hold the sabre, which was the weapon of choice and then how to salute your opponent before and after the fight, which seemed to hark back to a more chivalrous time. The stance, coupled with the attacking and retreating movements, followed. It was reminding me a little of boxing, getting the footwork just right. Then the sword was introduced and I moved forward a couple of paces and Jon encouraged me to tap him on the head with the sword. Other moves were introduced but inevitably it all went a bit wrong when I had to put it all together and co-ordinate the feet with the hand movements. It looks a lot easier in films and when you watch the Olympics, as the movements almost seem instinctive.

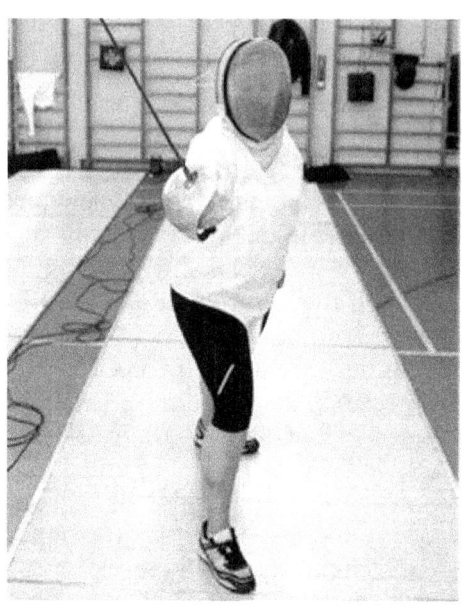

That is me under there!

The lesson culminated in a first to five point fight, where I could put all of my learning into a bout. To outside observers, it must have looked like a toddler attempting to swat a fly. Jon watched me for a few moments (most probably, stifling a grin under his mask) and then swiftly and deftly stepped in to tap me on the head. Jon was very kind and patiently waited for me to get it together enough to tap him for a couple of points, which he sweetly congratulated me for. The whole situation suddenly seemed hilarious and I dissolved into fits of giggles, as I tried to parry and then remember I had to attack as well as defend. My feet and brain started their own bout, which neither won.

It ended 5-4 to Jon. I was absolutely exhausted. I really hadn't expected it to be so physically demanding. The lesson was extremely enjoyable but I don't think they will be booking me a seat on the plane to Rio any time soon!

Powerhooping – Number 15

In my primary school playground, we had the skipping girls and the hula girls. Back in those days when I had a pelvic floor, I was a skipping girl. This wasn't a gang warfare situation: we all got on but we had a playground preference. I could never get the hang of hula hoop, so I avoided it. In private moments, I have had a few sneaky tries with my daughter's hoop, but to no avail. I would just get spotted by the family and ridiculed. I simply can't hula. However, I was made aware of a powerhoop class by Dianne from FunFit and in the spirit of relinquishing my dignity and facing childhood demons; I decided to give it a go.

The first challenge was Dianne told me to wear two tight fitting tops for the class. I avoid tight fitting tops as much as possible, so I had to go to the outer depths of my "tops drawer." It is a dark and desolate area of the wardrobe, which rarely sees the light of day. I pulled out a crumpled old gym top and discovered that if you don't wear a top for 4 or 5 years, it shrinks with isolation and neglect. It was never that tight before!

Dianne introduced me to the ladies in the class. They ranged in age and ability, with the younger, fitter, more able girls in the front, progressing to the back with the older and less fit ladies. I was familiarised with the powerhoop, which was a fairly heavy, thick and ridged hoop, with rainbow patterning that made it look inviting. But reading the disclaimer about mild bruising alerted my suspicions.

It was a hot evening, so the doors were opened and I tried a bit of practising before the class started. The idea was to get the right foot forward, heel on the floor, swing the hoop so it's level and then thrust back and forward. Off I went. Foot forward, swing and then air, dry-hump like mad; round once, round twice and then bang on the floor. This continued a few times and I had flashbacks to the playground and yearned for my skipping rope.

With all of my challenges, I go in determined to do my best and pay respect to whatever I take on but I couldn't shake the thought that I would never "get it." The class started with a warm-up, which was blatantly unnecessary as we were all sweating already. Part of the warm-up involved using our arms to hold the hoop in the air and I could really feel them ache as this point. Then on to the hooping part. Dianne encouraged me to continue practising as the others went through the steps, whilst I interrupted the music every 10 seconds with a loud bang as I lost the hoop to the floor. Thankfully, I wasn't the only one.

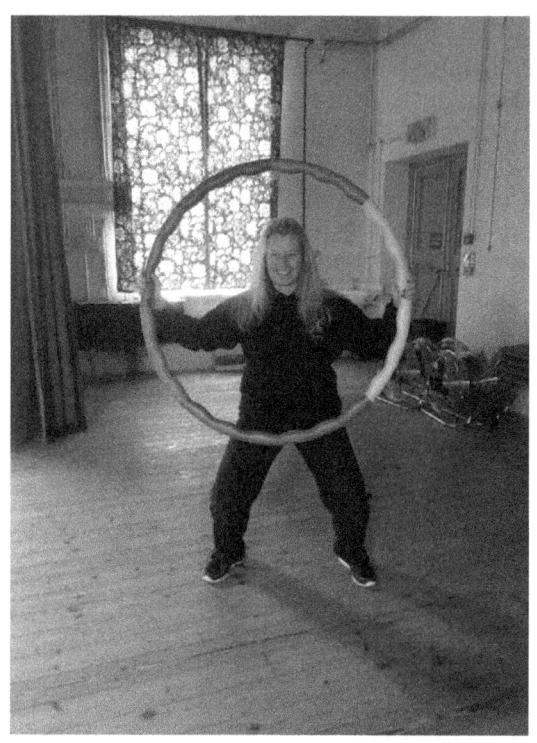

We then went through sequences which are recognisable in other gym classes and I was relieved that it wasn't all hooping. After some grapevines and steps, another hooping track came on and I awaited the inevitable hoop, hoop, bang. I swivelled the hoop the first time and roll the drums, toot the horns, it went round and around and around and then bang to the floor. Utter success, it went around three times! Immediately, I picked it up again and again I did a few more rotations. I got it! I couldn't believe it! Stuff the skipping rope, I was a hula girl!

Sometimes, the small wins are the great wins. I burnt some calories, met some nice people and I learnt to powerhoop. Give me a bit of mild bruising any day - I've smashed a croquet mallet into my own leg, I can deal with it!

Badminton – Number 16

My friend, Sugar, invited me on a no-strings lunch date, which automatically made me think she wanted a clandestine affair.

Before I could fully consider my orientation options, what I was going to wear and how long she had had these feelings for me, she made it clear that "no-strings" was Badminton's pay and play national initiative. Feeling spurned and hurriedly washing off my perfume, I agreed to join her for a spot of badminton and a sarnie after.

Sugar (as in Alan Sugar because she is so entrepreneurial) is not only a hockey player but also plays club badminton. She offered to take me along to St Austell Bay Badminton Club's lunchtime session. I occasionally play tennis and my adventures have already taught that I have hand-eye-ball coordination, but do I have hand-eye-shuttlecock coordination? Although, having written that last sentence, I see I do have an ability to resist the childish option on occasion!

I enjoy meeting new people and getting coached by all of the clubs I am visiting, but I was quite looking forward to having a knock about with a friend. No pressure. Experience the sport, take a picture and have a good old chinwag. The chinwag on the way there was successfully accomplished, so I assumed that the rest would slot nicely into place. I was incorrect.

I was introduced to Lyndon, the club secretary, who initially looked baffled by my presence but after an explanation and the back of the shirt inspection, I was included on the peg board for game play and immediately we were on court, playing doubles. Sugar introduced me to our opponents as a "newbie", which I thought was kind of her, as they would definitely give me a few pity shots to have a go at. Again, wrong. After a warm-up of approximately 90 seconds, we went into a full-on game.

These girls were good, Sugar was really good and my double-handed backhand didn't seem to be working! I do play hockey with Sugar, so I should know how competitive she is but even I was surprised. She was going to win, with or without me, dragging me along for the ride like a bemused child on a "quick shop" around a supermarket. I blinked again and she had almost single-handedly got us to 21 points and thus won the game by a point.

After handshakes, I had time to breathe, realign my new reality and meet the other players. The age range differed greatly but unlike other clubs I've visited, the standard was consistently high. Lyndon explained that badminton had varying levels of skill and if you wanted to go along to a club, you should definitely check whether beginners were accepted and what level you'd be playing with.

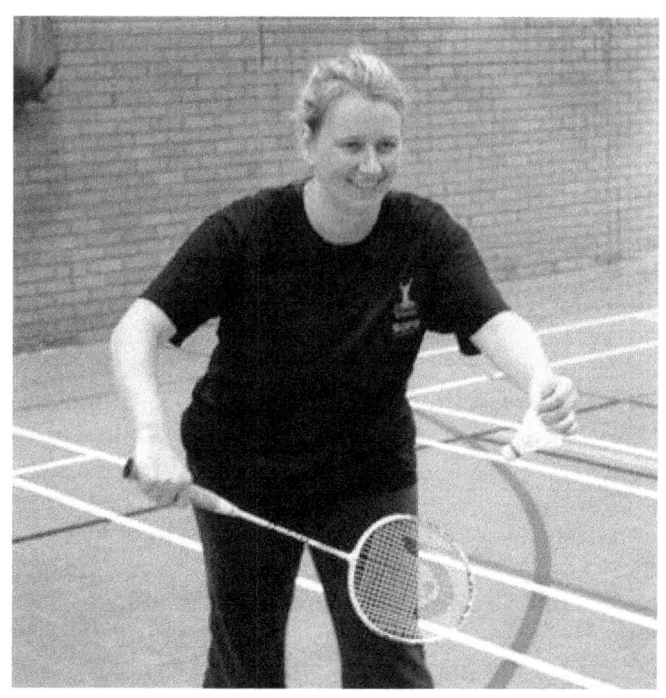

Serving it up

I was definitely out of my depth and Sugar was off playing on other courts, so I had to get it together, lose the double-handed backhand and focus. I played a further two games, the last one against Sugar. I am pleased to say that in one rally, I relentlessly hit the shuttlecock back, hitting it harder each time and finally wearing her down, I took a point. A treasured point, which went with my other 5 (out of a possible 63). With that scoring potential, I don't think she will have the nerve to invite me back on a second date anytime soon!

Canoeing – Number 17

The main objectives for my boat based challenges (canoeing, sailing and rowing) are firstly not to drown and secondly, not to capsize. Capsizing into the sea, in itself, isn't the worst thing that could happen but capsizing and then attempting to haul myself back into the boat, in the tightest fitting wetsuit known to man, in front of a group of strangers, is in the top 3 indignities which I am looking to avoid during this whole thing.

This was fresh in my mind as I made mental post-it notes driving down to Porthpean Beach to meet Kevin, the instructor at St Austell Canoe Club. He made the introductions and I was delighted to see a familiar face there, who was also having a go for the first time. Paperwork done, I went to my car to get into my wetsuit. After my Stand Up Paddle challenge, I chucked the wetsuit into the garage, where it usually festers until the next time I pluck up the courage to go back in the sea. I had obviously forgotten that I was now a professional athlete and need to take care of my stuff. I dusted off the cobwebs and then spent a good five minutes fighting to get into the damn thing.

Once in, I waddled my way over to the boat area, where I was given a life jacket and what can only be described as a fetching, waterproof kilt (or splashback). Whilst Kevin was explaining what it did, I was just thinking, whatever, it hides my bum! We had a quick briefing and then lugged the boats down to the beach. Kevin told me how to hold the paddle and how to sit in the boat. What Kevin didn't know is that I have already canoed a couple of years ago on my friend, Kat's hen party. Essentially, what happened was that at one point, as we moored up to the pub pontoon, we were accosted by a group of stags, who encouraged us to line up the boats. I was in the middle of the pack, when two alcohol-fuelled stags raced each other along the raft of boats, my paddle was sent flying into my face, causing a full-on nosebleed. I, therefore, viewed the paddle as my potential foe, to be treated with respect.

I managed to get in the water without capsizing, thankfully, as there were a number of families enjoying the remnants of the evening and we all know kids can be cruel. The launch was successfully accomplished. I can't tell you what a great feeling it was, bobbing around in the little boat, surrounded by the most beautiful stretch of coast. Then the whole club, about 20 boats, paddled a couple of inlets down on to Charlestown. I can't say that the paddling wasn't hard on the arms, but it was well worth the effort.

At Charlestown, we all paddled into the harbour and were greeted by a dozen teenagers bombing off the side of the harbour wall. As they got more confident, they started to take a run and then bomb, hoping to hit one of our boats. It was all done in good jest, but I had my objectives in mind and was not going to let one of those lemmings ruin it, so I swiftly made my way back out to sea.

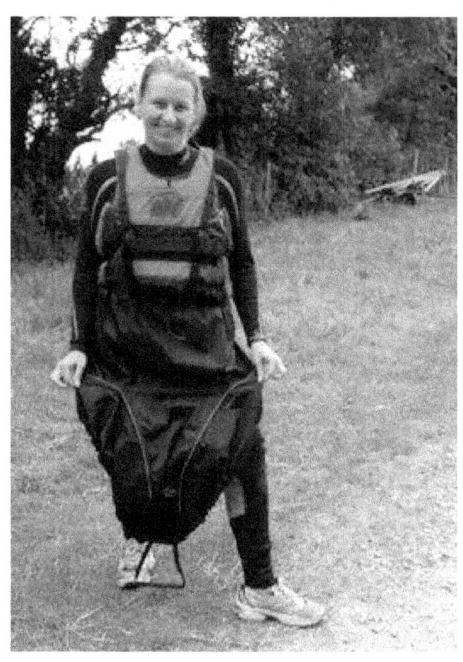

Fetching Sea Kilt/Nappy

Canoeing back was much easier, as we had the wind behind us. This gave me a chance for leisurely chats with a number of the group. Again, all ages and all abilities and it seemed like a very friendly and social club. Once we got back to the beach, we had a good half hour of what I can only describe as "titting about." There was titting about with balls, titting about by standing up and then the dreaded titting about in a raft formation. This tapped directly into the fears of capsizing and nosebleeds but I wasn't going to wimp out. I lined my boat up and clung to my neighbours' boats for dear life, as races went on up and down, before one competitor would fall into the sea. It was the best team bonding I've seen so far.

After saying my goodbyes, I left the rest of the club to enjoy a BBQ in the field, whilst I went back to my car and repeated the bout with my wetsuit; my new nemesis.

Trampolining – Number 18

In my last challenge, I named capsizing as one of the three indignities which I do not want to experience in my 100 challenge. Following hot on its heels in the chart is wetting myself, so as a mother of three, I classify trampolining in extreme sports. The kids have a trampoline in the garden - I've been on it, I know it's possible.

In the run up to the evening session, I limited myself to a few small sips of water from lunchtime onwards and regular toilet breaks. I felt like an athlete in competition. Another challenge trampolining posed was preventing self-inflicted black eyes, as I am amongst the larger mammary-ed of the species. So with my boobs scaffolded into place and an empty bladder, I trotted down to the Callywith Centre in Bodmin.

The one thing I love about this challenge is meeting so many different people, listening to their tales and for a short period of time, through osmosis, picking up their love and enthusiasm for their particular activity. Ann, the coach, is one such inspirational person. She coaches 7 days a week, in venues across the region; from little tots through to national contenders, one of whom she trains at 8am on a Sunday morning. If anybody was going to make me bounce, Ann can (I was determined to shoehorn that grammatically incorrect phrase in here somehow!).

She asked about my previous experience, and I self-congratulatory mentioned my preliminary trampolining badge when I was 11. Ann looked for a hint of irony in my eyes. She saw none. I still have that badge. Before we moved over to the trampoline, I moistened my dry, dehydrated lips with two drops of water on my fingers and excused myself to the ladies.

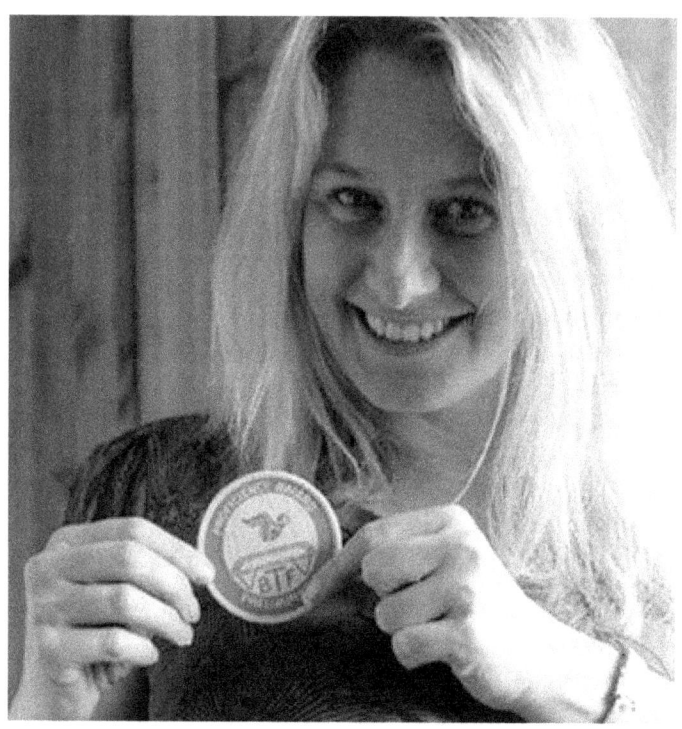

Yeah, I kept the badge-I found it sitting with my "Walked 20 Miles" certificate

When I commenced bouncing, I was surprised how much it differed from our one in the garden. Probably obvious, but it felt really different. Ann took me through the basic technique, as my arms were going off like a demented windmill. Next, was bouncing to sit and back up again and then sitting down and stay bouncing whilst sitting down. That was tough on the old abs! After a blast from the past, with pike, straddle and tuck jumps, we moved into putting it all into a sequence.

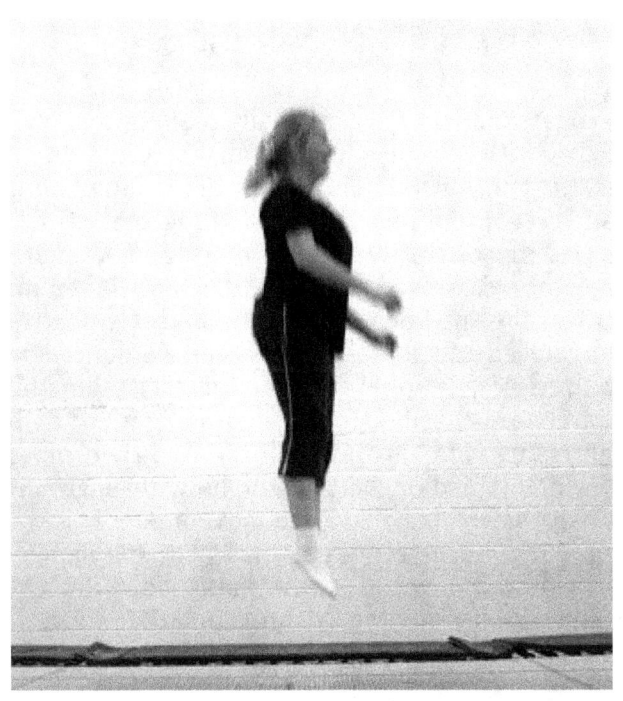

and bounce...

First things first though: off for a quick wee and back on for the sequence. I was in full self-achievement mode already, just by completing the moves individually and I wasn't confident I could pull off a routine. Usually I would find it quite funny, but there was no way I could risk a laugh - not even a smirk. I didn't manage to fully do the routine without mucking it up but I had a good go. Trampolining is a surprisingly exhausting sport, as you're literally working the whole body, especially the pelvic floor!

It's been a good few days all in all. No indignities have been made and I continue to meet the most inspirational people who keep me going on this adventure.

Tai Chi – Number 19

After my yoga experience, I was really looking forward to giving Tai Chi a try with Wal at Green Man Tai Chi. With all of my challenges, I try not to do too much research beforehand and go in without any preconceptions. The first thing that struck me with this class was that there were more men than women. Thinking back to my other class based activities, the only token male I have seen so far was the one I nearly kicked in Body Combat.

Wal introduced me to the group and we started with some loosening exercises. I think that "flopping" is something which does need to be practised, as my body was fighting tooth and nail to maintain some element of tenseness. We then moved onto a sequence, which joined one side of the body through to the other. They were very slow and considered movements. This was built on further and I felt a little bit like I was learning a dance routine. I think if you slowed down a 90s boyband video, (apart from the anatomy) it would be the style I seemed to be adopting.

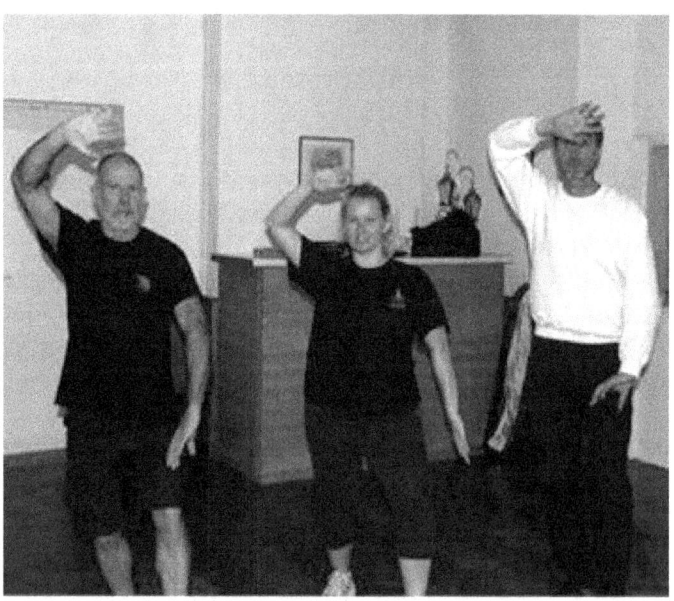

Tai Chi movements shown by Wal, whilst I adopt a mid-90s Take That pose

Next up was the focus on breathing and meditation, which I really enjoyed. Being mindful of your breathing is something which is proven to improve your mood and release stress and as with yoga, I feel it's something I'd like to explore further after the 100 challenge has finished.

We progressed onto developing the movements. A couple of minutes into this part of the class, it became apparent that my left side was way more uncoordinated than the right. The right is not good. The left is utterly useless. I started to panic. I hadn't noticed it before but I had flashbacks to other classes and a pattern started to emerge. Has this always been the case? I made a mental note to follow that up when I got home and hoped the right side of my brain was in charge of memory retention.

Wal tried to help me with my movements, but I declared that I'd just diagnosed myself with "Left-itis" and was almost beyond help. He moved my arms around a bit and moved on. Next up was "sticky hands". We were paired up, and led around the room with your eyes shut and your wrist resting on your partner's hand. You followed using Tai Chi principles of movement and breathing. I was paired with a gentleman who was a good foot taller than me. Thankfully, the picture couldn't imprint on my brain, as my eyes were shut.

Lastly, the room was divided into two, with the more experienced people on one side and me and the rest of the class on the other. We practised a movement which apparently takes a number of months to master. I had a good go at keeping up and everybody was really helpful and patient. I learnt that Tai Chi was derived from combat and the movements mirrored the blocking and punching of an opponent. It felt good to work on my breathing and I certainly came out refreshed. I even diverted on my journey home to take a picture over the moors, which I felt was very spiritual of me. Maybe the smell of incense was having an effect?

As soon as I got home, I rubbed my tummy and patted my head with one hand and then swapped to the other. Once accomplished, I went straight onto Google to diagnose my inability to coordinate on my left side. It turns out the right side of my brain controls this part of my body. I urgently looked up what the right brain controlled and what personality deficiencies this might explain. I am pleased to report that after completing an in-depth online questionnaire, both hemispheres of my brain are near enough equal and it just turns out I am rubbish at coordination!

Handball – Number 20

As I am writing my blog and taking on these 100 sports, in my mind, I am entitled to call myself either a wordsmith or a professional athlete if anybody asks me what I do. Professional athletes are not allowed to risk injury and this was the excuse I peddled out to the teachers when I was invited to line up for the mum's race at sports day. Still fresh in my memory was the dark time which was last year's sports day, when I was recovering from a hockey related ankle injury but still decided to participate, to show the kids that taking part was what mattered. As I was pity clapped to last place and the other mums were sticking on their prize badges, I glanced at my children, who were looking down in mortification at my efforts. This year, I had a prime excuse and I was happy to deploy it.

So, in tip top condition, I made my way down to Porth Beach to train with Newquay Handball Club. It was a beautiful evening as I walked over the golden sand to say hello. Geoff introduced me to the other players and gave me a brief description of the sport. It turned out that handball is an indoor game, so I was actually playing its sister sport, Sandball: a mixture of basketball, netball, football and much to my concern - rugby!

First up, we had a game of beach football. As the World Cup was on, we were used to seeing bronzed Brazilians playing skilfully on Copacabana beach; this was more like an un-skilled, free for all, with a pasty skinned, chubby girl running around like a headless chicken. I wasn't sure how I was going to last the whole session, as I was exhausted already.

We moved onto an actual game and were split into teams. My poor team had to work extra hard to carry me, as I clung to the hope that there was a goal hanging position in the sport. It soon became apparent that you had to defend from the front, so I attempted to get back to help out and then ready to help out on a break. At half time, it was 4-4, so it was time for penalties. This involved throwing the ball to the keeper, who like a quarterback threw it back to you as you ran to catch it. You then had to take three steps and throw it, at speed, past the defending keeper.

This had disaster written all over it and it transpired that running; catching and counting were far out of my reach, on all levels. However, I was fashioning a role for myself as a pivot and when the ball was passed to me, I would pass it back as they carried on running – in the coaching manual this is called the "hot potato" method of passing.

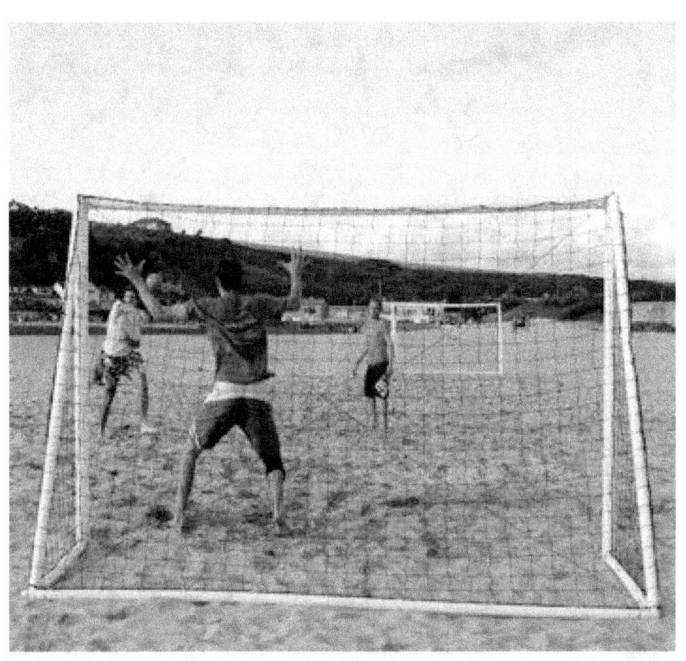

How it is supposed to be done

Half time gave me the opportunity to talk to the guys about their club, which is relatively newly formed and about the challenges they face: attracting new players to play and sponsors to help with the expense of travelling around for league fixtures. Not only are they the only handball club in Cornwall, they are the only handball club in Devon and have to travel to places like Oxford and Swindon to compete. They are coached by renowned handball coach Jürgen Koenen, who was coaching us that evening. He described the progress the club had already made and I really admired the enthusiasm they all showed to move forward.

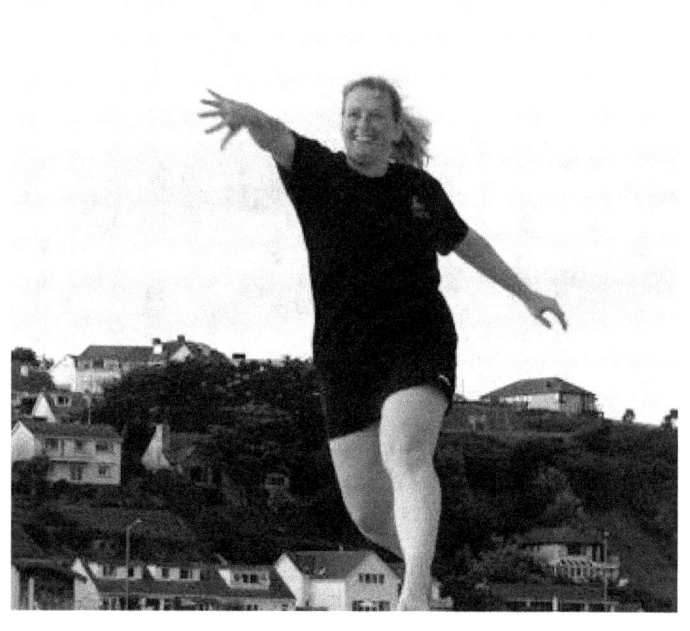

No, there is not a crane getting me that high!

In the second half, I offered to swap teams to even out the imbalance but the guys were lovely and insisted that I was fine as I was. I didn't manage to score a goal, or even get the technique of running three steps and throwing mid-air. I looked like a small, performing elephant in a zoo, waving a trunk around and tossing a ball but it didn't matter, I had a great evening, met a great team with loads of banter and all under the backdrop of the beautiful setting sun.

The Challenge So Far - Number 11 to 20

If my challenge was represented in years and not sports, my last 10 would have been the teenage years. A decade where you are thrust from the warm, comforting womb of primary school, into the daunting and scary world of "big school," where you attempt to find yourself, work hard, play harder and do a lot of growing up, ready for the big wide world. This analogy resonates with me a lot at the moment, as my daughter prepares for secondary school and I reminisce about being her age and wonder what the next few years hold for her.

The last ten challenges have certainly followed this course. I have really and I mean really pushed myself out there in some of the activities. Having being scared/suspicious of horses, I found myself galloping (plodding) along on one. I have attempted to conquer the pole in aerial fitness and fallen into the sea, an untold amount of times trying to unsuccessfully paddlesurf. I have tried my best to maintain my dignity in trampolining and canoeing and my stomach has found that it has another use, apart from storing my blubber, and has managed to rotate a powerhoop around it. I call these the difficult teenage years but in actual fact, as I inspect my "left to do list" I find that there is no easy retirement plan ahead, no downhill from here point. It still looks pretty damn daunting.

Beyond the sports, I am enjoying writing and in pursuit of excellence or a nose about how other people to do it and promote it, I took myself up to London to attend a blogging conference called BritMums. These ladies blog about anything from recipes to craft to travel to family matters. I also met a number of mothers who were looking to raise awareness of health conditions or start communities based around issues which they live with and share for mutual support. I was pretty in awe of what some of them were doing and how they were carving out successful careers in this field; the good ones were being chased by the big brands to associate themselves with their credibility.

The power of words has started to hit home a little with me. My challenge must have inspired someone, because I've been invited to speak on the radio a couple of times and interviewed for an article in the Western Morning News.

It seems that out of all this randomness, there is a headline. There is so much out there to try. I hate stats and I don't feel like I am the person to be wielding them out, but 80% of women do not do enough exercise to stay healthy. I am certainly still in this category, even though I do something sporty or active twice a week. The other times, I sit at the computer and work, which all contributes to a generally sedentary lifestyle and then I congratulate myself most days with a glass of wine, to celebrate getting through another day. Friends and family expect to see some sort of body shape change with all this extra effort but as there hasn't been any, congratulate me on my writing skills! A bit of exercise certainly isn't enough to make those kinds of changes and it does seem that fresh bread and wine need to be addressed if this challenge had anything to do with weight loss. But it isn't. The headline is to not be afraid of starting something new and trying things. Make yourself aware of what is out there and if you are a club or an instructor, put yourself in the shoes of somebody going for the first time and remember a warm welcome makes such a difference.

Chapter 4 - Challenge 21 - 30

Insanity – Number 21

It turns out there are a list of things which are unachievable the morning after an Insanity gym session: walking upstairs, walking down stairs, hanging the washing on the line, sitting down for the toilet and lastly bending to kiss a child on the head. As my three children and their un-kissed heads went off to school and with my wet washing sitting in the basket, I sat considering the warning signs.

The clues were all there. The name of the class in itself shouts "Insanity!" Another clue was talking to my gym-going friends (I have two of them and I am very proud of them). I tend to tell them what I am doing and gauge their reaction from what I call the wince-o-metre. This time, their response was off the chart. The "ooooo" was loud, the cheekbones pronounced and the eyebrows ventured north to the hairline. Yes, I didn't need to be Sherlock to know that this one would be a toughie.

Mike the instructor was extremely reassuring and told me that I was lucky to join that evening, as they were doing the Insanity fitness test. Oh, joy! I was handed a sheet with a list of moves which would be tested later. One was called Suicide Jumps. I signed the disclaimer, which felt like an omen. As I took myself off to the back of the class, the alarm bells were ringing at full power. I liked the actual venue, though, more village hall vibe than a gym with mirrors. Mirrors are bad.

So, to the warm-up. Bang, straight into it! Mike must have had springs in his shoes. He looked like a cross between Mr Motivator and Tigger after a vat full of Smarties, which was quite distracting in a good way and certainly made me smile. Warm-up done, we were on to the actual test. One minute to do as many of the moves as possible and then write down the score. I switch kicked, power jacked and planked my way through, unable to count my score; counting was not an ability I was able to harness while jumping around, wishing I had gone to the toilet beforehand.

Mike's enthusiasm started going through the roof, as the class wailed and groaned through the final stages of the test. It reminded me of childbirth; the pain of contractions and the accompanying sounds and then a 30 second respite to wipe the brow and take on fluids, before it started all over again. Mike bounded around the room, demonstrating each move and embracing the lactic acid. Another reason I like being in a mirrorless environment is that when the instructor's back is turned, you can be sneaky and stop and then resume the position when he/she turns back. Kind of reminiscent of the "What's the time Mr Wolf?" game.

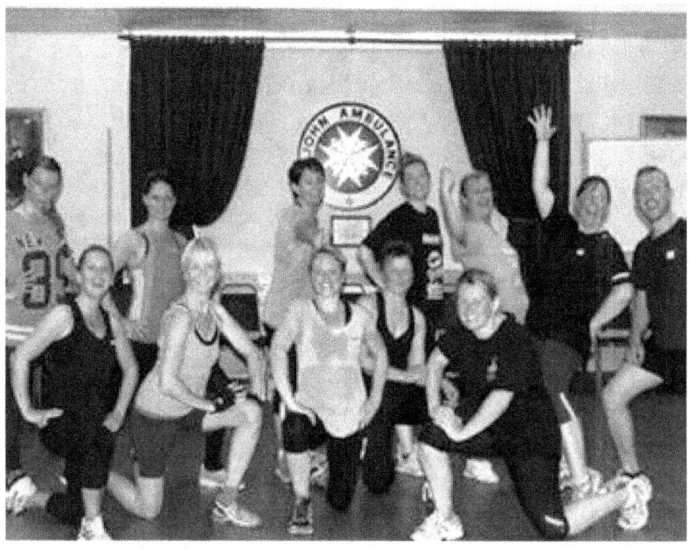

I am glad that I wear black and you can't see the sweat patches!

Once the test was finished, we moved onto a regular Insanity class and bounced about in different ways - working those glutes, abs and my favourite the core. Obviously, the class was physically demanding but you went at your own level and the moves could be simplified. Best of all though, you burn between 600-1000 calories! The other people in the class said the first class was always the toughest. It couldn't be that bad, though, as they had all returned and were glowing about the benefits. Maybe Monday is a good day to give your body a proper workout, to get over the excess of the weekend?

I considered this the following morning and thought about my next challenge tomorrow evening - rowing. I am not sure how I am going to get myself in the boat, pick up the oar or get myself in a sitting position. I considered my options and decided the best course of action is to run myself a hot bath and pop a dozen ice cubes from the ice cube tray into the bath. I know Andy Murray does something like that, so maybe it will do the trick?

Rowing – Number 22

There is no doubt Cornwall is beautiful, especially when the sun is out. So, even with my post-Insanity aching limbs, I was keen to join Robin from Castle Dore Rowing Club for a row on the river. Robin is the Cornwall Under-25 Coach of the Year for the work he does for his club's junior section, and we also play hockey for the same club, so he's just the person, a rowing rookie like myself, needs to show me the ropes. I considered bringing a couple of bottles of beer to enjoy over a natter, whilst Robin rowed me around in the sun and we caught up about hockey gossip.

When I turned up at Golant, the river looked stunning. Robin welcomed me to the club and showed me around the boatyard, explaining the different types of boats you could use. I couldn't believe the width of some of them, and there was no way my bum could fit into any of those. Robin reassured me I would be using a bum-appropriate boat. We went into the clubhouse, where I got the opportunity to hone my technique on the rowing machine. Robin said that apart from swimming, rowing was best for working out your whole body. He was impressed with my rowing action and mentioned that I was one of the better people he had seen. Turns out I am an excellent, land-based rower.

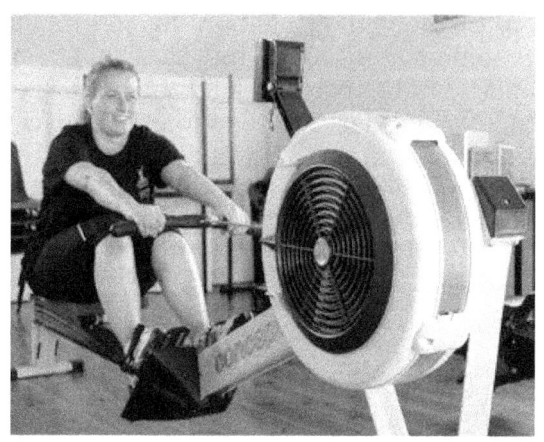

Skilful indoor rowing

As we walked down to get the boat, I was brimming with confidence. Robin picked me out a suitably large arsed boat, but there was only one seat. Naïvely, I asked where he would sit, thinking he might be a cox perched on the top but no, I was on my own. Worse still, I was on my own in a boat with a lead attached to it. I climbed in, concentrating as always on not capsizing. I put the oars into position, with my right hand in front of the left. I had seen this action many times, as I cheered on our Team GB Olympic rowers throughout the years. All I had to do was harness my inner Redgrave.

Robin told me whatever I do, I had to focus in front and not pay attention to the oars. Apparently, the oars misbehave if they are given attention. With a gentle push into the water, I was off. I waggled the attention seeking oars around a few times before being dragged back on my lead by Robin to start the sequence again. This happened three times and each time I tried to focus on the indoor row boat technique I had been shown in the club house.

Foolishly, Robin then decided that I was ready to go off the lead and told me to go upstream while he followed along on the bank. I felt alone and abandoned and I pined to be put back on the leash. Rowing in this type of boat is like reversing a car: you have to look over your shoulder, be spatially aware and know which way you will go if you steer one way. Living in the country, I haven't parallel parked since I left London 10 years ago.

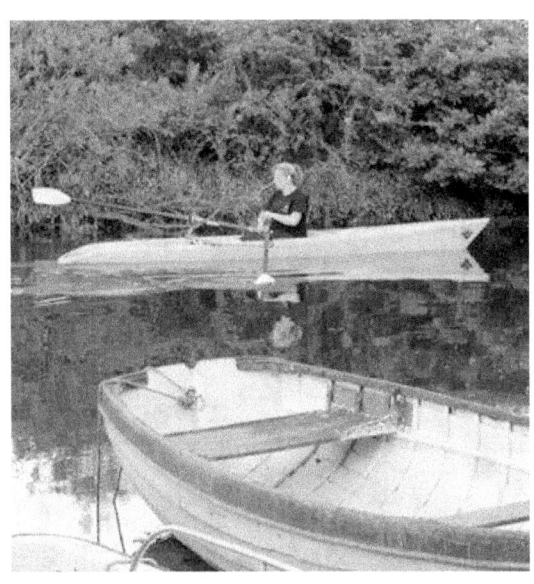

Damn bank in my way

Firstly, I veered straight into the wall to the left and it took a good while to work out how to get myself out of the flotsam and jetsam jungle I had managed to get myself tangled up in. Robin was calling encouragement from the side and telling me which oar to paddle. Once I straightened up, I started to go backwards and with a couple of strokes, I managed to move in the right direction. Hark though, what was the noise I could hear getting louder? Oh yes, that of course, would be the beer garden and yes, of course, it would be full, being such a beautiful evening. I zigzagged past them, summoning all the dignity I could muster.

Once past, Robin told me to turn and come back. Turning seemed to be ok and off I went again. I think the massive problem I had was that my boobs were too big and my action was halted mid-stroke as I bashed them, which made one of the oars go up and the other down. Back at the start, Robin gave me more instructions and encouraged me to do it again. I was starting to feel slightly more confident but unfortunately, somebody had left a pesky boat in the middle of the harbour and I went careering into it, not knowing how to stop.

In a pinball type motion, I then went into the other bank before I got it together and straightened up. I got a full 4 strokes of non-crashing, straight, strokes in and could feel the wind in my hair as I whistled gracefully past the beer garden. The oars felt I was being too confident, so started playing up again but I have had 3 toddlers and I was not going to be outdone by a bit of carbon fibre. Redgrave, I wasn't but I think if I had a few more attempts, I could get myself out of the harbour and onto the actual river, where the real action happened. Robin told me tales of salmon leaping into the boat and dolphins impishly jumping about as you rowed. I would love to experience that - maybe one day. For the moment, I had to contend with reversing out of my tight parking space to get home. Baby steps...

Aikido – Number 23

I feel a certain synergy with Superman at the moment. Not in terms of being a superhero, taking on dastardly villains, or saving the world but from the point of view of having an alter-ego. Superman's is Clark Kent, mine is more Clara Kent, who rocks up at various sports clubs and fitness classes and waggles about a bit. Like Clark, Clara has an outfit to change into – mine is my SofaDodger T-shirt and usually my flattering Lycra cycling shorts. Clark whizzes into a telephone box and comes out immaculately – Clara has to sniff the T-Shirt, apply a good amount of deodorant, ensure leg hair is minimal and that toenail varnish isn't overly chipped.

Last night, though, I didn't feel like playing along. I felt rubbish, the sun was shining and all I really wanted to do was catch up with my friend in the garden, having a cold drink. I made the fatal mistake of watching Aikido on YouTube and I wasn't looking forward to the first of my martial arts challenges. This, I guess, is where commitment and dedication start mentally prodding you. I bade farewell to the garden and went down to Camelford Leisure Centre to join Sensei Jack at TBBA Aikido Cornwall for a session. When I got there, Sensei Jack obviously knew that I was pondering about superheroes because he gave me a cape to wear. It was supposed to be a martial arts jacket, but it must have been for a child because it came up like a waistcoat on me. The rest of the class gave me a warm welcome.

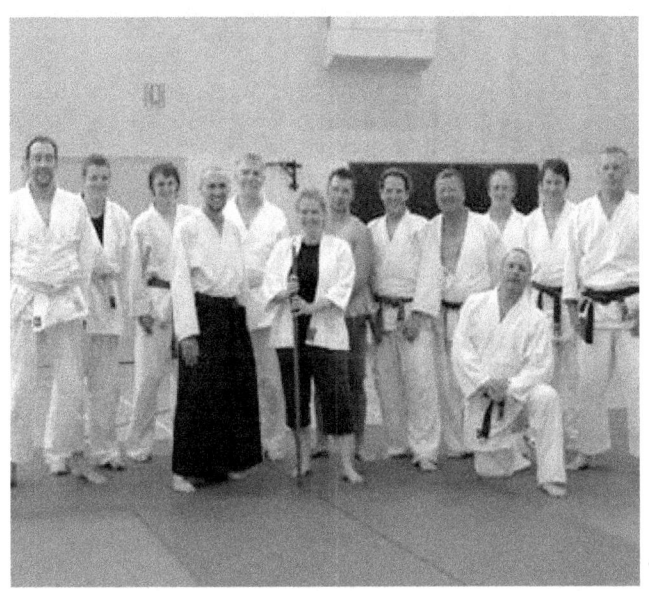

Don't mess with us lot!

Sensei Jack explained that Aikido derives from the Japanese for peaceful and that 95% of moves were actually defensive not offensive. I watched in awe as they glided and parried attacks, then swiftly and deftly turned them into offensive moves. This seemed not to be about attacking somebody and giving them a good beating, but more about taking control of an aggressor and giving a weighted response, fitting of the situation.

My first attempt was to parry a blow to the head by using footwork to shield and turn. I was assigned a carousel of babysitters in varying coloured belts, who were paired with me throughout the exercises. We moved on each time to different moves, which were demonstrated and then practised after in pairs. Sensei Jack, with his swishy black uniform, was reminiscent of Keanu Reeves in The Matrix. He made it look so easy. Thankfully, I was in good hands, as each of my babysitters helped me coordinate the move to the point where I completed each one, albeit to an extremely low level.

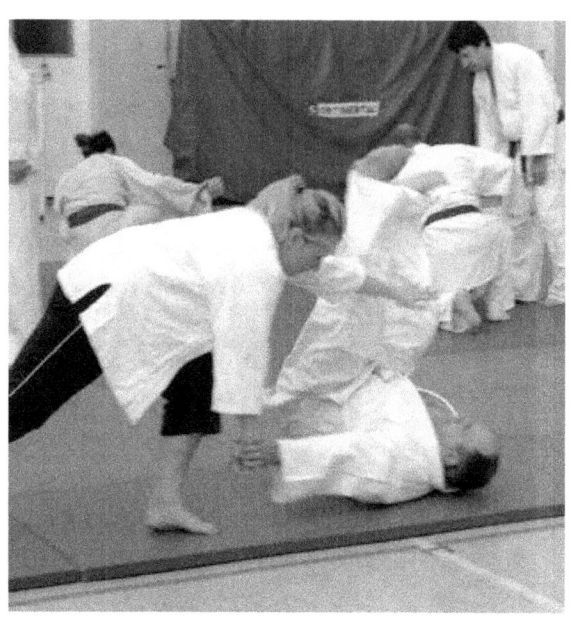

Take that...

We then progressed to taking down an assailant. Through fluid movement, I watched as an aggressor (one of the poor babysitters had to be thrown around in turn as a demonstration) was either unarmed or neutralised. This was absolutely the best bit: given that I was new, I was allowed to be the neutraliser not the neutralised, so I got to practise a range of take-down moves without having to be flung about myself. My babysitters obligingly prostrated their defeat by rolling around the floor after I had neutralised them – either by a headlock or a move which had the potential to break a wrist. I was feeling quite powerful and maybe I did have super-human strength? These tall, well-built, men were no match for me!

The session went by in a flash. After reluctantly giving back my cape, I was genuinely buzzing as I drove home. A great instructor, a great group of guys, and an insight into a martial art. It's something I would certainly encourage my children to attempt when they are older, as a means of looking after themselves.

When I got home, I was keen to show Paul what power I possessed and attempted to neutralise him as he was making a cup of tea. Unfortunately, he didn't get the memo and just stood still and batted me away. He didn't understand he had to approach in a certain way and move his hand where I told him before I could inflict the barrage of moves I had just learnt. He laughed, put his foot behind mine and (gently) pushed me to the floor. Either he was packing kryptonite or the powers had faded. I definitely should have kept the cape!

Rounders – Number 24

I don't know about you but my memories of playing rounders take me back to the school field on sunny days and the smell of freshly cut grass. I always enjoyed the PE lesson when the rounders bat appeared. The ones who didn't, would offer to field far away and set up a manufacturing line of daisy chains. Instead, I was one of those irritating children who would race to be first to pick up the bat and want to bagsy one of the key positions when fielding.

Apparently rounders is still played in 87% of schools across the country, which is a great statistic to hear. Unfortunately, though, I couldn't find a rounders team in Cornwall, so I joined my hockey team as we entered into a mixed rounders competition. My teammates are young, fit, competitive and enthusiastic; the first two of those powers have faded with me but I still possess remnants of the latter two. I am not quite ready to be put out to pasture, even if there are daisies there.

We met and whilst walking to the field, we brushed up on the rules. Only 1 attempt at batting? I don't remember that! Three no-balls are half a rounder and other various rules came back to me as we walked. We were one of a dozen teams and we immediately set about sizing up the competition. Apparently it could get quite competitive, so our team huddle consisted of whether we were going to high five, whether we could run in flip-flops and did we really need to wear shin pads.

Huddle over, we ran off to our positions. I had noticed in the previous game, 3rd post didn't get up to much and didn't seem to be a pressure position, so I deposited myself there and hoped my team would carry me, as I remembered my limitations from the cricket challenge: I can't bowl or catch a hard ball. Our back stop Hugh and Scott on first base worked well to get 4 people out and with Sugar's consistent bowling, we managed to limit the opposition to set ourselves a manageable target. Once into bat, the boys and Sugar (our token good female player) scored a number of rounders and then it was my turn to bat. One ball faced, one ball missed - damn it!

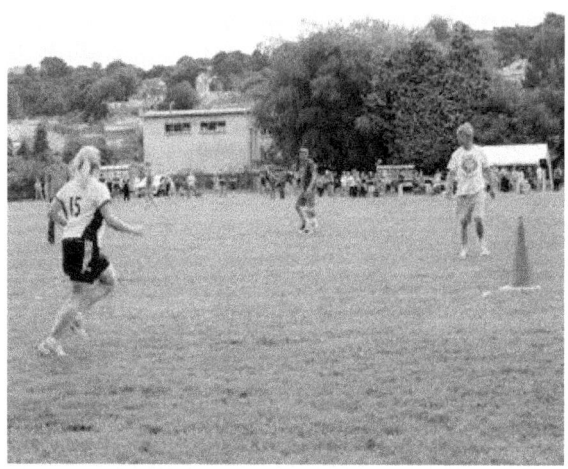

Missed the ball, so could only run to first base

The allotted time was up and we lodged a comfortable win. We then had a beverage to aid team morale and confidently went into the next match. What transpired in this match went against all my views on how a game should be played and the spirit it should be played in, but as I've always recorded all the good things, I have to report on the bad; there was cheating, time wasting and arguments from the opposition and after the match had finished (which we narrowly lost) there were no handshakes, just a festering sense of ill feeling. We marched off in protest to the nearest pub to reconcile the wrong doings we had experienced.

I can't stand unsportsmanlike behaviour. I wince when I see overly competitive parents on the sidelines shouting down the umpire or worse still, the opposition. It is rare but it happens. It's a game and it should be fun, even if it is competitive.

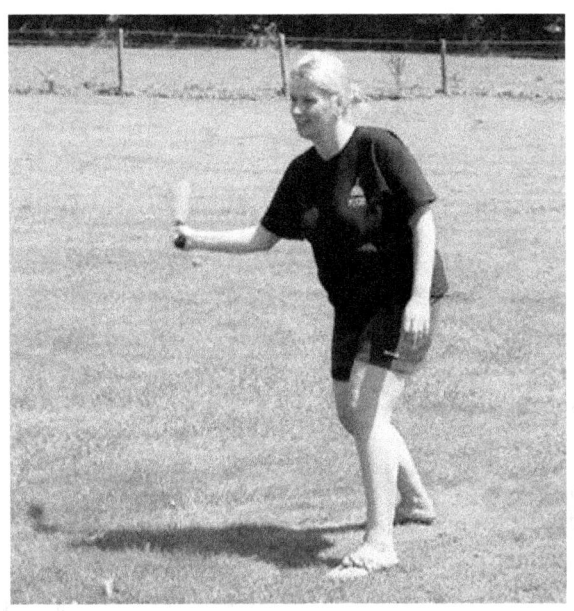

A happy ending in the garden

These instances don't happen very often but I didn't want to write negatively about my experience with one particular sport, which I hold in such high regard. So I decided to get a bat and a ball and set up a game in the garden with the kids and a few friends. The kids had an absolute ball, whilst I managed to hit a ball. I am a firm believer that you can craft your own happy ending.

Wild Swimming – Number 25

As I hadn't swum in the sea for years, I decided to get in a little practise the weekend before my wild swim challenge, so I trooped the family down to Hemmick Beach on the South Coast. I had my usual struggle with the wetsuit. Having already identified it as my nemesis, each tussle is pitched in my mind as mortal combat – good against evil, rubber versus blubber. My eldest shattered this illusion by nonchalantly remarking "Mum, it just doesn't fit you anymore."

Feeling deflated, I wobbled into the sea as the kids opted to play on the beach. This winter wetsuit was very buoyant and as the kids walked, I swam in the same direction but it soon became evident that I wasn't actually going anywhere. I tried the breaststroke with front crawl kicks and then opted for full on doggy paddle then onto backstroke. By the time I caught up with the family in the next cove, they had climbed rocks, built sandcastles and set up camp.

That was it, the final straw; the wetsuit had to go! It had been cramping my style for too many challenges now – maybe that's why I was so bad at Stand Up Paddle? So for the swim with the Cornwall and Devon Wild Swim Club at Porthpean, I was newly togged up in a summer wetsuit, which wasn't as judgemental and clingy as its predecessor.

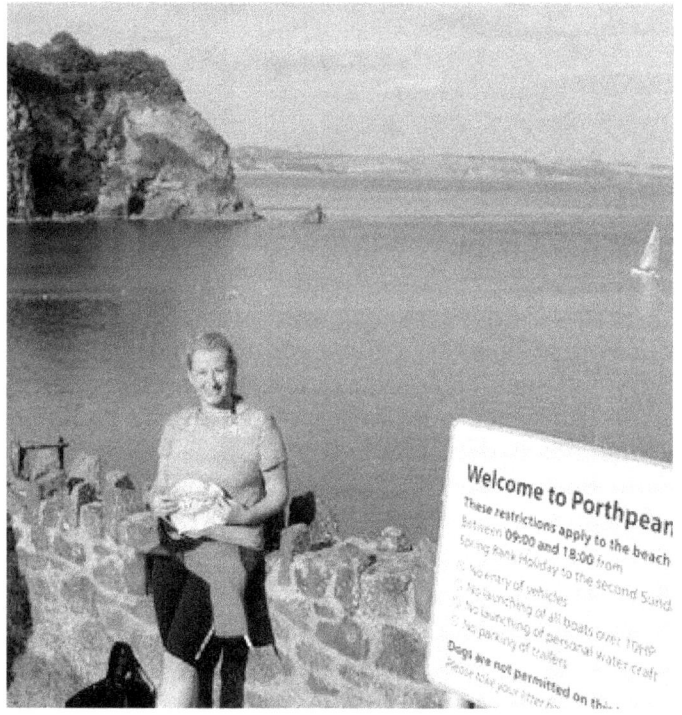

Beautiful evening at Porthpean

I went along with Lin, a family friend, and her friend Oriel, who are part of the group. The sea looked absolutely stunning – apparently the warmest it has been in a decade. There were about a dozen swimmers and Lin assured me that she was a "pootler" not a full on fast swimmer (the difference seems to be whether you were a front crawler or a breaststroker). The water was certainly bracing but after a count of three, I held my breath and launched myself into the water. The non-pootlers were off in a flash and Lin and I took a gentle pace, as I tried to coordinate my doggy/crawl/running on the spot action.

I was worried I would slow her down, but she assured me that people at the club went at varying paces and she swam for the noticeable health benefits she had experienced. I have to say, some things feel like exercise and some things are exercise disguised as play. I am definitely of the persuasion that you should get active whilst having fun. It makes you more likely to get out and do something and if you have kids, it is something which you can share. Plus, of course, the fact if you live by the sea (and it is clean), it's free.

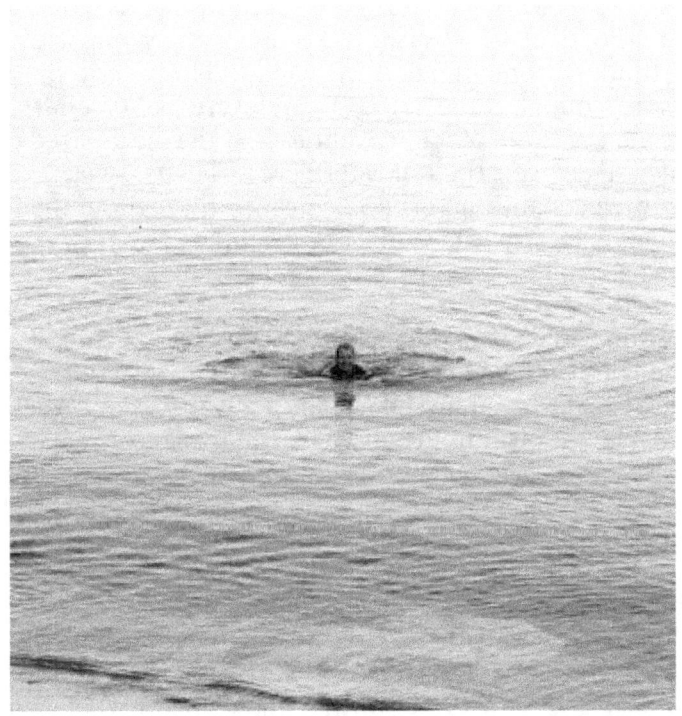

However, there are definite benefits of finding a club to swim with: the safety in numbers adage certainly applies but you also have the social side as well (after the swim, there was cake and hot Ribena). As we made our way to the destination rock, then headed back, as the speedier group went on further. The sun was shining, the water was clear and glistening and I felt really blessed. Sounds very corny, but I am guilty of thinking of a million things at once and always juggling life. This challenge is certainly teaching me to take time out, to look and wonder and to appreciate.

When we got close to shore, Lin went off to practise her front crawl. I lay on my back, and shut my eyes, taking in the full sensory moment and as I lay there in a fully tranquil state, I pondered what the protocol was about wee-ing in the sea with a wetsuit on...I didn't.

American Football – Number 26

My next adventure was to join the Cornish Sharks to play American Football. This was a full Sunday afternoon session, so I had to think of something which would help occupy the kids to help Daddy out. On the table, I put every bit of craft I could muster, all 3 drawers of it and went to find the mega-sized card for the kids to use for their masterpiece. The A1 sized card only appears occasionally and is used sparingly throughout the year for such emergencies as weekend work deadlines or hangovers. Their brief was a familiar one: A picture of anything but don't swirl the paints together and don't rush it! I waved goodbye to my budding artists (who couldn't see me behind the fortress of stickers, paints and glue pots) and made my way down to Truro.

I hadn't really given myself a chance to think about what was in store, so on the 40-minute drive, I tried to recall what I knew about the sport. When I was little, my dad used to watch it on Channel 4 on a Sunday evening. I would have my bath and then go and snuggle in, pretending I was interested, when really I was on bed-avoidance duty. I remember the full gear they wore and the crunching tackles that used to come flying in. I started to think about the tackles and the claustrophobic helmet on a warm day and my own lack of fitness and for the first time in this challenge, I had butterflies. Not just one flitting about, but a whole swarm of them.

When I arrived I was met by Brian, who put me at ease immediately by enthusiastically engaging with me about my challenge. I was so flustered, though, I forgot what I had done already and what number I was on and which was the best/worst I had done so far. Be calm, damned butterflies. I composed myself further and met the other guys who were there. Brian gave me my helmet, shirt and pads to put on after fitness.

Whilst the rest of the team arrived, Brian talked animatedly about the club and the sport in general and it soon became apparent the club had got to national league status mainly through Brian's tenacity and ambition. The lads seem to treat him in a patriarchal way and I could sense a lot of mutual respect. I tried to continue the questioning, like some sort of renegade reporter, in the hope of buying time before the inevitable showdown with the helmet.

First up though was fitness, which was really well drilled and included jumping in and out of big tyres and traversing cones - backwards. It was a hot day and we have already established my fitness is that of an asthmatic slug, so I was pleased to move onto the drills. I excused myself to the changing room to put on my shoulder pads under my shirt. This was not without struggle but finally, and feeling properly ridiculous, I was ready.

At the level these guys play, I was aware they needed to practise without me hampering training, so I was taken away for a few drills on how to catch. Catching in American Football isn't static, as I found whilst going through various types of offensive and defensive moves. My catching was mediocre but I was enjoying myself away from the main action. Brian's comfort zone radar must have bleeped because he hollered for me to join the defensive backs. Here, I was given the task of trying to get past an opponent by blocking him and essentially roughing him up and getting past him. I am not sure what the opposite of comfort zone is, but that was where I was currently residing!

After a few attempts at swatting my opponent, I joined a new group to become a running back. The positional play was described to me in number codes and my job was to run through the defensive line, when the quarterback passed me the ball. "Hut hut," off I went. I excelled in this role, as I didn't have to throw, catch or get in a fracas; I was just handed the ball as I ran past, with my armed guard pushing away the opposition.

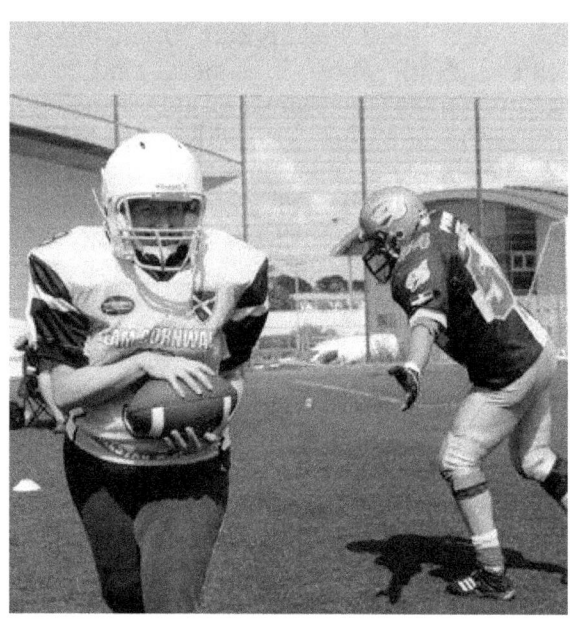

I've got the ball

I really enjoyed the camaraderie and found the game itself fascinating. One of the guys referred to the sport as "angry chess" and I think that succinctly describes it - strategic, fast moving and very combative. In the States, American Football is their number one sport, with an average attendance of 70,000 per game. The NFL league pulls in a revenue of $9 billion dollars but in the UK, it is a lightly funded, minority sport, which takes unpaid volunteers like Brian to drive it. I admire what has happened with the club and how the sport is being developed in the county.

I wished the lads luck for their final games of the season and I drove home; glad to be rid of the shoulder pads and eager to jump into the bath. When I got back my daughter proudly showed off her afternoon's work: a big beautiful butterfly!

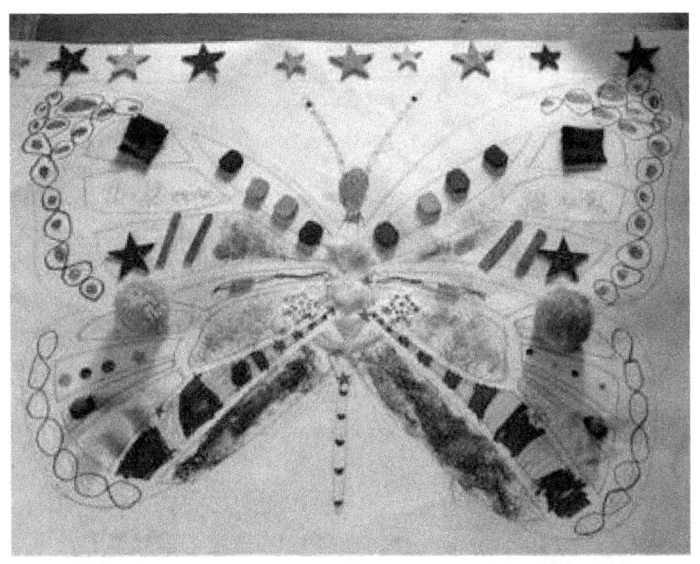

She Must Have Known Mummy Had Butterflies!

Running - Number 27

I hate running. Running just isn't my thing. Sure, I have gone for runs when trying to get fit but as I live just outside of Bodmin Moor, there are damned hills everywhere. You can't go more than a minute before you hit an incline. As soon as I see a sign for an incline, I bow down to its superiority and meekly reduce the pacc to a walk. Once an incline is conquered, I jog, until the next one. This makes me not a runner, but a jogger/walker or a jalker or wogger if you prefer?

Another reason, (apart from my size and shape), as to why I am incompatible with running is that I have nobody to talk to and even if I had a running buddy, I would be so out of breath I wouldn't be able to chat with them anyway. When we do a warm-up around the pitch before hockey, I get all my questions and conversation into the first bit, knowing I will be out of puff by half way.

So, off I went with a head full of grumbling resentment and pessimism about my next challenge of going for a dreaded run with East Cornwall Harriers. I was met by an array of different Karens, who in turn welcomed me. We were split into three different groups; one for runners, one for joggers and one for social/beginner runners. The last group was explained as slow jogging and walking with a lot of nattering. Yes, I was with the Woggers!

I was still unconvinced that I would be able to keep up, but Debs explained she was in the same boat as me and not to worry. Off we went, around the town of Liskeard. The pace was slow and very manageable but then on reflection, it was completely downhill at that point. I managed to get my nattering in without losing too much breath and was feeling OK. In this case, what goes down inevitably had to go up but as soon as we hit the incline, we walked. Apparently, running doesn't get in the way of the chatting. Fantastic.

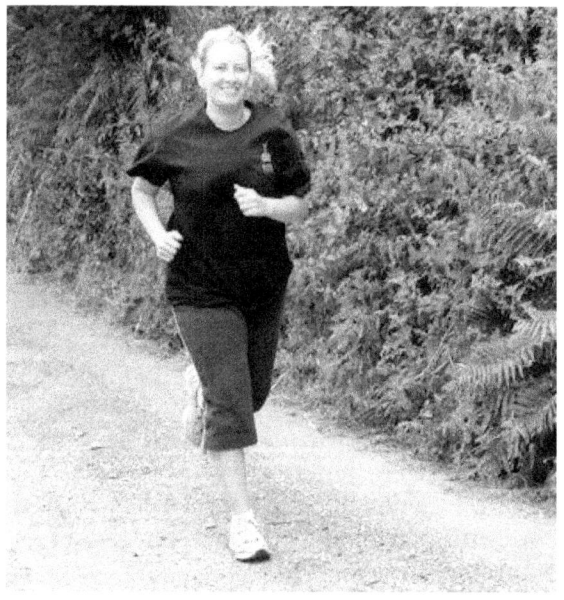

Wogging

It was a beautiful evening as we jalked our way back to the start. I asked questions about running in general and Amanda told me there were a lot of social runners in the club, and not everyone wanted to run fast. Again, I definitely felt happier running in a group and would certainly be more motivated to go for a run if I was meeting people and running at a manageable pace together.

As we neared the end, I asked how far we had gone and the reply was "about 4." I didn't ask for clarification if that was 4 miles or 4 kilometres. To me, I had done a solid 4 miles. At the end, I felt refreshed and invigorated, and my legs ached slightly in recognition of my efforts.

There is a lot written about how to run and why to run in the first place. Running, like any sport, is not elitist. If you can run and you want to run, no matter what size or shape, you can just run. Like anything, I guess the first hurdle is just trying. If you do feel a bit self-conscious or that it's something you can't do, I came across a site called Too Fat Too Run, which gives great advice and motivation to people who aren't sure. As for me, I have firmly put running clubs in my "After the Challenge" list. Although I'm worried that this is filling up quite rapidly and I'm not even a third of the way through - it joins sea swimming, yoga, cricket and badminton. I would hate to think I'm not going to come across anything else which I want to continue, but at the moment the list is getting out of hand!

Tang Soo Do – Number 28

This week is martial arts week, where I am going off to try the Korean art of Tang Soo Do (or as my son impishly remarked, Scooby Do) and Krav Maga. First up was Tang Soo Do with ISK Martial Arts.

With all of my challenges, I like to find myself in the newbie/beginners class, where I can usually find an equally clueless kindred spirit, but somehow, in a gargantuan administrative error on my part, I had found myself booked into the advanced black belt class. Clearly, I am more a white or peachy colour - anything but black.

I was welcomed to the club by Master Rob James who runs the club and holds an impressive CV, which includes being the British and European Champion numerous times and competing in the World Championship. It sounds really cheesy, but I have a huge amount of respect for people at the pinnacle of whatever they achieve and felt privileged to be literally learning from the Master.

Master Rob's favourite saying is: "The more you sweat in training the less you bleed in battle." Initially when I read that, I baulked slightly at the literal interpretation but thinking about it, this is all about hard work and preparation and can be related to

85

anything in life. My mantra is more: "The more you chat in training the less you have to talk about in battle" – maybe I need to revisit that?

So preparing to sweat, I joined the black belts. Master Rob explained that the class would be going back to basics, which I guess is good to do occasionally in all sports and disciplines. Warm-up started with gentle jogging and stretching, which was fine. The stretches then went to a new level, which my body is unaccustomed with. When I stretch and it tweaks, I stop. When you stretch with a partner, you can't cheat and my partner, Xena ensured that all cobwebs were dusted off my hamstrings and quads.

Next up, Master Rob went through a variety of moves. Similar to Aikido, I learnt the best self-defence is to be able to run fast but if that is not an option, there are techniques which can negate an assailant's assaults. We practised a number of them with rotating partners. However, unlike Aikido where I got to beat people up at will, the black belts respected me enough to equally share out the pain with me.

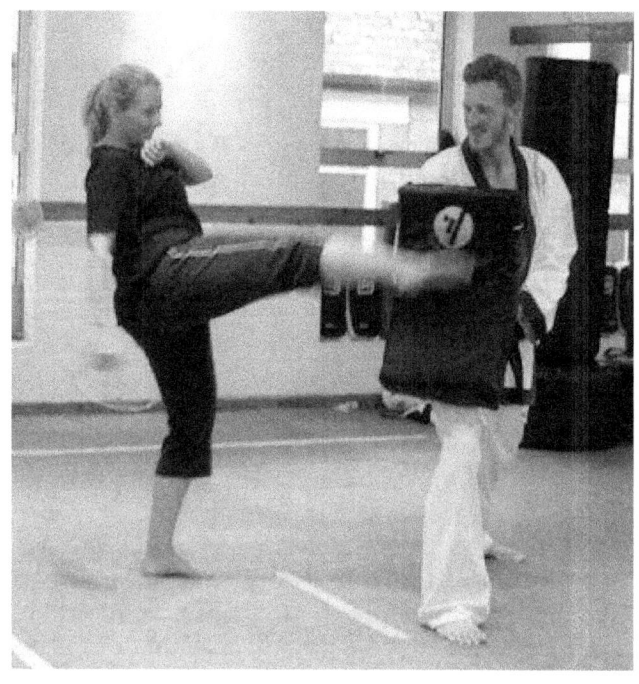

Getting the stress out

86

One tip I learnt is that the internationally recognised gesture for "ouch that hurts, let go!" is to tap yourself on the leg. I did not have this knowledge for my first two takedowns, as I found my arm twisted around my head. We finished with kicking. Who knew that round house kicking a padded mat releases pent-up kids off school/summer holiday/too much work to do stressful tension so well?

I really enjoyed my time with the advanced class. I like the discipline and respect which is shown in the martial arts classes I have tried so far; something which can be lacking in some mainstream sports. I found Tang Soo Do to be a defensive art, with measured aggression that was founded on technique, rather than brute force and that these Eastern philosophies are definitely piquing my interest.

Krav Maga – Number 29

Not twenty-four hours had passed before I was back getting another mock beating in a martial arts class. This time, it was Krav Maga at Kernow Martial Arts.

Owner and Chief Instructor James explained that Krav Maga had derived from the Israeli army and had since been adopted by the likes of the SAS. I was introduced to the class and we started the warm-up - my back was creaking from my exertions the previous day. After the warm-up, we put on our pads and started practising hitting. There was no punching but a kind of padding up of the assailant and then slapping hard around the ears (pads) with the intention of perforating an ear drum.

I was paired up with young Aiden, who looked pretty harmless as assailants go - definitely one of the more manageable varieties. He wore the gloves and took my blows, as I kept resorting to a boxing stance instead of the Krav position. Then it was my turn to wear the pads. Aiden obviously hadn't been given the script and set about pummelling me for a solid three minutes, as James turned off the lights and put on some music to reflect a real life situation. If somebody had been vomiting in the corner, I would have thought I was in the local nightclub.

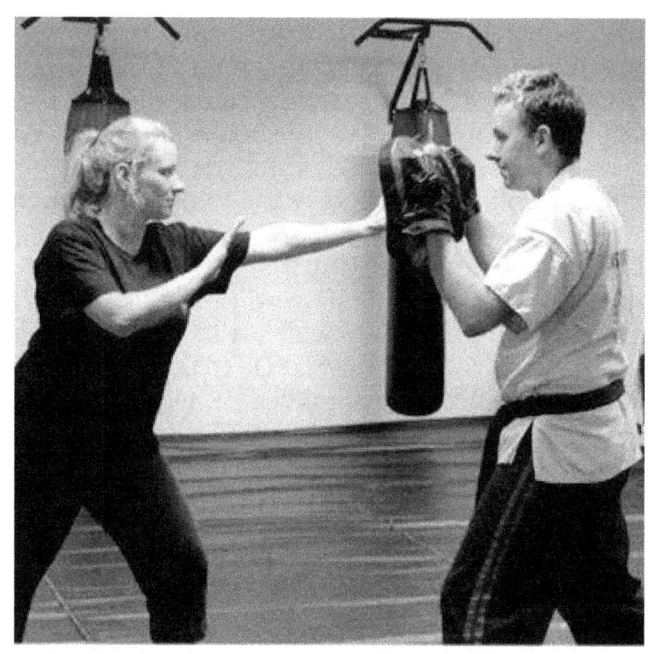

James holding the pads and me looking fierce!

If Aikido was slick and flowing and Tang Soo Do was fast and furious, Krav Maga was dark and menacing. Minimal moves are learnt for maximum impact - it's certainly not meant to be pretty, just effective. James said he sometimes teaches the class outside, in alleyways or even in the toilets - anywhere where it reflects real life.

The next real life situation I found myself in was being pinned up against a wall with a knife (piece of wood). Thankfully Aiden refrained from beating me with the mock-knife and observed restraint whilst demanding money from me. As the victim, I had to confuse him by asking a random question to cause a split second of confusion before I deftly unarmed him by grabbing his arm and poking him quickly in the windpipe, dragging down his elbow, and kicking him in my choice of head, abdomen or groin.

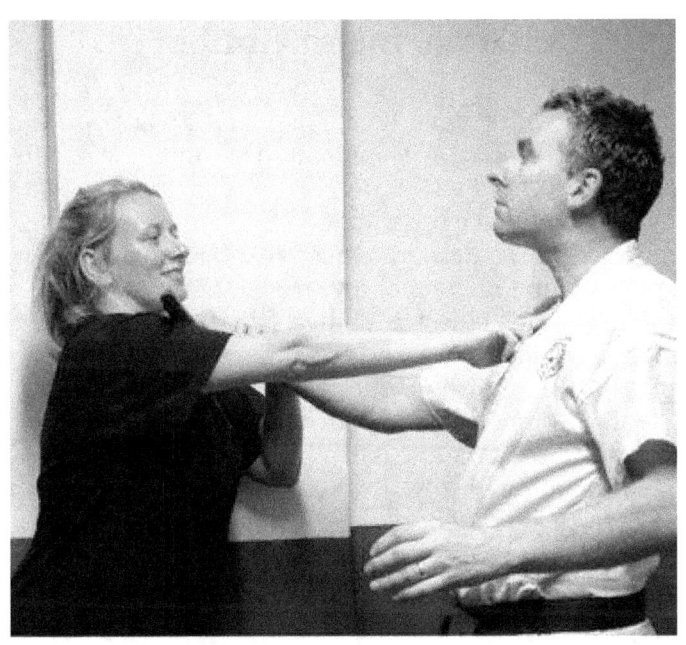

Right in the windpipe...

In terms of self-defence, this martial art seemed to be very instinctive, set against the backdrop of real life and James confirmed that it would be ideal for girls to learn, as a means of protecting themselves. It's the sort of thing I'd like my daughters to learn as they get older and more independent.

Keen as always to put my skills into practice, I rushed home to Paul and immediately weaponised him with a courgette. He was initially reticent to get off the sofa, having just got the kids to bed but remembering the joy he got by nullifying my moves after Aikido, I managed to persuade him up to hold the dangerous vegetable. I adopted the Krav stance, told him "I didn't want any trouble" and put my hands up submissively (with the cunning intent of luring him into a false sense of security before I unleashed the barrage of moves I'd just learnt). He took one look at me, looked at the courgette, smacked me over the head with it and sat back down. Foiled again...

I've got angling down as my next sport – maybe a fish will be something I can batter.

Orienteering – Number 30

It's been over a week since Krav Maga and Tang Soo Do and the combined effort managed to put my back out. Two visits to my Chiropractor later and having to postpone my angling last week, I finally feel ready to take on orienteering. Paul decided to prioritise DIY, which left me in desperate need of a teammate who would be able to read a map - not one of my strong points.

I drafted in my eldest and her friend Lily. I guessed that orienteering would require you to be fleet of foot and cunning in equal measure. Lauren is cunning and Lily is both cunning and fleet of foot, so I emotionally blackmailed them into participating, with me as the token adult patrolling for bears or other hidden dangers. Although with my strained back, I was the one who was most likely to be bear fodder.

The weather forecast spelled doom and gloom, so without imparting this information to them, I encouraged them both to take waterproofs "just in case." Luckily, pre-teens have an obsession with loom bands, which means they were concentrating on little bits of elastic and not the looming rain clouds.

When we arrived at Lanhydrock, we went to the tent to register and were given instructions as to what it was all about. Basically, there were 13 checkpoints, which required you to enter your key into a letterbox type marker to register the fact you have hit that checkpoint. We were given an OS map, with our targets marked out - some worth one point and others worth five. The hazards on the map were pointed out and we were encouraged to go to the start point. Then the rain started and to precipitate the moaning about precipitation, we detoured to the National Trust cafe for some sugary treats. The girls picked up a packet of fudge and we agreed that if they got to a marker and hadn't moaned, they would be allowed one fudge each.

Ironically, it took us twenty minutes to actually find the start line and thoroughly disorientated, we started the course. We had one hour exactly to get as many points as possible. We saw other contenders zigzagging the course and the girls' first strategy was to follow other people. No, I said. That wasn't the spirit of the game. Fast forward 10 minutes later and trekking through a field of ferns and mud divots, we stalked a luminous contender who led us to our first checkout. Bingo! The fudge packet was opened and we set off for the next one full of confidence and sugar.

Between Lauren and Lily, they confidently found a further 4 checkout points, with me mainly acting as a mobile fudge dispensing unit. We reconvened to talk strategy about the next checkpoint: should we go for the easy 1 pointer or, with 20 minutes left, go for the trickier 5 pointer? At this point, I should have maintained my role of guardian; instead, I took the map. Things rapidly went downhill as I took the "as the crow flies" approach, dragging them through bogs, brambles and getting them to traverse fallen trees to get over streams. Like a crazed contender in the Crystal Maze with the impending door closing, I was determined to find the elusive 5 pointer that was "around the next corner."

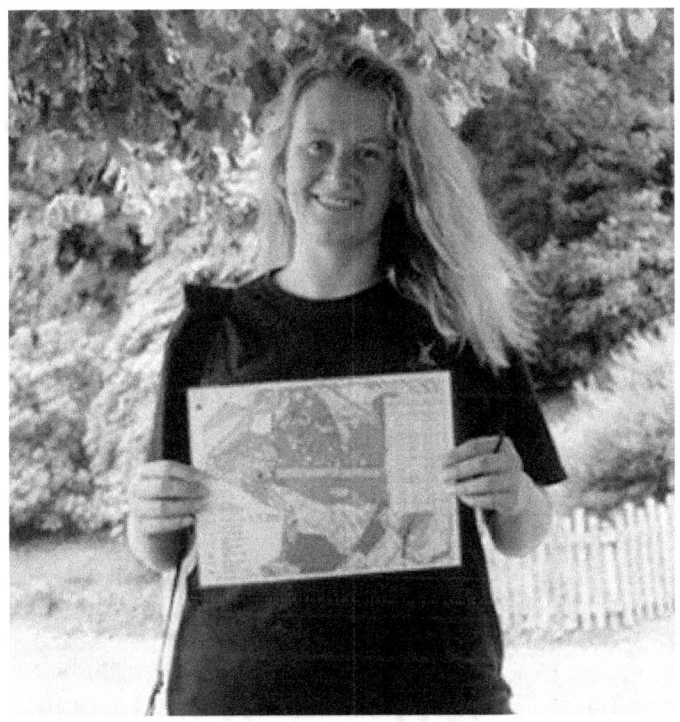

Do not let me hold one of these again

Lily started to complain about blisters. Lauren started to whine about her legs getting too tired. I offered them a fudge, they declined - we were in trouble. There were five minutes left. Should I sacrifice the kids to the elements and make a dash for it? If we went over the hour, we would incur penalty points. My feet were sodden and the kids were thoroughly disillusioned with my team leading skills. Damn it, the time was up! We meandered back pondering what we would have done differently: apparently giving me the map was the main problem.

Our key was handed back at the finish line and the scores fed into the system. Out of 28 teams, we came 25th. Not bad given that we started the day fairly clueless. We agreed that with our new found knowledge, we would come back again but with a different strategy. My little ones would also love the smaller courses, so I decided to keep an eye out for any more events. Now, it was time to go home for a bath and the chance to consider what on Earth happened to number 26, 27 and 28 – they must have been eaten by the bears to come behind us.

The Challenge So Far - Number 21 to 30

The inevitable happened in my recent ten and I picked up a back sprain. It turns out now I have hit the latter part of the mid-thirties; I need to warm-up to warm-up. The knock-on effect meant that I had to cancel a couple of sports, as I literally spent two days bent over like an old lady. On one occasion as I went to visit Liz, my chiropractor, I felt my back seize up in the car park and I had to take deep breaths bending over the bonnet of the car to steady myself, whereby a lovely lady came up to me to enquire whether "I was going into labour?"

To a non-pregnant lady, there is no sentence which is more cutting and hurtful than to be asked: "when is it due?" or as I have found to be worse still: "are you going into labour?" I bent myself back as straight as I could, so I could see the full remorse in her eyes as I told her I was just a little sore in the back area. She apologised and trotted off to find somebody else to "help."

Having had to postpone some of the sports I had lined up, I frantically started to think about my schedule and pro-rata up what number I should be at if I am to finish on May 1st next year. I'm two sports down on where I should be – or a week out. If I had an injury once a week every 3 months, it would mean me doing a challenge every day in the last week. I am a low-level, wannabe, sports-tryer; what must professional sportspeople go through when an injury wreaks havoc with their timetable? I can't think of that. I need to stay focused and get fully acquainted with my new best friend, Biofreeze.

However, yet again the evenings are drawing in and as I type, there is a chill in the air, so I have to keep focused and motivated.

My next sports include archery, netball, coasteering, wakeboarding, cardio tennis, korfball, surf life-saving and ice skating. If the previous ten had a martial arts feel about them, the next ten have an adrenaline/water sports vibe going on. I am not exaggerating when I tell you I'm petrified of the idea of coasteering and wakeboarding, but I have tried to be strategic in doing them at the end of August/early September, when the tourists have gone home, so there are fewer people to point at me and laugh and the water is still relatively warm. So essentially, I am trying to limit the cold - the cold and the bitter humiliation.

Chapter 5 - Challenge 31 – 40

Archery – Number 31

Next up was archery at St Austell Bay Archery club. In the morning, I managed to accessorise my backache with a swollen and bruised stubbed toe. However, I'd already postponed archery on account of my back last week, so I strapped up the toe, carried on with painkillers and made my way down to the club, to family choruses of "if you were a horse, we would take you to the knackers' yard!"

Knackers' yard? I'll show them! I had a good feeling about archery – it didn't primarily focus on my weak points of balance or coordination and I went in feeling fully Maid Marian about it all.

After being introduced to the club members, Chris the club secretary took me off to get kitted up. First up, Chris asked if I was stronger in the right eye or left - "right," I confidently replied. These previous 30 sports have enabled me to gain insights into the inner workings of my body and as discovered in Tai Chi, the left side of my body is un-coordinated and frankly, a bit rubbish. To confirm this, Chris rolled up a bit of A4 paper and handed it to me and instructed me to look through and tell me the number at the far end. I held the paper to my left eye and peered through. A general chortle went up, as it was confirmed that I preferred the left and was immediately labelled "Cack-Eyed."

My tuition for the evening was left to Kevin, an accidental archer, who took it up with his son 18 months ago and continued with it whilst his son moved on to other pursuits. I was given the safety instructions based on various whistle toots. I was fully attentive to the advice, as these arrows travelled and I didn't want to re-enact the Bayeux tapestry.

After putting on my protective gear, I held up the bow and stood right-angled to the target, as instructed and fired my first arrow. The first three arrows landed out of the scoring range but bang on in pretty much the same place. Consistency was there, just not accuracy.

I really enjoyed firing off the arrows and when Kev started scoring me, the competitive side came out and I scored a 27, which I was pretty pleased about. I should have packed up there and then, as I didn't reach those heady heights again. I was surprised that, after an hour, my hand started to shake as I got tired and new muscles were awakened.

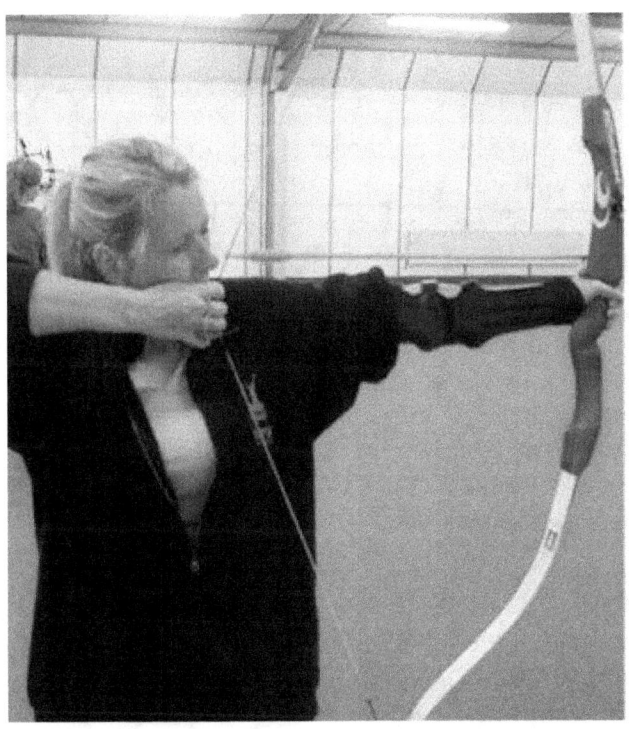

Looking through my "cack-eye"

After everybody started to pack away, I asked if I could have a go on the proper target (up until now my target was half way from the actual target). This target looked a long way away and with three arrows, I didn't manage to score but I can see that this would be quite addictive as a sport. I don't think I could walk away until I had scored well.

Archery was very enjoyable, but I have now discovered a new area of personal weakness - cack-eyeness - which completes the head to toe look I am currently rocking.

Coasteering – Number 32

I have learnt something new while doing this challenge. I thought a fear of heights was called Vertigo, but Wikipedia enlightened me to the fact that Vertigo relates to dizziness; what I have is called Acrophobia. To give you an idea on how much I hate heights, I met some girlfriends in Bristol a few months ago and Paul was travelling back with the kids from London, so we agreed to meet on the M4 services, where he would pick me up to go home. All I had to do was cross the bridge over the motorway. As I stood and looked at the other side, my heart started pounding. I started to sweat and thought the only way I could get across would be to crawl (whilst dragging a small suitcase behind me). The only way I managed to get over was to think that my children were in a burning building over the other side and I had to get to them - without crawling over a public bridge looking like a prat! So, the thought of jumping off rocks into the sea, makes coasteering the biggest challenge I've faced so far.

To take the focus off me and dilute the very real prospect of having a public breakdown, I asked if any of the hockey lot would like to join me. I had 8 other takers - most of whom are at least 10 years younger than me and full of adventure. We met at the car park; three of the girls who agreed to come didn't actually know what coasteering was and thought they were kayaking! Not a great start.

When we got to Fistral beach in Newquay, we joined about 15 other people. I immediately scanned the crowd to see if I could spot a fellow Nancy to befriend. The safety instructions were led by Mark of Mad Ferret Adventures, but unfortunately I managed to position myself on the corner, where the prevailing wind meant that I could only hear every other word, which isn't great when you hear the words "Don't do...." or "Definitely don't......" and then miss the relevant information which followed.

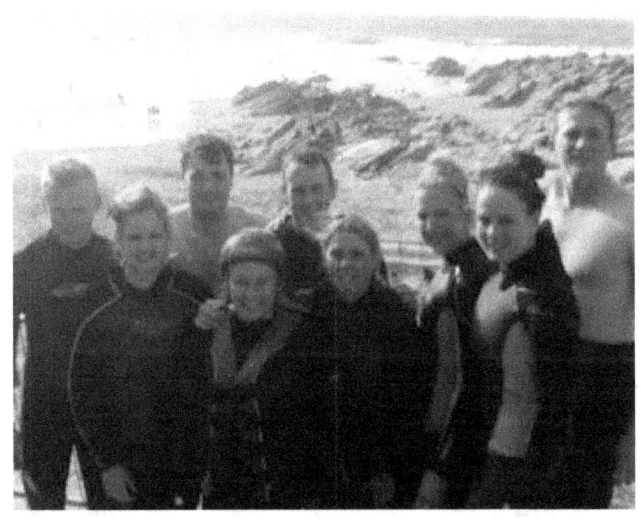

The nutters who actually wanted to jump off high rocks

We kitted up in wetsuits, lifejackets, helmets, shorts and jackets and set off to the unknown. After about 10 minutes, we climbed down some rocks to a collection of massive pools. Thankfully the safety tips were repeated and that was it; we were invited to choose the level we would like to jump from. Ummmm, I don't want to jump off either of them! My lot, without reservation, went to the top and started hurling themselves off like a bunch of lemmings, whilst I scrambled to a shelf halfway down with a few others.

My turn to jump. The irrational fear gripped me and every part of me tensed with utter terror. My heart was pounding and sheer panic coursed through me. Several aborted countdowns went by before I finally made the leap. I bobbed back up and I can't tell you the relief I felt. The lady behind me made a full belly flop into the water and I decided that my job was to emotionally nurse her back to health and thus avoid repeating the exercise.

I never felt inclined to repeat that initial achievement, so whilst everybody else went to higher points, with some adding dives and backward flips, I entered the sea via the "grandma route" - going to the lowest point and shuffling in on my bottom. We got to swim in awesome swells and powerful whirlpools, but no part of me felt like I wanted to repeat the jump. I achieved what I wanted to get out of coasteering and I was really proud of myself.

As we sat eating cheesy chips overlooking over the sea, I pondered why some people crave the adrenaline rush. I guess it must be addictive but give me the tea-cup ride on the fairground any day. I am pleased to say that is the end of my height based challenges - even riding Spot the bloody horse made me fearful. I'm relieved I didn't add abseiling or paragliding to the list; I don't think Wikipedia has a definition for what my reaction to that would be.

Aqua Aerobics – Number 33

As the modern day poet Jay-Z eloquently declared in his recent sonnet, there are generally a total of 99 problems and I think he was referring to swimming in a local pool. I can empathise with Mr Z, as I too have the same quantity of issues when considering getting into a swimsuit. From cellulite, to body image, to lighting, to being a fashion philistine with my choice of swimwear, to fear of floaters; there are indeed 99 problems, which equates to 99 reasons why I generally avoid the pool.

My existing swimsuit possesses no powers to keep my rather large boobs into position and thus a breaststroke is usually self-fulfilling. My friend, Sugar is a retailer of swimsuits for the over mammary-ed amongst us, so I trotted down for her counsel on the subject. Sugar presented me with a range of revolutionary swimsuits, which had an inbuilt bra inside - amazing! She found it almost incomprehensible that I had gone through my life without this knowledge. Her disparaging remarks went on deaf ears, as I was busy falling in love with a tankini which ruffled at the tummy.

Once purchased, I took myself, my ruffle at the tummy, boob-holding tankini, and my eldest down to try Aqua Aerobics at Atlantic Reach (the scene of the pole-dancing debacle). My back is still proving a bit of a problem, so I had hurriedly substituted wakeboarding for the gentler aqua class. That particular nightmare can wait for another day.

I met Frances, the instructor, who initially looked bemused by my challenge and then once she realised I wasn't an outpatient, enthusiastically questioned me about it all. She also said the class would be perfect for my back and that I could put in as much or as little effort as I felt comfortable with. She didn't mention my tankini.

After scanning the water for floaters as I eyed up the vacating toddlers, I waded into the pool, which felt pleasantly warm after all of my sea challenges. The music began and I splashed my way through "I'm Sexy and I Know It" and other equally bouncing music and at no bounce was there a slip of any kind. It was a pleasant change not to be constantly worried about if I had preserved my modesty.

The good thing about the class is that coordination was not a massive requirement, as you could freestyle if you mucked it up and nobody could see what blunders you were making with your lower limbs. My back felt comfortable, even though I was exercising; certainly, it was something everyone could do.

My aqua prancing was over and I had a great time. Maybe the land based fitness classes make me focus too much on my lack of coordination and rhythm. In aqua aerobics, no one will win an award for timing: that is best left to synchronised swimming, which isn't one of my 100 sports. Best of all, I managed to stay all in one place for the duration – I may have 99 problems but the t*ts ain't one!

Ice Skating – Number 34

Ice skating falls into my list of "not looking forward to" sports. I remember ice-skating when I was a young teenager and it not going particularly well. Plus, I am still suffering a little with the back, so it may not be the best idea but I figured if I fell, at least I would have an immediate ice-pack. The whole family were going to join me for this challenge down at Pavilions in Plymouth.

Plymouth Ice Skating Club meets every week and families are welcomed, so despite my deep reservations, we booted up and got on the ice. Now, being new to ice, you would appreciate a bit of time to acclimatise to the new surface and get your bearings, focusing mainly on poise and balance. What you don't need is your 6-year-old son trying to use running motion between your legs, in a cartoon type style. He went through the following stages - excitement, anticipation, frustration, panic and disconsolate tears. Please, take in the mental image as the five of us clung to the wall, shuffling our way around.

We were welcomed over the speakers by Shirley, who introduced us to the club and encouraged people to find and welcome us – we weren't difficult to locate, as we looked like a family of newborn giraffes. All I needed to do was to get Oliver off the ice-rink and calm him down. He sat down and munched on some penny sweets. My girls were off and skating... well, more fast clinging to the wall. The problem is when you are highly dependent on the wall to keep you balanced, if somebody else is there already, you have to let go and skirt around them. Maybe a traffic light system could be introduced?

My own confidence started to grow as I tentatively let go of my lifeline and shakily made my way around. Other club members came up to talk to me about my challenge and to see if I needed any help. When Olly decided he was ready to get back on the ice, a couple of ladies helped him around until he got the right motion and I was thankful that he hadn't sulked and given up. He fell a few times more and one of the little girls (who was 8 and could hold her skate behind her back) came over to ask if he was alright and whether he would like some cake. He coyly accepted.

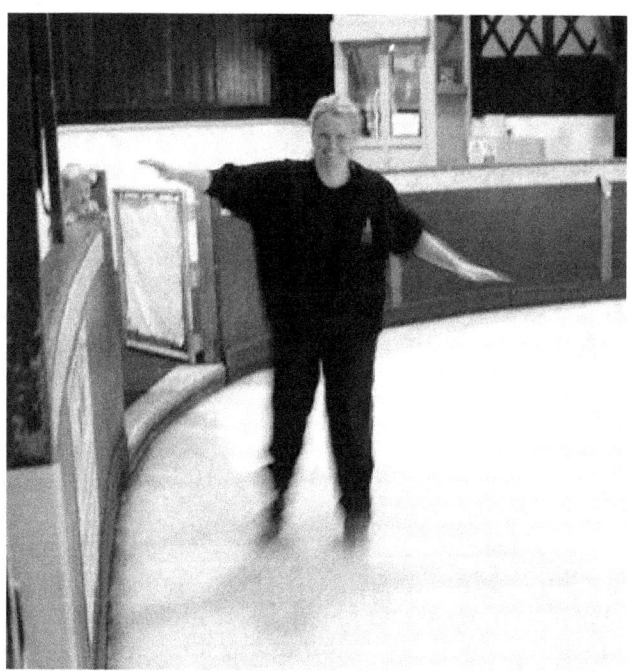

Look, no hands!

The standard varied, from our family on the bottom rung, right through to very twirly people but everybody was friendly and welcoming and we didn't feel out of place at all. I guess everybody starts in the same way. After singing happy birthday to Shirley and enjoying some cake, we went back on the ice, where there was the opportunity to play some games.

Finally, there was a "show off" spot, where everybody stood around the edge and over the tannoy, a name was called out and they would show their moves to everybody's approval. It was great for the kids to see what could be achieved with hard work and dedication. Then over the tannoy, I heard "and the family from Bodmin, would you like to show what you have learnt?" Rising dread and humiliation started to fill my whole body as Shirley couldn't hear me shout back "No, we're good" or see me shaking my head. I looked around to see general pity and sympathy in people's eyes, as my children (and a smirking Paul) willed me to do something fancy. I shuffled a metre from the wall and back and received a resounding round of applause, as Shirley, again over the loud speaker, congratulated me for "getting off the wall." Pure mortification!

The time was up and despite a few falls, the kids had a great time. They relayed every one of their achievements while they mock skated back to the car. Apparently, I had better get used to it, as they want to go back as soon as they can. It looks like I'll have to improve my skating if I want to keep up.

Angling – Number 35

Next up on my list is angling. After all of my recent escapades, I was looking forward to a gentle afternoon in the sun, being at one with nature. I met Alex of Roche Angling Club at one of the club's lakes on a beautifully sunny day. Admittedly, there were a few trepidations around meeting a random stranger in a remote location, having been told to look out for his blue Mondeo. When I arrived, Alex looked as relieved as I was not to come face-to-face with a loony!

As we approached the lake, I felt a lovely feeling of serenity, which I often get being around water. Even looking at a puddle long enough can de-stress me in moments of distress. The swallows danced on the water and the lake looked tranquil and peaceful. Alex brought down a range of rods and fishing paraphernalia and started me off with a basic Huckleberry Finn type rod. I am not a fisherwoman, but my understanding is that fish bait is usually something disgusting and I was ready to wince. Instead, it was a value bag of sweetcorn.

Alex fished around in his box of gubbins and pulled out various weights and tied them on to the end of the line. Once we had found the perfect spot, he showed me how to cast out. I followed suit, whilst Alex sprinkled some fish cat-nip out to entice them to the tempting kernel. The idea of fishing is to keep an attentive eye on the bobby thing, which alerts you to the fact you have a taker. My job would then be to "strike" at which point you have to go into full overdrive and commence the ritual wrestle to land the whopper!

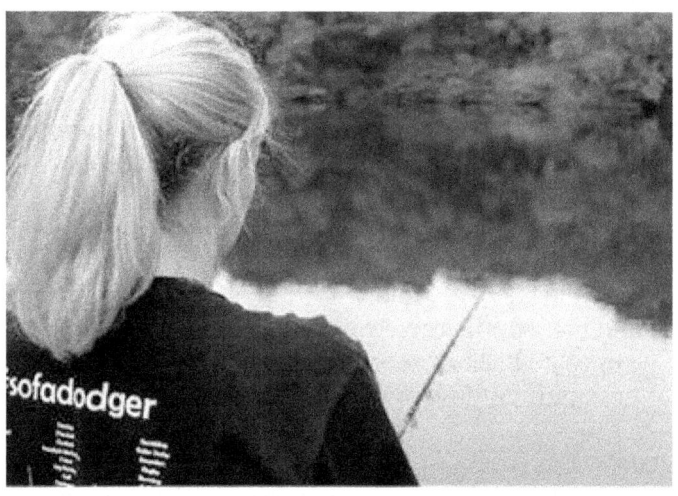

and so the wait begins....

All around the line, we could see the perpetual circles of ripples being made by the inquisitive creatures. We waited and we watched. It gave me a chance to talk to Alex about his hobby and the club. As a practitioner of communication techniques, I tend to try and make eye contact in conversation, which in angling is a fatal mistake. I twice missed the bobby thing sinking, which meant I was a split second too slow in successfully striking. Each time, as I pulled in the line, a solitary sweetcorn kernel waved back at me. I was starting to get frustrated.

I threw the line out again and managed to hook myself in the finger, which dislodged the sweetcorn. Out again and more waiting. Alex said he was pleased I was getting the full experience of what fishing is actually like. A cormorant swooped down and picked off a fish in a mocking display to further test my patience. I started to complain about the brand of sweetcorn. Surely, Green Giant had to be the corn of choice? Then...hark, what was this? Mid-moan, the bobby thing submerged....strike! I bloody striked alright! I yanked the fish out of the water, screamed as I saw its flappy, wet body hurtling towards my face and in the confusion, the little critter managed to dislodge himself and make a leap for freedom.

Nobody told me angling was an adrenaline sport. That tussle certainly sent my blood pressure rocketing. With continued frustration but with renewed hope, the jousting continued. However, there had to be a happy ending i.e. me beaming, holding a fish. I asked Alex whether maybe he could catch the fish for me to hold up (turns out that I have little to no pride). He answered by getting out a new rod; one with a reel and everything. I practised the technique of casting and fully loaded with bait, I set about reeling in the sucker. After a couple of near misses, the bobby thing bobbed and strike, I reeled. What appeared was probably the smallest fish which could have been feasibly snared in the whole lake but to me, he was a whopper.

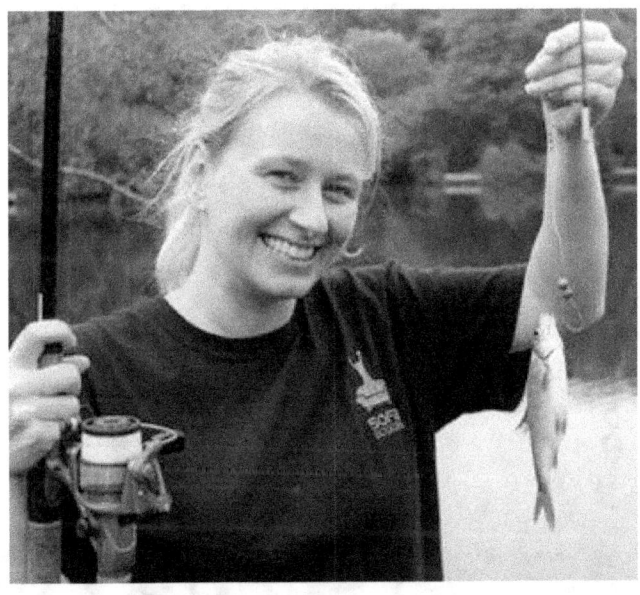

I hereby name him Jaws!

Alex took the necessary picture and then unhooked it and encouraged me to hold it for a further shot. I was very reticent to be forming that kind of friendship with the fish but my reluctance was stopping him getting back in the water, so I quickly posed with him and chucked him back, leaving me to deal with the residual slime and what turned out to be a lingering odour.

Korfball – Number 36

There are a lot of ball sports in my challenge: netball, basketball, handball, dodgeball, floorball, stoolball and the recently identified Wallball. Also on the list is korfball. Last week, I switched over to the BBC programme Pointless, which was on this exact topic and it turns out 5 of these sports were pointless (according to the programme). Not only do I have a new layer of knowledge through this challenge, but in an alternate reality, I would have won £6,000 on a game show.

There are no korfball clubs in Cornwall, so I dusted off my passport and made a second foray in a week over the Tamar Bridge to Devon, and a meeting with Exeter Korfball club. The club were putting on an open session for beginners to experience the sport. Being surrounded by newbies was a new experience for me, as I usually have a fleet of babysitters to take me through the sport but last night I was strangely anonymous around people who were as clueless as I was.

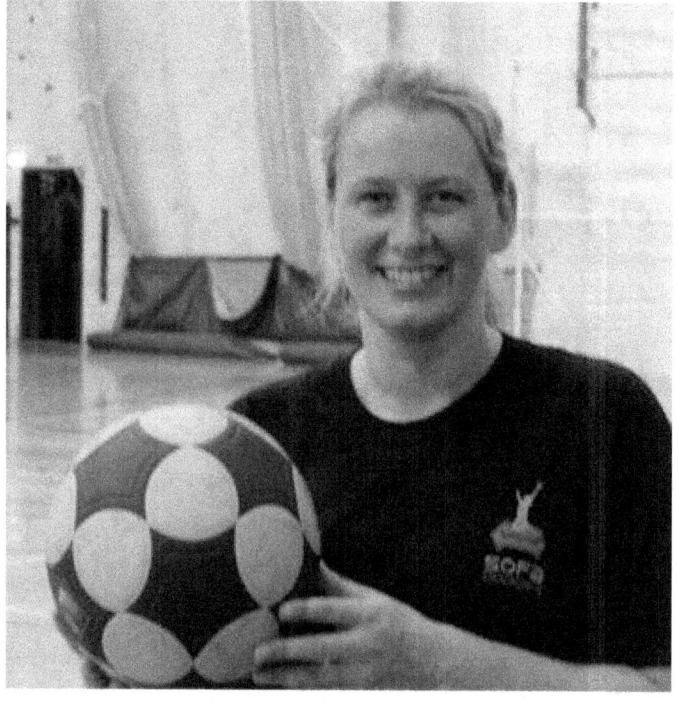

Me and a korfball...

Korfball is a mixed team sport: 4 girls and 4 boys and off the top of my head, is unique amongst other sports in that regard. As previously noted, I like team sports and I like blokey banter, so this had the potential to be right up my street. However, I became alarmed by the size of the basket which was wheeled out - at over 11ft high it looked like a netball hoop on steroids. I couldn't even imagine a possibility where my short self could score with something that high up.

We warmed up in a circle throwing the ball to each other, and once we were comfortable with our throwing and catching we sat down to watch the team actually play a game. The match was played at a fast pace and had similarities with netball, apart from the fact that I have never seen a man play netball...maybe more should, these guys were good. Play could go around the hoop as it wasn't stuck on a back line, but the main difference was that if you were being closely marked, you couldn't take a shot, so there was a lot of movement to free yourself from your defender.

The pros started to come off and give their bibs to us rookies to take over in their positions. There were quite a few newbies and I suddenly felt the need to get a drink of water, which happened to be at the back of the line. When my wimpery was exposed, I was given a bib and went on the court. Girls can only mark girls but unfortunately, my opponent was a good number of inches taller than me, so fleet of foot and cunning were the order of the day. The game was relentless and I was kicking myself for wearing my tracky bottoms, as I was quickly turning the colour of a newly hatched lobster.

The match finished and we split into four groups to practise shooting. We threw the ball to a teammate and then ran to pick up their pass and hoist it into the basket. Technique is everything. You can forget the one handed netball shot; what was encouraged was a two-handed lob into the air. Six attempts later, I perfected the technique to bag myself a basket. There were no cheerleaders to whoop at my achievement but internally, I was high fiving myself.

After, it was back to the game and I was far keener for the bib. The match was fast, hot and frenetic but thoroughly enjoyable. One of the girls had played for Holland and I watched how she played the game. I tried to master watching the opponent like she did and not the ball, which was slightly disorientating, and I did get hit on the head by random fire but I shook it off and continued.

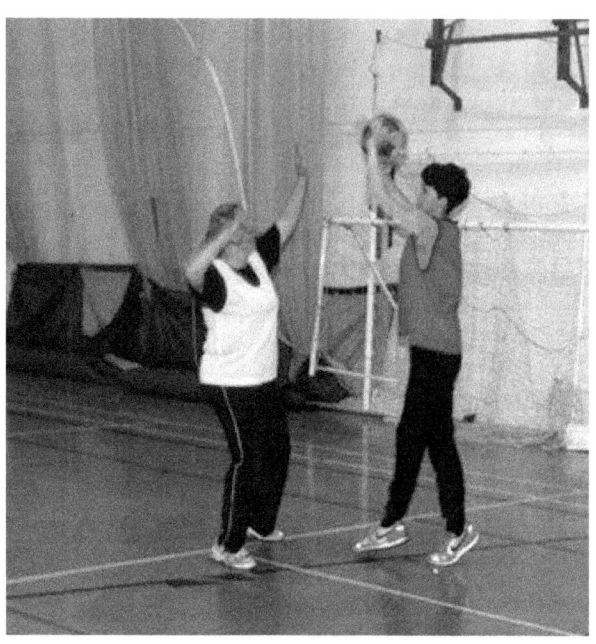

I am such a short-arse!

Korfball was a thoroughly enjoyable game and although reminiscent of my netball days, it also felt very different with the male dynamic included. Definitely worth a try if you're local to a Korfball club.

Surf Life-Saving – Number 37

I finally felt my back was getting back to normal, so I am ready to resume my challenge. My friend, Maxine is a coach at Polzeath Surf Lifesaving club, so I took myself down to Polzeath beach on a sunny Sunday morning to give it a go. I wasn't sure what it was all about, so looked it up and apparently surf life-saving clubs "provide beach lifeguard training, where they practise rescue techniques and provide a greater understanding of safety in and around the water, whilst getting fit and having fun." This smacks of Baywatch to me but unfortunately, I looked more like a fat Pamela Anderson, whose roots need doing and thanks to sitting outside in the week and failing to put on any bug spray, my legs were dotted in bites. In fact, Paul had remarked that I looked like a "medieval, plague-ridden, wench." So as much as I wanted to evoke my inner Pammy, it was just the usual, must-try-harder, Sammy.

Maxine quite rightly put in me in the nippers class – or Under 9s. They looked at me suspiciously as I was the only adult playing flag games with them and generally fully participating. I am not sure why I had to get so competitive with them but I was determined to give it my all, no matter that they were half my size.

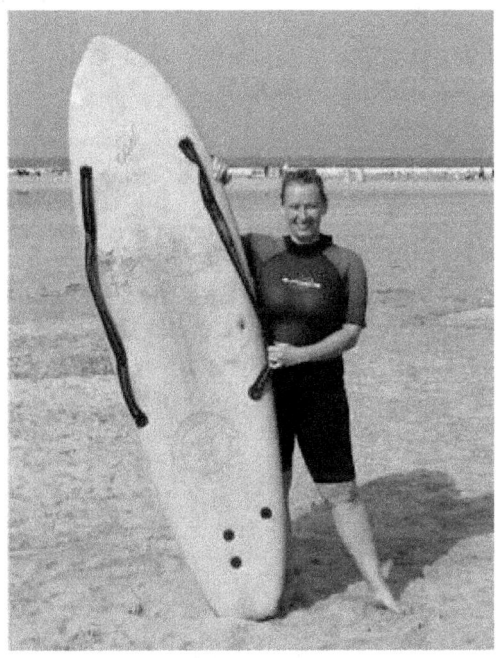

Me and the board....

Once fully warmed up, we took our boards down to the water's edge for further instruction on safety. We started our water based fun by running into the surf, past two markers and back to the beach. This was not a pretty sight and in no way reminiscent of Baywatch. My little classmates turned into dolphins as they hit the water and cruised back to the start with puff to spare. I must say that in everything I have done, this had to be one of the most physically demanding. Repeatedly running through water, with the resistance that entailed, certainly gave you that burning feeling in the legs.

As a reader of this book, you will know by now that not one of my challenges goes past without me incurring some sort of humiliation. It is now a given that I will collect a new mortification badge. I thought I had already ticked that box by stepping out in my summer wetsuit with all the previously described issues but no, more was yet to come. As we teamed up to repeat the circuit, I was put with three of the children. Jack, who I later learned was six, turned and looked at me, shrivelled his face in disappointment and nudged his mate and said: "Oh no, look who's on our team!" The race began but I couldn't focus, as I was mentally regaling all the things that I could probably do better than Jack. He didn't even cheer me back to the finishing line. I decided not to make Jack my nemesis, given his tender age, but things were frosty between us.

It was time for the boards and I was allocated a slab of finned polystyrene to master. Maxine helpfully instructed me to get on the board, paddle out, turn and catch a wave. I could do each separately but not together, so I decided to focus just on the headline grabbing wave catching. Maxine helped me to catch the first few and then I was left to my own devices to practise.

It was a real joy to watch these kids riding in the waves, as they screamed with sheer joy and excitement. Living close to the coast, I can really appreciate the need to get our kids confident and safe in the sea and they were absolutely having a ball. I caught a couple of my own waves and felt a semblance of their exhilaration, before I inevitably beached myself in unflattering poses at the feet of random paddlers.

It was time to get back to the clubhouse. I had a fantastic morning and would certainly consider sacrificing my sacred Sunday morning lie in when my little ones are older and would like to try it out in the future. As for me, I will now go into full training to ensure that Jack begs me to go on his team if that day ever happens!

Pilates – Number 38

I have a friend who is a Pilates' instructor and she has a bottom which looks like it belongs to an 18 year old (her bottom's actual age is nearly 25 years older than that). She looks good - very good. I have never gone along to a class, as I assumed I wouldn't be able to follow the moves and although having a bottom that small would be lovely, I just didn't feel it is achievable, given that my bottom looks like it belongs to an 18 year old elephant who needs to lay off the hay! I'm over a third of the way through this challenge; I now know that, although it's normal to feel intimidated when going into a class for the first time, there is no need to worry. People don't judge and everybody has to start somewhere. Therefore, I have high hopes for Pilates.

I joined Dianne at FunFit Fitness for a Monday morning session. I was introduced to the class and came up to the front to explain why I was there and a little bit about the challenge so far. There was a flurry of questions before we found our mats and began our warm-up. As we continued, Dianne asked the group why they were unusually quiet and one gentleman piped up "It's like having Ofsted in the room!" I've previously been called a journalist and now an Ofsted Inspector - what next? Estate agent? Banker?!

After slow, considered movements for the warm-up, we moved on to other postures and movements, whilst continuing to be mindful of our stance and breathing. With some of the moves, I had to opt for the more basic postures, as I'm still being massively mindful of my back. I've only just been able to start putting the washing out without wincing, so I want to be careful. However, Dianne told me that Pilates would be excellent for strengthening my lower back.

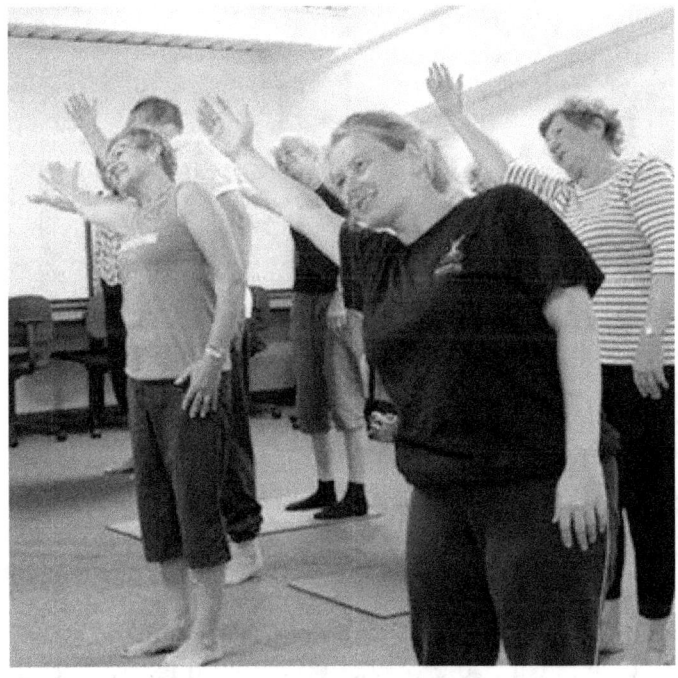

The warm-up

Most movements were more than achievable and the more difficult ones were always pre-empted by a class full of groans, which I found very amusing. Pilates is supposed to incorporate elements of yoga, martial arts and Western forms of exercise to achieve greater muscle strength, balance and flexibility. This leads onto the second fact I already knew about Pilates: never ask what the difference is between Pilates and Yoga and certainly Never, Ever ask which is better. Although amusing to watch your Pilates instructor friend and your yoga instructor friend having this heated debate outside of the school gates of an afternoon, I have learnt that one must find less flammable questions to ask whilst passing the time!

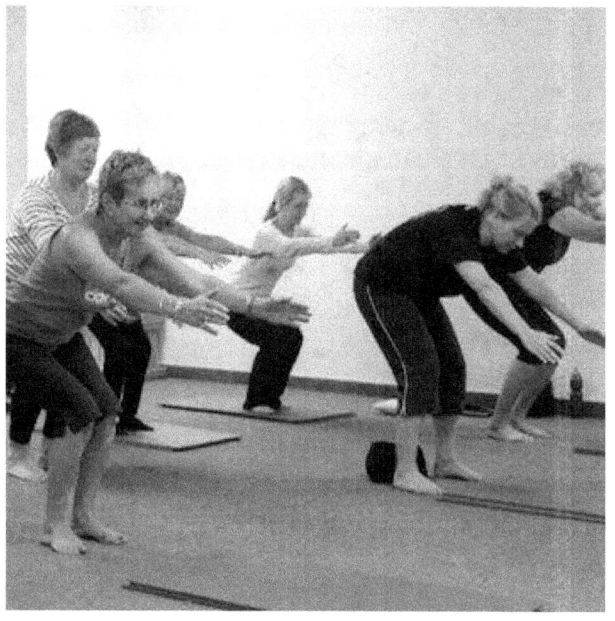

Monkey swing!

Back to the class and Dianne proceeded to shut the door, dim the lights and put on some ultra-relaxing music as we settled into quiet reflection. I remember really enjoying this element in yoga. I found coordinating the breathing with the earlier movements tricky as I consistently inhaled and exhaled out of time, but left with the focus on breathing, whilst listening to Dianne's melodic tone, I started to get into a nice rhythm. However, the by-product of doing this challenge is that I find it difficult to switch off, as my brain is always ticking, thinking of things that I can write about. I guess being constantly alert to a "story" does make me into a bit of a journalist after all. That's another job title to add to the list!

Dianne then told us to think about our toes. A friend of mine also taught me this a few years ago: "when your head is full, think about your toes," he said. It sounds strange but I've found that it does actually work and following Dianne's instructions, I immediately started to release a bit of my internal typewriter and felt my shoulders un-tense as I refocused my thoughts. The lights came on as we slowly readjusted from our dreamy state to reality. The class filed out, along with a lot of well-wishing from my class mates. I really do like this sort of exercise and as I said before with yoga, something which I feel would not only strengthen and tone me but would also help me to wind down from my busy life. It feels good to stop and breathe.

I said goodbye to Dianne and caught myself in the mirror on the way out. If I am honest, I was a little disappointed not to see Kate Moss's derrière looking back at me, but I guess it would take more than one one-hour class!

FitSteps – Number 39

As a kid, I had myself down as a bit of a dancer. In my bedroom, I would get my groove on to whatever Madonna album I could get my hands on and with hairbrush in hand, what looked back in the mirror, to me, was a right little mover. This delusion stayed with me throughout secondary school, when at 11, me and three of my friends danced in assembly, in front of the whole year to Salt N'Pepa's Push It (still a signature move). In my latter teens, the dancing involved either grunge - jumping on the spot, feet together with one hand in the air or rave - standing still, with a wiggle, using the hands to build and stack elaborate, invisible boxes.

As I progressed into my early twenties, my dancing partner was Stella Artois. Stella and I ripped up the dance floor in a number of Central London venues throughout the late 90s and early Naughties and I saw no reason to think I was anything other than an undiscovered Spice Girl. As I entered my late twenties and became a mum, I became more responsible and Stella and I went our separate ways as I struck up an occasional friendship with Pinot Grigio. When Pinot and I went out and had a boogie together, it dawned on me one day that, if I was honest, I was quite out of time to the beat. This revelation came as quite a shock and ever since, I have adopted more of a shuffle, unless my signature tunes come on (Vanilla Ice being another favourite) and then it's carnage.

Strictly Come Dancing is the pinnacle of dancing prowess and due to the popularity of the programme; the idea has been adapted to a fitness class called FitSteps. Although it sounded fun, the thought of shaking my booty without as much as a white wine spritzer sounded daunting but nevertheless, I joined Mike Truscott from Iconik to give it a go.

When I got there, the ladies were very friendly and I was relieved to see people of all ages and shapes and sizes. I placed myself at the back, out of the glare of the mirror, as the music started. Ironically, the first track was "Dancing Queen." I shimmied along to it, following the moves as best I could and trying desperately to mimic the lady in front of me. My shambolic efforts made me smile. Smiling went to laughing as we moved on to a Grease track and Shoobop sha wadda wadda yippity boom de boomed around, copying the iconic moves of that final number.

I was loving it and pleased to see that I wasn't the only person out of time, but that made everybody giggle all the more. Next came the cha-cha and more bottom wiggling and then onto the Samba or as I have renamed it, the Sham-ba. I probably got about 10% of those moves. It didn't matter though; I was probably burning twice as many calories as everybody else, trying to keep up. Next up was the waltz which had moves I actually followed. My arms swung elegantly around and my posture kept straight. Who knew that this could actually be my type of dance?

The cheese factor was high but I love cheese. The cheesier the better as far as I am concerned. To finish off, we warmed down to "She's Like the Wind" from Dirty Dancing. Damn, I love that song! As we clapped Mike and ourselves at the end, I looked around and there wasn't one person, who wasn't smiling. Makes you wonder why people go to the gym if they don't enjoy it? Get fit with a smile on your face has to be my new mantra, I think.

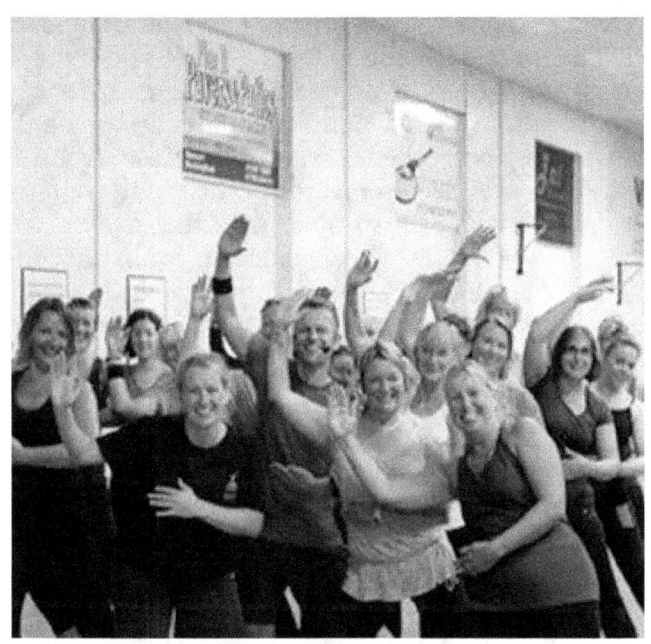

We've been Tangoed!

Some of the steps were tricky for me to pick up but Mike did say that it takes about 3 sessions before you get confident with them. I would certainly recommend this class as a social and fun way of getting active. When I got home, I cha-cha'd in the door, declared to a bemused Paul that "Nobody Puts Baby In The Corner" and then collapsed on the settee (in the corner), humming Dancing Queen and smiling. Maybe I'll book us into Waltzing lessons at some point – he'll love that!

Circuit Training – Number 40

Friday 26th September heralded National Fitness Day and although this challenge isn't necessarily about getting fit and more about trying activities, I thought I would go along anyway to my local leisure centre to give it a go. The idea of the day was to get people trying an activity for free. Clubs, parks and leisure centres up and down the country opened their doors to encourage people to turn up and have a bit of fun, while enjoying all the benefits exercise can bring.

I coaxed my friend, Sarah (of my previous Bums, Tums and Thighs challenge) to come along with me. We selected a half hour circuits' class at 5.30pm. Unfortunately, when we booked on the phone, the receptionist knew nothing about it and when we turned up, there was only one other person in the class. It felt kind of a shame that more people either weren't aware of the opportunity or chose not to take it up. If I'm honest, I think it may be the first reason, which was really why I came up with the SofaDodger website in the first place. I really wanted a website where people could see what was going on around them and where you could register your interest in certain activities and get notified directly if something was going on that might float your boat.

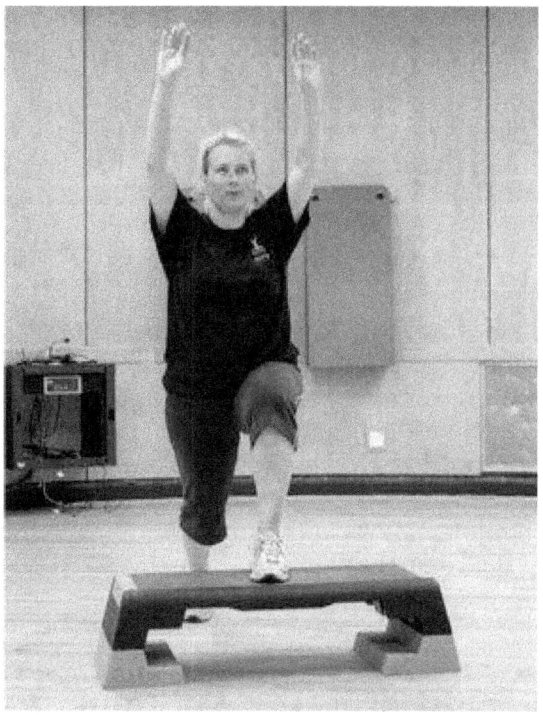

and step....

Anyway, I put that soapbox away for another day as Sarah and I prepared for our 'Power Half Hour.' The idea of circuits is to provide an all over body workout, whilst being timed on each station. I did go to a circuit class about 5 years ago and it currently holds my title of "Most Stuck At Fitness Class:" I attended 6 sessions before I found an excuse to not go anymore. It appealed to me, as the stations were hard but as you only had to do each one for a minute it felt manageable. I always approached it a bit like going into labour; you had one minute of painful contractions, with somebody egging you on to keep going, then a chance to breathe before it started again. It hurt like hell but was ultimately worth it in the end!

This class was a cut-down version given that it was half an hour, so we both felt confident it would be fine. We started with a warm-up before we moved on to various squats and lunges on and off the step. I started to feel that not unfamiliar burn in the quads and was pleased when the big fans were put on. Sarah and I gritted our teeth to the 10 second countdown on each exercise.

Steps away and we moved to our mats and worked on our core. Thankfully my back held up to the crunches, as I simplified them to ensure I didn't do any further damage. Our instructor was lovely and really motivated and encouraged us to keep going. Next up was the infamous kettlebells. I've heard a lot about these fellas. One of my future challenges will be a full class of these, so I was keen to try them out, if only for a few minutes. I speak to a lot of people who rave about them, so I'm looking forward to that class.

The half an hour was up but it did feel like a full hour. My legs felt like jelly and my bingo wings were complaining about being woken up. After, Sarah and I spoke after about an interesting dilemma this pleasure vs. pain approach to exercise poses. Not 24 hours ago, I was boogieing on down in a FitSteps class and having a ball. Today's class was tough and I ache. Ultimately, I guess I would have burnt more calories and probably strengthened and toned more in the circuits' class but it was hard. Maybe burning fewer calories but having fun would keep the enthusiasm up, on a cold raining evening, to visit a class. I don't know really. Each to their own. As long as you are being active, I guess it doesn't matter. People have their own goals and own preferences and as I have found out at number 40 of my challenge, there is enough out there to try, for you to find exactly what suits you and which can fit into your own lifestyle.

The Challenge So Far - Number 31 to 40

I have reached the 40 milestone and the last 10 have been a bit of a slog in places, as I recovered from my back sprain. I have completed archery, the dreaded coasteering, aqua aerobics, ice-skating, angling, korfball, surf life-saving, pilates, FitSteps and a circuit training class.

Due to the back injury, I did have to take a fortnight's time out between korfball and surf lifesaving, which did send me into a bit of a panic, as I scanned my list of activities, desperate to find some low impact classes or sports that I could manage. My halfway point is at the end of October, so I was starting to get concerned about missing that milestone.

Because of the high potential of me getting injured and further impacting on the challenge, I have decided to stop playing hockey this season, which for me is a big decision. I've played competitive hockey ever since I was thirteen and bar the odd injury and my three pregnancies, I've never missed a season out of choice. However, hockey can be a rough game and I know that all the knocks, bumps and bruises would definitely have an effect on my challenge. However, the main reason is not having enough time to fit it all in. The family have been very patient and supportive with me but to then have Saturdays away for a game and another night on top of that for training seemed a little bit selfish. My seven year daughter started junior hockey this season and I go down to help out with the coaching, so I am not totally bereft of holding a stick. I will follow the team throughout the season and be their number one supporter!

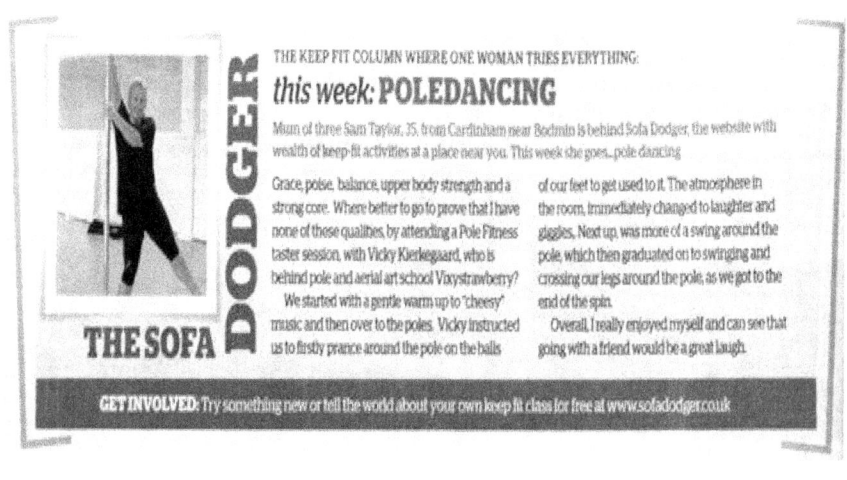

THE KEEP FIT COLUMN WHERE ONE WOMAN TRIES EVERYTHING:

this week: POLEDANCING

Mum of three Sam Taylor, 35, from Cardinham near Bodmin is behind Sofa Dodger, the website with wealth of keep-fit activities at a place near you. This week she goes...pole dancing

Grace, poise, balance, upper body strength and a strong core. Where better to go to prove that I have none of these qualities, by attending a Pole Fitness taster session, with Vicky Kierkegaard, who is behind pole and aerial art school Vixystrawberry? We started with a gentle warm up to 'cheesy' music and then over to the poles. Vicky instructed us to firstly prance around the pole on the balls of our feet to get used to it. The atmosphere in the room, immediately changed to laughter and giggles. Next up, was more of a swing around the pole, which then graduated on to swinging and crossing our legs around the pole, as we got to the end of the spin.

Overall, I really enjoyed myself and can see that going with a friend would be a great laugh.

THE SOFA DODGER

GET INVOLVED: Try something new or tell the world about your own keep fit class for free at www.sofadodger.co.uk

The Western Morning News has also started taking my blog on as a weekly article in their Sunday Supplement which is nice. Due to the word count, it has been slightly edited and certain words which I have used have been watered down, so as not to offend. Apparently, Spot the Farting Horse in my horse riding challenge was deemed a little too windy for print. Another interesting development has been my children's primary school teacher approaching me to discuss a possible "Mini SofaDodger Challenge" for the kids to try; possibly 20 different sports and an award at the end of it. I absolutely love this idea. I'm sure we've all watched and got acquainted with minority sports at the Olympics and wondered how the athletes stumbled across these non-mainstream sports. I'm really keen to explore this further and work with some of the instructors and clubs I have already visited to put something together. Who knows, maybe this is something which could develop further? I think it is important for children to try as many activities as possible as not everybody is going to be good at the standard football or netball. The enthusiasm of children, mixed with opportunity, must equal potential?

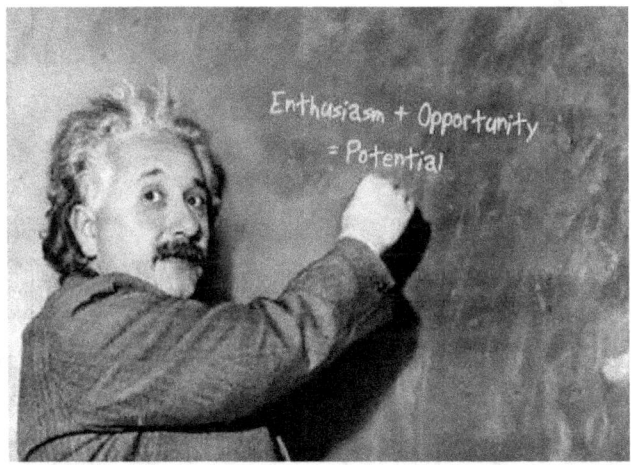

Doesn't take Einstein to come up with that formula!

As for me, the challenge sees me take on some of the following activities; Volleyball, Cardio Tennis, Special Olympics, Segway, Football, Judo and Barre Concept. I look forward to taking the challenge up to half way and as we all know, life begins at 40!

Chapter 6 - Challenge 41 - 50

Segway – Number 41

For those of you who don't know what segwaying is, it is like walking but in the future. I'm not going to lie: I have slipped in this challenge, blatantly going against the list on the back of my shirt. Why? Two reasons: firstly, it looks like a lot of fun and secondly because I had to swap out wakeboarding, as I am a chicken! Yes, I've said it, I'm a chicken and I think my back would literally snap in two if I tried wakeboarding, so I've made a tactical substitution nearly half way through my season. Several people have questioned whether Segway is a sport, but apparently you can play Segway Polo and joust on a Segway. Not sure how the horses feel about that but in my eyes, I can justify its inclusion.

Cornwall Segway are based in the Hendra Holiday Park, just outside of Newquay. I met Chris the instructor and joined a group of two couples. One lady was there with her boyfriend as part of a 21st birthday treat (on my 21st, I was tied to a tree and shot at with paintballs but that is a different story) and the other couple were eager to try it on their children's recommendation. We were handed out our protective gear, which included a helmet, gloves, knee and elbow protectors, and once in our get-up, we made our way outside to the training area. Word of advice: it is impossible to look stylish on a Segway!

Chris took us through a background about the Segway, as we ooooed at the cost and gasped at the demise of the previous owner of the Segway company, who reversed himself 70ft down a cliff, a few days after buying the company for $50 million. At this point, we all furtively looked around for cliffs. The safety instruction included not running yourself over or using them as dodgems. Birthday Girl was first to go and as I watched her zoom off in the distance, I started to feel a bit anxious. This looked like balance would be a key requirement.

After a slight wobble, I tentatively moved forward. Segways do not have a brake or accelerator. To go forward, you just have to lean forward and to slow down, you lean back - it is that simple. I see myself as a barometer as to what is easy to pick up, given that I am useless at these type of things and although I wasn't fast, I was manoeuvring around quite happily. We spent 10 minutes weaving in and out of cones, as we familiarised ourselves with this new mode of transport before Chris removed our speed limiters and allowed us to "run free."

I like to think of myself as a bit of a cautious driver, so I was never going to go full pelt but I was really enjoying whizzing about. Chris then invited us to leave the safe, grassy womb of the training area and into the big wide world of the holiday park. The speed signs around the site stated a maximum speed of 5mph but as I didn't have a brake, I felt slightly alarmed about the prospect of meeting any kind of traffic and so it came to pass. As the last person in the procession, I looked right at the crossroads and saw a ride-on mower coming towards me. In a panic, I leaned forward to try to out-race the mower and like a crazed mad woman in a mobility scooter, I cut up and outflanked the nonchalant gardener.

Once we had circumnavigated the holiday park, we ventured to the race area, where we relay raced each other through various obstacles. We then moved on to off-road Segways, which had monster truck type wheels. As we hurtled at speed through the field and then traversed the trees in the forest part, it sounded and felt like a scene out of Star Wars. We ended the session with another assault course and one more relay race.

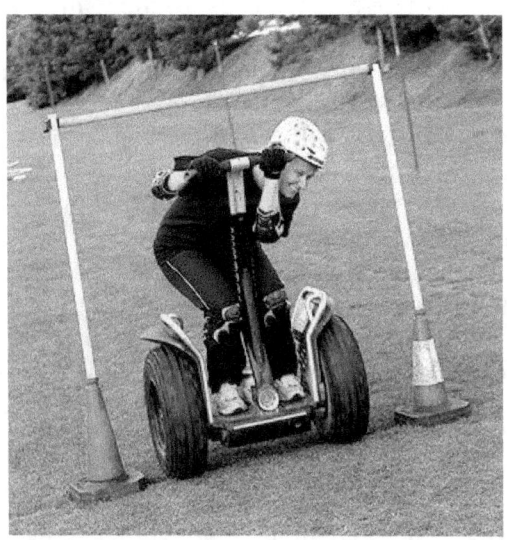

A Segway limbo to end the day

The Segway session was really good and I would thoroughly recommend it. I've decided that walking is rubbish. I want my own Segway and I want to pootle around the streets on one and failing that, I would like one of those Princess Leia sit on things to get around. That's the thing about the future; it's very frustrating that it isn't now. So whilst I wait impatiently for the future to hurry up and happen, I will try and persuade Paul to join me for another Segway session, so I can go back to the future. Maybe I need a DeLoreon as well?

Special Olympics – Number 42

Momentarily in my teenage years, I decided that I would like to go to the Olympics; not as a spectator but as a participant. Hockey would be my route in but quite frankly, I would have tried anything to get to the Atlanta games in 1996. As with all unrealistic dreams, my hopes faded but I remained an avid supporter of all sports. So to my intense joy, I was invited to the Special Olympics Cornwall, to join people with learning difficulties to get a chance to try a range of different sports at Truro College. I was invited to play boccia (pronounced Bot-cha), a Paralympic sport which allows players to throw, kick or use a ramp to propel a ball into the court with the aim of getting it closest to the white "jack" ball.

When I arrived, I entered a large sports hall rammed with people trying various types of sports, which included badminton, bowls, archery, basketball, tennis and apparently a very competitive game of football outside - which I decided to avoid. The club meets every month and although it only started this year, it's proving to be extremely popular, with people coming from all over the county. Participants ranged from the social, just give it a go person, right through to the eager beaver, competition hungry person. As I made my way over to the Boccia court, I was hoping I wouldn't be next to that person!

Karenza, a volunteer and specialist in the sport of Boccia, explained the rules. Basically, you had to stay seated and throw your ball to get to the jack ball. The team with the most balls nearest to the jack won the corresponding number of points. I took my seat and eyed up my competition. Everybody was keen to win but I knew that I was a distinct advantage, given that I have already played bowls and petanque as part of my previous challenges. We played half a dozen games, with me bemoaning that I had the unlucky blue balls, as my team got trounced by the opposition.

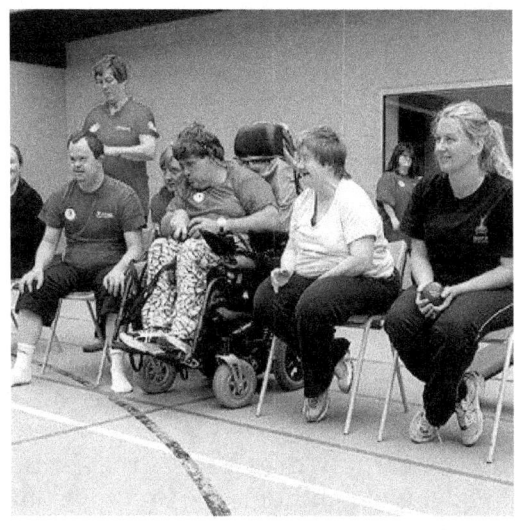

Learning the ropes

The atmosphere was very friendly, with laughter permeating and echoing around the hall, as people experienced the highs and lows of the sport they were trying at the time. Various people would come over to me and ask about my T-Shirt and my challenge, and I enjoyed talking about the various sports I'd tried already. There was a lot of enthusiasm from some of the participants about the possibility of actually competing within the Special Olympic movement, with specific training happening to prepare for a full competition.

It was inspiring to see so many people out and enjoying themselves but for me, it was the number of volunteers who were there, helping and encouraging people with the activities, which was the most impressive. Being a club secretary myself, I understand the need sport has for volunteers who are willing to give up their time to drive things forward.

After an interlude, I went back to the game and was pleased to see new teammates and opposition. First blood went to my team and as we prepared to repeat our victory, a gentleman came and sat down in the vacant chair and picked up the balls. I told him he would have to be good to beat us, as we were on a roll. Every ball he threw literally landed on or near the white ball. At one point, he was actually turning to smile at someone as he threw the ball, which landed perfectly yet again by the jack. I might have yet again been foiled in my Olympic aspirations but somebody needs to sign that guy up.

Judo – Number 43

My back has felt better for approximately 48 hours but I am not sure that 48 hours is enough time to give it before I go to my next challenge of judo. As a reminder for those of you who have forgotten; judo is the sport where you are thrown about, with the aim of landing your opponent on their back. Possibly not the best challenge to be doing right now but I have run out of seat based, low impact sports to try.

As I got into my car, my misgivings were set to the ominous backdrop of thunder and lightning. The first song on the radio was "Please Don't Go" by KWS, which I took as a sign that my back was mystically voicing its appeal through the medium of Heart FM radio. "Hush, lower vertebras. I am booked in and together, we will get through this," I beseeched.

I was meeting Sensei Jack from my Aikido challenge and I was comforted that I had somebody kind there to look after me. So, another day, another Dojo! I met Jack, who introduced me to our instructor, Roger Tarrant and the rest of the Camelford Judo Club. We started with a very quick fire warm-up and so far, so good – just a slight bit of creaking, which I put down as normal.

We moved on to practising the various throws and holds. With all my martial arts challenges to date, there's always one person who is used to demonstrate on and I watch these poor people getting ritually pummelled, as I undulate between a wince and a grimace. Usually, the person used is rotated but it wasn't the case this time. My maternal instincts were evoked, as I mentally renamed this guy "poor lamb." I am not sure there is a place for such sentiment in mortal combat or, indeed, a judo bout, but I felt sorry for him nevertheless.

To my relief and probably everybody else's, I was paired with Jack for the whole evening and it seemed like he was willing to be the one who got flung about, without returning the favour. This was excellent news for me, given his track record in martial arts excellence! It started off a little like twister, as I was instructed to "put your hand there," "now put your leg there" and "grab that."

Some of the throws induced a fit of giggles, as we ended up in a tangle of knotted limbs when I misplaced a foot or an arm.

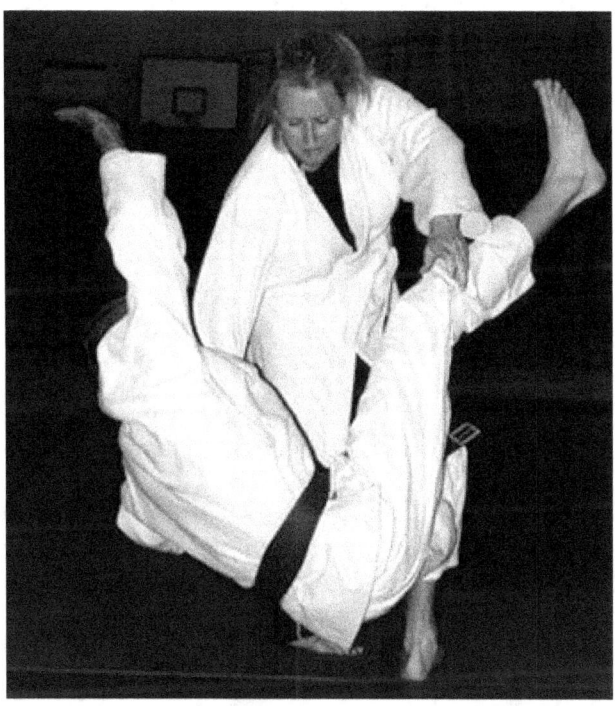

Don't I look strong?!

Jack was extremely patient with me, as I built up my confidence and attempted different grabs and throws. I appreciated his over-elaborate falls as he allowed me to chuck him around like a rag doll. It was all very good for my ego, as I was congratulated each time on my technique.

Then we moved on to the choking. We weren't re-enacting a Homer throttling Bart scene; the movements were deft, quick and ultimately effective. Again, a compliant Jack (who is no way resembled a realistic assailant), instructed me to cross my hands and grab his collar and in one pincer movement pull down with one arm and pull up with the other to effect a strangle. You never know if you have any effect on your opponent; they are always very accommodating with my efforts but I think that it must feel like they're playing with an eager little toddler, with my moves having little to no effect on them. But this one was achieving the desired result, as Jack's face went red and his eyes started popping out! I released my grip and offered a flurry of apologies.

Judo was great and I enjoyed the fast pace of moving from one thing to another. The guys were very encouraging and thankfully my back held up – not that it had to do an awful lot. I felt empowered leaving the class and really needed a Beyoncé track to come on the radio and embody this girl power coursing through me. Although actually thinking about it, Take That's "Back for Good" would probably be more apt.

Dodgeball – Number 44

My next challenge lay nearly 300 miles away in the distant shire of Bedford. No matter how good (or probably bad) I was going to be at this, I would at least win the accolade of most Dedicated Dodgeball Dude of the Day. It warmed my cockles to think that probably nobody in the whole of the land would be going to such an effort to get to a dodgeball training session, or maybe any training session, as I was today.

My co-pilot for this epic journey was a third of a pack of Oreo biscuits. As dodgeball is really popular in America, I felt that Oreos would be in keeping with the theme. With the strange feeling of just getting myself out on a road trip, without having to pack and think about my whole tribe, I waved goodbye with a mixture of excitement and anticipation as I braved the journey to the fabled "Up Country."

Five and a half hour hours later, after two traffic incidents, one standstill, one misreading of the sat-nav and with my biscuits long since consumed, I pulled up at the venue, feeling exhausted and disillusioned about the whole thing. Usually when a traveller makes such an arduous journey, they are greeted at a warm hearth as they seek refuge and refreshment. I was stepping into the bloody unknown, in the dark, to get battered with balls.

When I eventually located my teammates for the evening, I found them in the gym doing some pre-training weights. I'm not sure what I was expecting but if I'm honest, I was kind of hoping for a community club, just chucking some balls about and having a bit of a giggle. It turns out that what I had stumbled across was England's elite dodgeball club, with both men and ladies representing the country and incidentally becoming European champions. Fantastic and there was little old me; unfit, an extra-large target to aim at and with Oreo crumbs on my T-shirt!

Initially, I was worried this would be like paintball but with bigger balls, so it came as a relief to feel how light they were. We started practising, with the aim of throwing the ball at the opponent's feet. If they caught the ball, you were out, so the idea was to get it in the area where it would be difficult to catch.

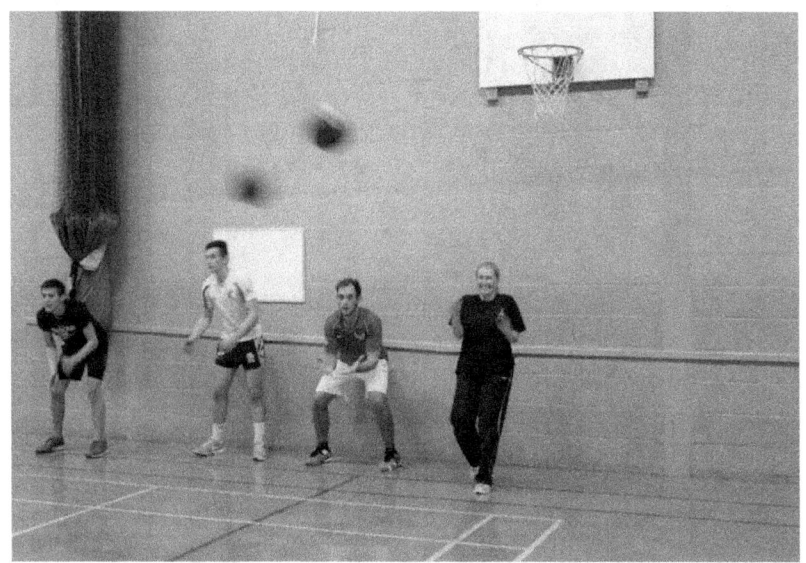

Reminiscent of a firing squad!

Then it was a match play situation, where two teams faced each other over the width of the hall. Three balls were in play and the idea would be to hit an opponent for them to be out. They, in turn, had to dodge the ball, hence the name. The game commenced as we ran to try and pick up the balls in the middle first. What happened next was reminiscent of a World War I trench warfare re-enactment, as the balls were launched at an average speed of 60-70mph. I screamed. I swore. I hid. I then repeated those three in order for the duration of the game.

I am a hockey player and I have now tried 44 sports and apart from coasteering tapping into my fear of heights, I like to think that I am able to handle myself, especially in ball sports but this was different. These guys were different. I guess you don't represent your country at a sport without being good and this lot were damned good.

The rest of the training focused on fitness, technique and game play, as I tried my best to keep up and to stop being such a wuss. Maybe I could invent a new ball sport - Screamball or maybe Swearball - where you have to shout as many different expletives as possible whilst bouncing a ball. More points would be given to foreign swear-words, so a kind of mixture between a dark version of Countdown and basketball. I will keep that on the back burner for further development. When the session finished, I thanked the guys for hosting me and wished them the best of luck with their season. I am not sure, after what I have seen, they will need it, though. I then set off the 50 miles down the M1 to my friend's house, knowing that she would have a bottle of wine in the fridge, a warm hearth and hopefully some more biscuits.

Lacrosse – Number 45

Part II of my epic journey to the Home Counties was to play Lacrosse with the Hatch End Hawks in Watford. It took me an hour and a half in London rush hour traffic to cover the 17 miles to the Sports Centre. The rain was heaving down so badly, I could barely make out the road markings at some points and I started to panic at the possibility that it might be cancelled. The fact I hadn't packed anything which constituted waterproofs didn't register until I stepped out of the car.

In my eagerness not to be late, my first foot out of the car went straight into a puddle, followed shortly after by the other. My feet were soaking already and the only thing I could wear to ward off the sheet rain was my M&S rain mac! I looked ridiculous and cursed myself for packing so optimistically. Never mind, I told myself. I am a hockey player and used to training in this weather.

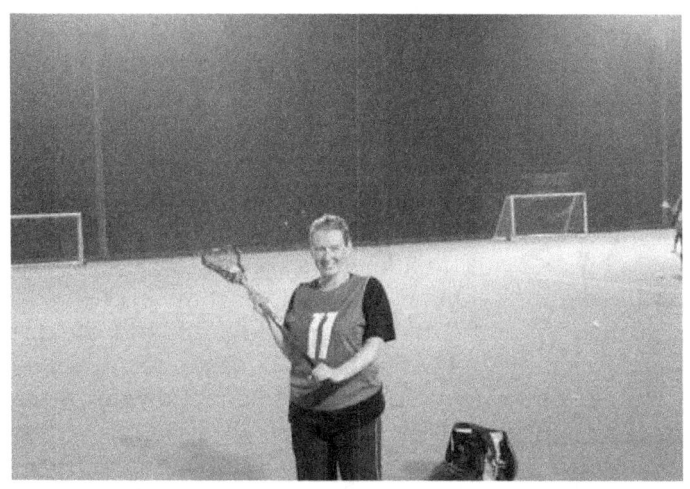

Dedicated to the cause in the rain

After being introduced to the club and completing the warm-up, I was sent off with John the coach to try some of the techniques as the heavens opened even further than before. Being a hockey player, it did feel a bit alien to lift the stick above shoulder height but I got the hang of the having the ball in the net bit and I seemed fairly OK at catapulting the ball out. However, just like baseball and catching with the mitt, I had a bit of difficulty catching the ball properly. We moved on to picking up the ball off the ground and that went well, so it was just the catching to work on.

Once the girls felt I'd got the basics, I was invited to take part in one of the training drills, which involved attack against defence in the last third. I opted to watch for five minutes to get the feel of what was going on. Lacrosse is an 11 a side game and the idea, like in hockey or football, is to score a goal. Defenders marked their assigned player and I watched in amazement as an attacker made a "cut" into the scoring area and almost like a rugby player dodged past several defenders, whilst shielding the ball, to score. At this point, defence would shout "RED!" and if you were a defender, you had to run to that attacker, like bees to honey, to block a shot.

I was subbed on into defence and given the task of man-to-man marking my player. In hockey, you do not leave this player to follow the ball. If you do, you get shouted at by your sweeper, so I missed the first call of "RED!" and was dutifully told off by my team. This logged, I carried on chasing my player around the pitch and when there was a bolt from the attackers, I sprinted into the melee. I wasn't sure how to tackle, so I waved my stick about in the air and considered coupling it with an aggressive noise but realised I would look a complete fool, so stuck to waggling it instead.

This chasing was hard work, so I was delighted when we changed to attack. This was my time. I have spatial awareness. I understand field sports, making runs and calling for the ball. What I forgot was that I couldn't catch the damn thing, so any good positional play and call I made was a complete waste of my team's effort, as the damned thing went sailing past my head.

We finished up and I said goodbye to John and the girls, who were very welcoming. Lots of them questioned me about my challenge and took a few pictures of the back of my T-shirt. The fact that I was driving back to Cornwall afterwards must have made them think I was a particularly odd individual.

When I got in the car, my tracky bottoms, top and trainers were sopping wet and when I typed in my postcode, it emphatically relayed the information that I wouldn't get home until 1am. Maybe I am strange? This behaviour can't be normal. I'm minded to liken my quest to Frodo travelling to Mordor. I'm sure people pointed at him and said: "Oi Frodo, you're an idiot, what are you up to, messing about on a quest? Go and do some housework!" I can't exactly remember how that all ended but I am sure he probably trudged about in the rain, meeting loads of new people, miles from home. I'm still not sure how my ultimate quest will end but the journey is certainly an interesting one!

BarreConcept – Number 46

Please believe me when I tell you that I am not purposely looking for ways of making a prat of myself but it does just seem to be a theme running throughout this challenge. I have developed a slight immunity to it and if anything, I am embracing my inner prat. Therefore, when I heard about a class called BarreConcept and found out that it was a mixture of Pilates, yoga and ballet; I rushed to find my tutu. Yes, I have a tutu.

I arrived at Cornwall College and met the ladies who mostly worked at the college and come to the class after work. My heart dropped as I saw the floor-to-ceiling mirrors on each of the walls. As previously noted, I find mirrors judgemental and overly honest, which is why I spend my life avoiding such encounters. I prefer the company of disinterested and non-judgemental walls. Our lovely instructor, Jess glided in, looking poised and graceful and advised me how to ensure that I don't hurt my back further, which was kind of her.

The class got underway and, boom, straight into some Pliés. I was feeling a bit ouchy in my legs already and there I was thinking that there would just be a lot of frolicking! We moved to the ballet bar at the side of the room. This isn't my usual type of bar and I disliked it intensely, especially as it was placed right next to my nemesis, the mirror.

We faced forward and extended out our legs, pointing them and then back to Plié and instead of having the backing music of Swan Lake, we were working in time to some fantastic 90s tunes, which I was really enjoying. You can see in their physique how hard ballerinas train: they're lean and toned but their grace belies the power and strength they possess and my God, wasn't it becoming clear to me how hard they must train!

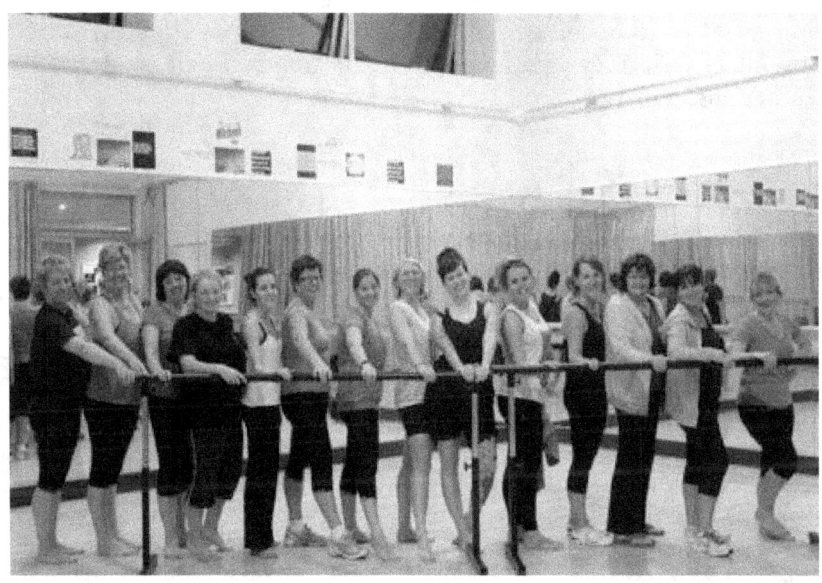

The lovely ladies of the BarreConcept Class

In all of the classes I've taken so far and I include Insanity in that, I don't think my legs have burnt like this. Jess shouted encouragement to us as we all gritted our teeth and shook it out after the set had finished. She demonstrated an exercise whereby your knees went together and then you bent one leg and moved it out to the side. It all looked very elegant. We faced the mirror and tried to replicate the move. Unfortunately, I got to stare at my beetroot-red face, as I attempted to mimic the move and looked like a dog cocking its leg.

Next, we worked on our arms, as we pushed forward on the bar and back and repeat, then hold and then pause. The burn factor was high and everybody had a groan throughout. It was pleasing to see everybody wincing - not just me - as we moved to the floor and the dreaded core. I had a get out of jail card, on account of my back. So when everybody else was crunching, I followed without raising my head far off the floor.

Once the core was fully worked on, we got to our feet for a warm-down to a chill-out track. We ended with some yoga poses and the downward dog (not the previously adopted "urinating dog" position.)

I found the class to be very challenging but the girls said that the first one or two sessions were hard and to have a hot bath after. I didn't wear my tutu in the end, as I felt that quite rightly, it would flatter to deceive and this class proves that I am no Darcey Bussell. Give it a few classes though and maybe I will be up for The Nutcracker... or not!

Climbing – Number 47

With so many challenges to get through, I've almost trained myself to not think about what is going to happen until I get in the car to the venue. In this case, I was only going a few miles up the road to Magic Wood Climbing in St Neot. Somebody pointed out on Twitter that I didn't have any kind of climbing on my list and probably against my better judgement, given my fear of heights, I looked to rectify that and ensure I was being representative of all activities. Aside from aeroplane based activities, of course; frankly, they can do one!

As I entered the converted barn, it pretty much took my breath away. Everywhere I looked there were walls of various shapes and sizes. I met Simon, who invited me upstairs to sit in front of the wood burner with a drink, as we talked about his love for the sport and why I was doing what I was doing. I think you would need a posse of psychiatrists to unpick that particular question.

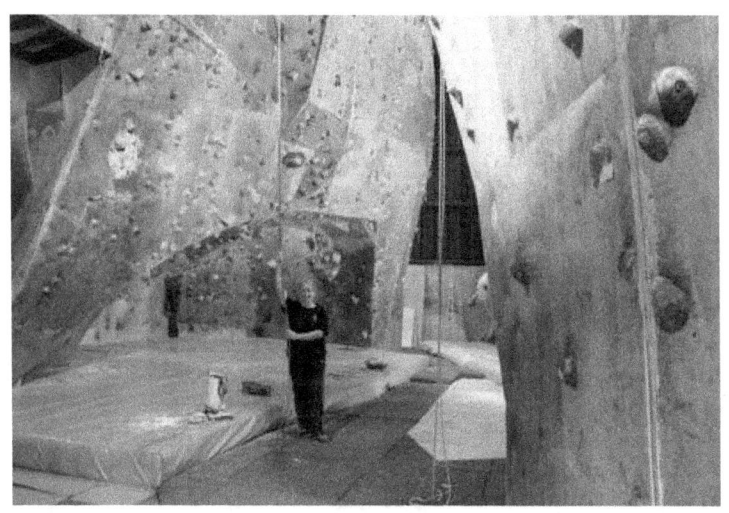

Lots of walls to climb

We were having a lovely chat but Simon probably sensed I was stalling, as he invited me downstairs to take a further look at his self-built creations. Not unlike Peter Pan, he flew up a stepladder to show me a better view of the place and beckoned me to follow. I managed about 6 steps, before looking down and with pulse racing, stopped mid-climb and let out a whimpering noise. Simon obviously didn't realise how pathetic I was about heights until this point, as he held out an almost disbelieving hand and encouraged me up. Once up, I felt a great sense of achievement to even manage a small stepladder.

I warmed up by tackling some bouldering. This involved manoeuvring around a small but angled series of walls. Problem two soon became evident: how an earth was I going to pull my own body weight around with my lack of upper body strength? I think even Spiderman would have issues with this. To me, it seemed almost impossible.

Simon wandered over with a harness and various ropes. My face fell as I looked up to a 30ft wall. Several knots were tied (which I repeatedly checked were tied correctly) and then after a lesson in technique, I took a breath and harnessed my inner Yazz: The Only Way is (indeed) Up! I tentatively tried to find my footing and the first bit was OK, as I fought against all of my thoughts of falling. Just under halfway up, I went into a full-on panic. I couldn't find anything to grip to and forward momentum seemed impossible as I clung like an overly needy limpet to the wall.

I was lowered down on the rope. I went into moaning overdrive and I became insistent that it would be impossible to do. All I wanted to do was to run away. I had THE FEAR. Simon was not having any of it and like someone dealing with a petulant child, soothed away my negativity and encouraged me to try again. Against all my better judgement, I put my leg up and then groped to find a ledge for my hand and I repeated it. I felt better knowing that my rope could actually take my weight but still I didn't look down. Half way up and the swearing started – apparently a common place for such outbursts.

I wavered. Surely I had gone far enough? "Keep going!" I heard from below. Damn, he was like the Alex Ferguson of climbing. I willed myself up a few more feet until I got to the top (or near enough for me). Even writing it up later and recalling it made my heart race and my hands sweat. I did it, though! I actually did it! The exhilaration I felt when I got down was quite overwhelming.

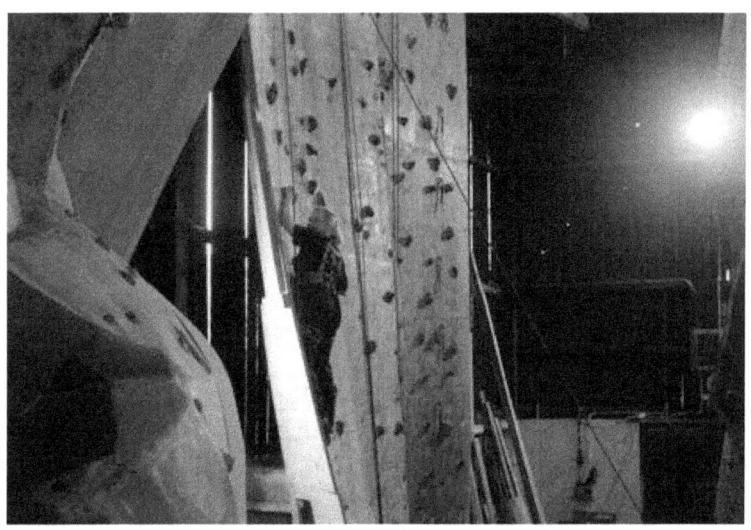

Go me, climbing to the top!

Simon beamed a knowing smile as I thanked him for making me continue. It would have been so easy to give up. I am a grown woman; if I didn't want to do it, I would be in my rights to decline the incline. That's what makes it so sweet. I stuck with it and the buzz stayed with me for hours after.

I am learning that sometimes, pushing yourself out of your comfort zone is good for you. Charles Atlas once said: "Step by step and the thing is done." I am not going to be climbing Mount

Everest anytime soon, but I got a lot from this and I might just carry on trying to surprise myself by pushing myself that little bit further. Who knows where it might lead?

Karting – Number 48

I was talking to a lady this week and when I told her about my challenge/quest, she declared that I must be some kind of "daredevil." I chortled outwardly, knowing inwardly that I had deceitfully allowed myself to be portrayed as something I am not. The reality of the situation is that I am a bit of a wimp. When I think about when my wimpiness first became apparent, I am pretty sure I can pinpoint it down to the day I became a mother. Suddenly, you have to consider the risks you take and consider them I do.

Saying all of that, I climbed a 30ft wall a few days ago, so I may actually be on a roll and although karting on paper is a risky business, who knows...I could turn out to be a bit of a Lewis *Sam*ilton!

It didn't take much persuasion to convince Paul to join me on the track and on the journey there, he seemed to be relishing the potential competition. He tried to initiate wagers, which I wasn't responding to. We arrived at St Eval Kart Circuit and got dressed in our racing boiler suits. This was not a good look at all and every time I bent down, 2 buttons would pop open in an embarrassing fashion.

The karts looked harmless enough. They were two pedal affairs and kids of 7 years old could drive them, so they couldn't be that complicated. Once we received a safety briefing and found a helmet, we made our way to our allotted cars. I ignored Paul's attempts to playfully intimidate me and wafted away the invisible clouds of testosterone emanating from the pit area, as I witnessed friends challenge friends and dads challenge sons. Yes, even the 7-year-olds!

The first lap would be a controlled one, where there would be no overtaking, just single file following of the pace setter. Then we were off! Paul raced off immediately, whilst I tried to work the accelerator. I sensed that I wasn't that fast because I couldn't see Paul and then after a lap, I had obviously been the bottleneck because half a dozen cars raced past me at the earliest opportunity, as I tried forlornly to locate the "racing line".

Two laps in and I was making Driving Miss Daisy look like a high-speed police chase. This was not good. I started to get paranoid that the stewards were smirking at me as I watched one little tot after another speed past me, leaving a cloud of engine fumes in their wake. I tried to muster a bit more speed on the straights and went full pelt, only to slow to near standstill as I tried to navigate the chicane.

The chequered flag waved and as I entered the pit lane, I saw people in my race already with helmets off, walking to the exit. I parked up to find Paul grinning at me and then excitedly recounting the racing foes he had duelled along the track. I was just glad to be out and doubly glad I had a helmet on, so I couldn't be recognised as the "rubbish one who kept getting lapped."

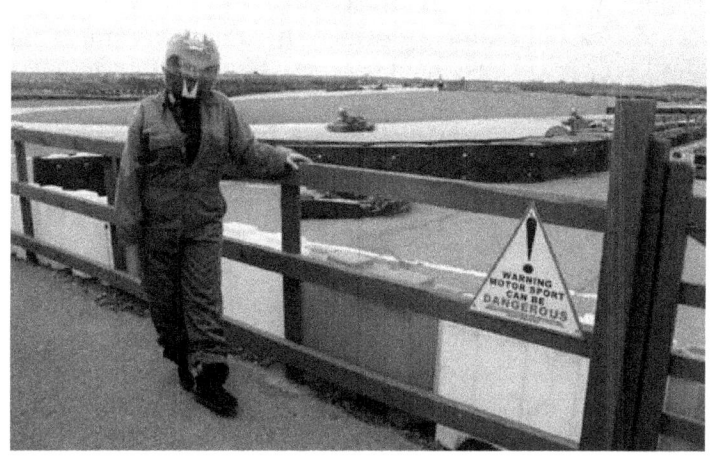

Maintaining anonymity behind the helmet...

I try to invoke the parable of the Hare and the Tortoise to make myself feel better but in this instance, it doesn't really work. In this case, all the hares were high-fiving each other at the end, cheering their feats, whilst the tortoise pretended it didn't matter and sloped off quietly.

I shall resume the challenge and gain confidence trying...oh wait....football! This is not going to be a good week for the old ego, is it?

Football – Number 49

The next challenge is football. My six year old son looked at me with all the concern he could muster and pointedly said, "but Mummy, you can't play football." It was true that, by the age of 4, my little boy could tackle me and get past me when playing football in the garden. When I travel to most sports, I have no idea how it is going to go, as I inevitably haven't tried it before but football is different. I have a proven track record of being rubbish. It's a shame really, as I love the game and like nothing better than cuddling up on a Saturday night to watch Match of the Day.

With my son's reality check ringing in my ears, I headed off to Saltash to train with Dobwalls Ladies FC. After the Lacrosse debacle, where I failed to dress for the conditions, I decided not to take any chances and wrapped myself up like a polar bear, with my under-layer, big socks, tracky bottoms and my huge hockey shin pads. All of which seemed a huge mistake after just the warm-up.

We started with a simple passing drill, which actually felt quite comfortable. It turns out that you need a decent ball and wearing appropriate footwear helps, unlike my flip-flops in the garden. Maybe this is why I am usually so bad? I was gaining a little bit of confidence with the passing as we moved on to a two-on-one exercise. My spatial awareness, movement and calling were OK but my control was ropey and any time a defender approached me, I panicked as the tackle came in. I did manage to somehow dink the ball through the legs of the defender and then shout: "Nuts!"

We moved on to three-on-three, and my lack of fitness was starting to show. I felt like a boil in the bag fish with all of my get up on. I decided that my job in this exercise was to "create space," which involved me running up and down the wing, in a pass avoidance mission. The drill developed into a 5-a-side game. Suddenly my teammates started putting on some skills, as my powers started to wane.

Obviously with so many names to recall, I shall have to use my imagination to describe the play. Within minutes Angela Di Maria stormed up the wing and deftly passed to Lauren Messi to score. In hockey, I myself have a few game plays I like to employ; the main one, which brings me a fair amount of success, is to shimmy to the right, shimmy to the left and then goal hang. I missed out the shimmying and went straight to the goal line and called for the ball. It then occurred to me the offside rule would preclude this strategy, so I sloped back a bit.

Amidst my indecision, the blokes' team, who were playing after us, filed in and started watching. I made a few runs and called for the ball and my team, bless them, indulgently passed me the ball, only for me to let out a pterodactyl shriek as the ball ran away from me. One time, a looping ball came to me, which I tried to control with my chest, to which I wailed, "it hit me on the boob!!" The men were sniggering and I really wanted a time-out to fully explain to them that it was my first time properly playing football but I sensed that stopping the game for such a parley was inappropriate.

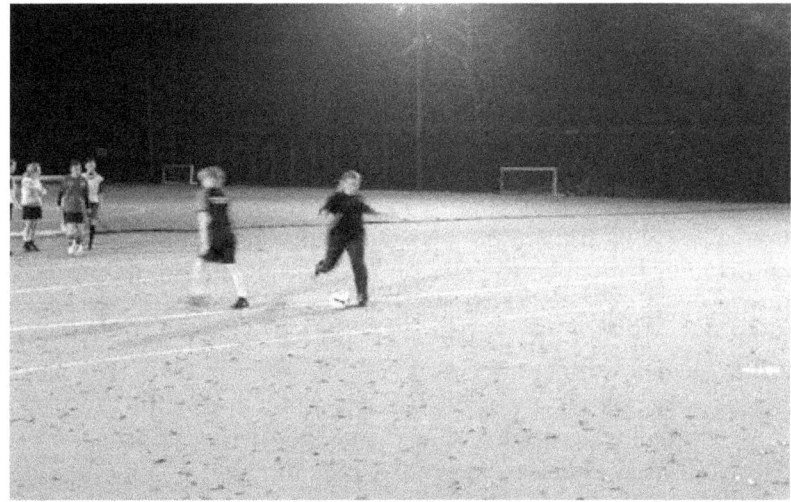

Toe punts are hugely underrated in penalty shoots

We finished on some shooting. Compared to a hockey goal, a football goal is a huge area and if it wasn't for the pesky goalkeeper cramping my style, I think I would have scored a bagful!

The session finished and it went really well. I had enjoyed my time with the girls but it made me miss the banter of being part of a team. One of the girls asked if I would consider playing - apparently they were short on numbers and I detected desperation. However, when I recount this to my son in the morning, I will exclude that detail and tell him that a team wanted to sign me but couldn't afford the transfer fee - I still have a few a years left before he works out Mummy's fabricated web of lies.

Roller Skating – Number 50

There are a few roller sports that I could try, but it seemed like a wise idea to learn how to skate before I embark on anything ambitious. Every week in Plymouth, you can learn how to skate and as it was Halloween, they were putting on a spooktacular roller disco. I dragged along my little girl, Izzy, who was up for giving it a go. However, she declared that she was "Halloweened out" and refused to put on a costume. After drawn-out negotiations, she agreed to bring some vampire teeth. Having no costume myself and being heavily reliant on Izzy providing the scare factor, I asked Paul to hurriedly draw a cobweb on my cheek, as a token gesture.

When we got to the YMCA in Plymouth, it was full of super speedy, skating spooks. Their dressing up efforts made ours look even more pathetic. As we waited, we could only watch in awe as various skaters, ranging for little minis to teenagers and adults, circumnavigated the hall. This added to our apprehension, as we couldn't spot any fellow "wall clingers" or "shufflers."

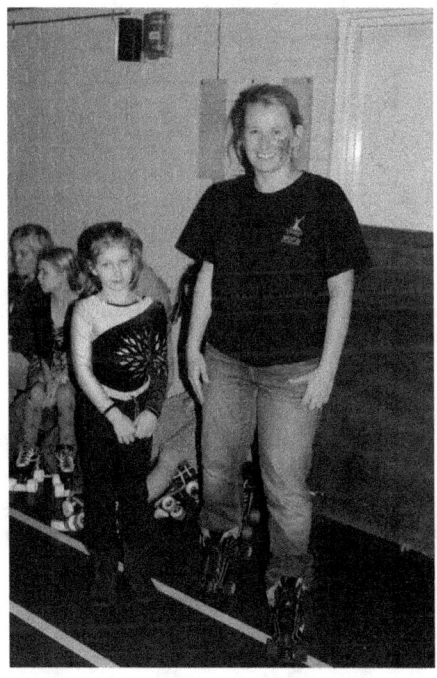

Booted up with a token cobweb on my face

Thankfully, as we were booting up, we spotted a few rookies. The lights went off and the music belted out, accompanied by a fluorescent light show. As soon as I stood up, I started to feel very shaky. Some of the helpers guided Izzy around the first few circuits, as I was abandoned to my own devices. My deficiencies on wheels were amplified by the various ghouls whizzing in and around me.

After one shuffle around, I sat down to regroup. I started to focus on everybody else's technique. I stood up again and once I steadied myself, I adopted my own skating style; essentially that of a demented bull. I thought it best to work on one leg at a time and once I had perfected one leg, I would move on to the other. So, this involved keeping my left foot on the floor and my right foot, making a pawing of the ground, like a bull before a charge. I got into a sequence, which I managed to get into time to the music. Paw, paw, roll... (Travel about 6 feet) - paw, paw, roll and repeat.

This strategy was getting me around the room but it was bloody well hurting my left foot, as it stayed rigid to the floor. Izzy and I regrouped again. She herself was adopting her own technique but I could tell she was getting a little frustrated. She is a determined little thing though and after we had watched a game of bulldog (which we sat out) she was off again in no time.

Next circuit and I focused on getting my left foot to do something of use. I initiated the shuffle, progressed to the pawing technique and then attempted to lift my left foot. My foot was not complying though and I physically found that I couldn't lift the damn thing. It stayed rooted to the floor. No matter what I tried, I couldn't seem to lift it.

I wondered how long it would take to get to the level some of these guys were at. It seemed so effortless and graceful. I would love to be able to skate like that. I gave it my best but I was knackered by my efforts, as was Izzy. Neither of us fell over, which was an achievement but we would need to put in a lot of practise to get confident on wheels. Izzy asked for skates from Santa but I may need to reconsider street hockey and roller derby, based on this performance. Maybe I should have dressed as a full-on witch and rowed myself around with a broomstick, kind of like a Venetian gondolier...

Chapter 7 - Challenge 51 – 60

Netball – Number 51

Like most girls, I played netball at school and for the first year, played as Goal Defence, which proved a fruitful position for me. That was until the Goal Shooters continued growing and I didn't. I was swiftly moved into the centre position, as I was fairly nifty back in the day. However, at the same time as honing my netballing skills, I was also getting into hockey. Hockey and netball aren't great bedfellows as they are both winter sports and school fixtures started to clash. In the 3rd year my teacher Miss Sheppard, who I considered my Yoda at the time, took me aside and said something like: "The decision is nigh my child and you must choose your path – hockey or netball. Choose it you must but choose wisely, as once the choice is made, you cannot go back (apart from the odd house match)".

I considered my options and went with hockey, on the basis that it didn't seem so height reliant, I was quite good at it and also boys played hockey as well. In another dimension, I could be a mediocre netball player now, instead of a mediocre hockey player. Sometimes you can only ponder the fork in the road of one's destiny.

Anyway, I shuffled into the local leisure centre, so as to avoid eye contact with any of the staff who know me from hockey, and made my way down to the court. I was greeted by the club and I was introduced to a familiar face. It turned out that it was one of the girls from football the previous week. She looked at me as if I was stalking her and probably mentally calculated the cost of a restraining order.

We warmed up with a few good exercises, which I am going to promptly steal and use at junior hockey practise. I felt like a spy infiltrating enemy lines. Unfortunately for me, I'd managed to come down on "fitness week" as circuit training stations were laid out. This varied from planking to shooting to footwork exercises. Damn, netball is tougher than you'd think!

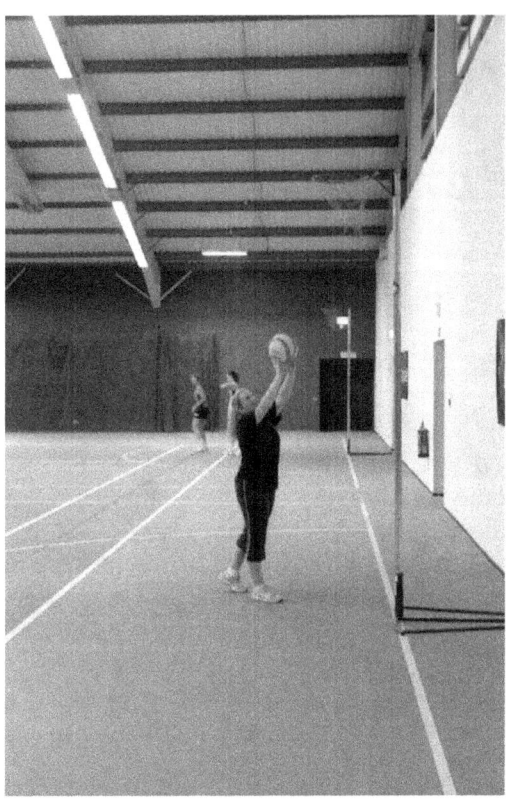

Shooting is not where my skills lie

Finally, after a thorough but enjoyable workout, we got into a game situation and I managed to land the coveted centre position. The bib was handed over on the proviso that I would have to run around. When the whistle blew, I gave it my all and run about I did. It was like riding a bike; the pivot was still there. My favourite, the old bounce pass was deployed but unlike 20 (plus) years ago, I was knackered after 5-6 minutes, so subbed myself off for a breather.

When I came on again, I was playing Goal Defence and my Goal Attack, (who I subsequently named "Zippy") did the same play every single time and although I knew what was coming, I was way too slow and short to have any impact at all. It was like having two dogs chasing after a stick – the young puppy always getting there first, with the old dog trailing behind, thinking, *That used to be me!*

The session tweaked some nostalgia in me and I know that England Netball run nationwide "Back to Netball" programmes. If

I didn't have all these sports to try, I think I would go back and play non-competitively, as it was good fun, the team were welcoming and if nothing else, the fitness was good. I would just have to make sure I went in disguise though, so none of the hockey lot would see me.

Karate – Number 52

Apparently Beyoncé embodies an alter-ego when she goes out on stage and she has named her Sasha Fierce. Sasha is a bad-ass diva and as her name suggests, she is fierce. As I sat in front of the fire, looking out on the dark evening, I knew I needed to rouse myself off the sofa (as this is the SofaDodger challenge) and embody an alter-ego for my looming karate class. As I kissed goodbye to my roaring fire and a potential glass of wine, I felt more like Sasha Farce.

My Olly has been going to Karate at the Byrne Black Belt Academy for over a year now and Master Ed was more than happy for me to come down and give it a go with them. Thankfully it was not the same class as Olly's. He may not have dealt with the embarrassment very well and I didn't want to see that ashamed look in his eyes either.

This challenge has given me the fortunate position to have trained with a number of World Champions and an Olympian. This particular class was rammed full of World Champions – 6 of them in fact. I find that pretty amazing to think that in a village hall on the North coast of Cornwall, there was such a concentration of elite athletes...and me!

We started off with a warm-up. A light jog around the hall, adding in some air punches. Master Ed then called out a body part that had to touch the floor. Left hand, right hand, bottom.....nose, tummy! Thankfully my tummy didn't have as far to travel to the ground as the others, so that actually proved to be a bit of an advantage. Next we partnered up and started progressing through sparring sequences.

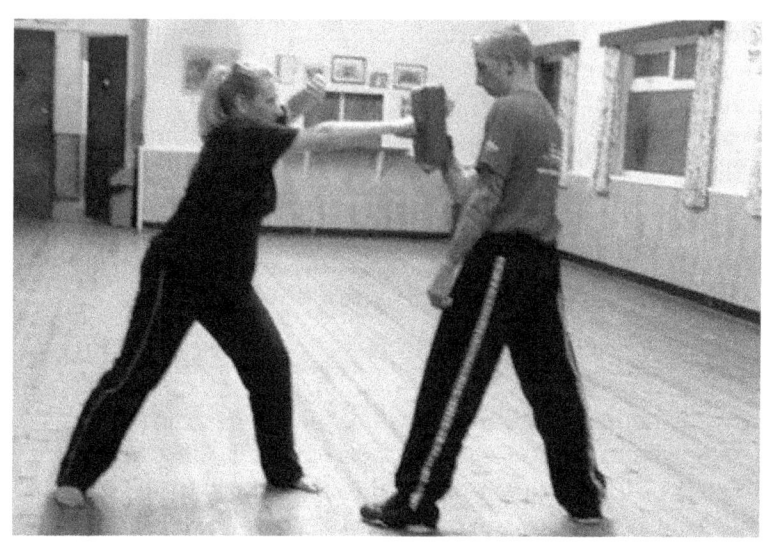

Ouchy knuckles!

I tightened my fist into a ball and prepared my two knuckles to rain down a volley of blows, in groups of 10 punches – then a rest – then again for a minute. After, as I uncoiled my fists to take the pads, I saw that I had left nail marks in the centre of my palm and my knuckles were starting to glow. At least, I could rest and hold the pads. Billy, my partner and World Champion in his class, went about speed punching to the point it became a bit of a blur, as I tried to maintain an upright position while being progressively pushed backwards. So much for a rest!

I've found in my other martial arts challenges that I really like a bit of a kick, specifically a roundhouse kick. I have tried to incorporate this into my general life and as it is called a roundhouse, I have literally started doing it "round the house." I could be hanging out the washing and then roundhouse the washing machine or better still, give the sofa a good kicking. Maybe Father Christmas will bring me one of those hang from the ceiling punch bags to practise on – if somebody had said I would type that sentence a year ago, I would have had them down as doo-lally!

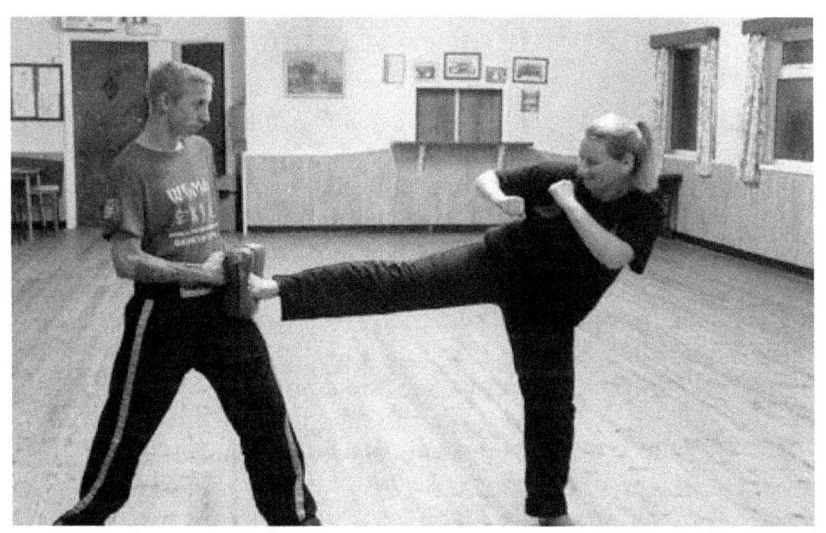

Love a bit of a kick!

The only other thing about trying so many other types of combat sports is that I do start mixing up things I have learnt previously. So for instance, when presented with a pad to hit, I adopt a boxing technique and when I have to reverse punch, I seem to want to go in with an elbow, as taught in Krav Maga. This has moulded me into a fighter with no discernible skills and unclassified in my mode of combat. If my fighting style was to be compared, it would be to a bag of Liquorish Allsorts – you never know quite what you are going to get.

I don't have a name for my alter-ego yet and these things should not be lightly considered, (especially as I can only think of the name Nancy Ninja) but I do have a mantra for this challenge and it is "Fake it Till You Make It." I think Sir Richard Branson once said that and my interpretation is to be enthusiastic and give everything your all. I am not going to "make it" as a Karate champion but I was certainly happy to pretend that I could for one hour, especially around those particular classmates.

Spinning – Number 53

Bikes and I have a very distrustful relationship, ever since I fell off my bike riding to school when I was 8. Soon after, we moved and wheels were no longer an essential part of my life, so I avoided them up to this present day (aside a family day's cycling up the cycle trail 10 years ago). So if I'm honest, I wasn't really looking forward to my Spinning Class at The Retallack Resort.

On paper though, it should be OK. My (now fashionable) Kim Kardashian sized arse would act as a nice cushion on the seat and the bike is stationary in a gym, so there wouldn't be big lorries to worry about. The only thing which seemed to be an issue would be if I was strapped into a bike and placed in front of a full-length mirror. Luckily, when I got there the bikes were facing a screen, which were simulating a biking experience on various North American roads.

I noted the small, shapely bottoms of my classmates and I smirked to myself at the cushion advantage I clearly had. I mounted my bike and Darren, the instructor, took me through the control pad and showed me where the resistance knob was to control tension. I had a premonition that me and this knob were not going to get on.

We sat on our bikes and started cycling and immediately my bum started to hurt, as I tried to find the most comfortable position. Ouch, that hurts. It really hurts! I carried on and winced through the first song and then the second. I put my towel on my seat to see if that would help. The poor guy behind me must have had a horrible view of my adjustments. I am not going to lie; the first fifteen minutes of the class were some of the longest minutes of my life, as I struggled on.

Thankfully, we then moved onto standing up and peddling. This was much better and I started to feel far happier about life. Darren shouted encouragement and urged us to turn the resistance up either by half or a full rotation to make it harder. At this point, I decided to go Lance Armstrong and started cheating by halving the rotation, which was hollered out to us. If Darren said a full turn, I only turned it half way. Lance would be proud of me.

As the class went on, I found it got easier in terms of my bum and after the initial shock; I managed to get into some sort of rhythm, as I focused on the screen and imagined myself cycling along the roads in Washington State Park. If the class was representative of an actual road race, my classmates would be the ones racing ahead and I would be the one with a basket on the front of my bike, meandering along and looking at the scenery

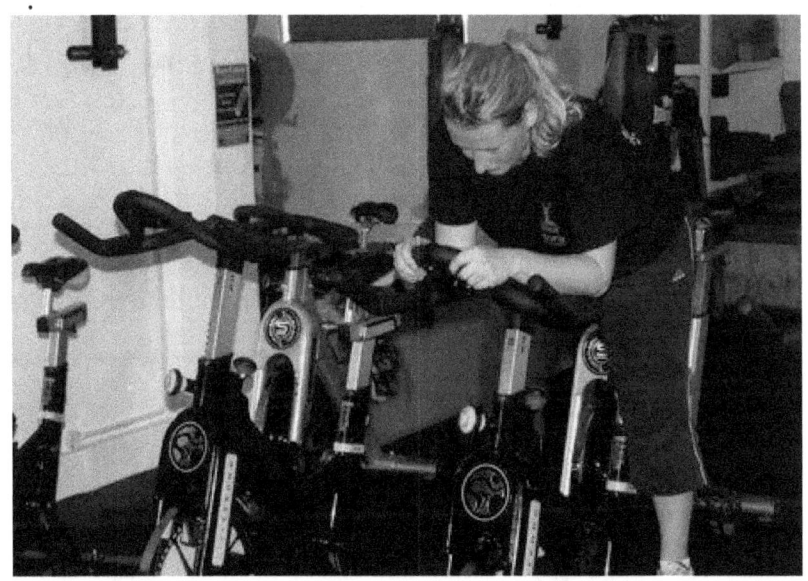

Putting it in!

Darren's instructions popped my dream bubble as we "put it in" for the last quarter of an hour. At points, my legs felt jelly-like so I focused on the calorie counter as I gritted my teeth through the sprints. Finally, the warm down came and slowed to a standstill. I dismounted and immediately found I had the John Wayne walk before I shook it out.

The class was tough for me but looking at the physiques of my classmates, it would be worth it. I have recently read about the use of virtual reality in spin classes, where you can pop on a headset and take a ride in space or anywhere in the world. I think I might come back for that class but until that time, I am off to spend the 200 calories I burnt on a hot chocolate in the café. Life is all about balance after all.

Piloxing – Number 54

With both my girls having suffered from the lurgy in the past week, I was keen to get out of the house for a few hours. I helped out at the junior hockey club to start with but, aware that I had a mild sore throat, I opted for the quieter and smiley approach instead of my usual "shouty encouragement" for the kids. It seemed to suitably unnerve them. After the club session finished, I went to join Tara of Versatile Fitness Choice for a Pilloxing Class.

Pilloxing is a fitness class based on a mixture of Pilates, Boxing and Dancing and as I have already tried all three of those on my previous challenges; I went in with full confidence. Once Tara had provided us all with our resistance giving gloves (which had a faint whiff of cheese and onion crisps), she explained that the class would be non-stop and to grab a drink when necessary. Once I pitched up camp at my standard back of the room, boom - we went straight into the high octane dance music.

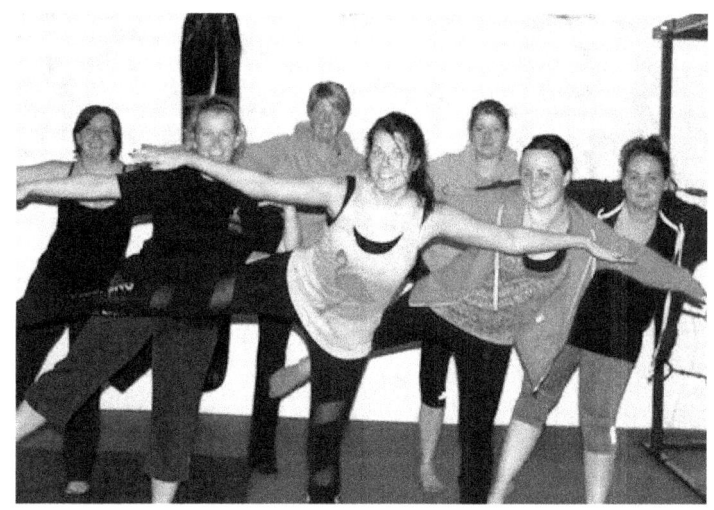

Balance and clench!

This class was sassy and Tara's charisma was magnetic. I found the moves easy to follow and I especially enjoyed the boxing aspect to the class. Tara encouraged us to dig deep and when sufficiently sweaty we were rewarded with a "woop woop." The next set of moves involved us incorporating some Cha-Cha. Since my foray into FitSteps, I am all about the Cha-Cha. We developed the movement to include a skip and a reach to the air and to the side. I went up on the skip, with a smile on my face, full of enthusiasm and energy but by the time I landed, I had a wave of pain convulse from my back, which quickly spread through the whole of my body.

I looked up to see if anybody else had suffered this invisible debilitation but as I looked around, everybody else was still laughing and shaking their booties in time to the music. My throat started to tighten in pain and my body felt heavy as I tried to maintain the rhythm and follow the moves. I felt like a car which had broken down on the fast lane of the motorway and I had to try and limp to the hard shoulder.

The clock said we had twenty minutes to go. I had to finish the class, so I opted for the smaller movements and I tried to steer my boat from the rocks. I was feeling the burn in my legs, as we worked on toning our tushes but unfortunately, I was also feeling the burn in my cheeks, while my body started to feel cold. I have never experienced anything quite like it. The end of the class ended with us shouting "Sleek! Sexy! Powerful!" in a unison of feminine, exercise-induced endorphins but for me it was more "Sham! Sickly! Pitiful!"

I got through that and the girls stood for the obligatory "I was there" photo. I thanked Tara and apologised for my lack of exertions in the latter part of the class before making a quick exit, as I felt completely gripped by a terrible ache all over. I made it home and went to bed, where I stayed for 48 hours, with no lights and barely any food. I have renamed my illness Wotsit-it is, as everything smelt of a variation of crisp to me.

Really, I should count Pilloxing as half and not a full challenge down but I do want to return to do a full class, after I finish my challenge, as I really enjoyed it up until the lurgy stuck me down. It certainly had everything I enjoy in a class: sassiness, girl power, cardio, punching, toning and high energy – definitely worth giving a go, just make sure you aren't borderline flu-like before you attend and you'll be fine.

Cheerleading – Number 55

Due to the virus I had gone down with mid Cha-Cha in Piloxing, I'd spent a few days in bed and even had to postpone my rugby and volleyball challenges. I was pleased to get back into things with what I had assumed would be a gentle class of cheerleading. Yes, a bit of pompom jiggling would be just the ticket I needed to ease myself back into things. Paul had helpfully offered to come and take photos for this challenge, but I found his motives questionable and declined.

I arrived at West Coast Cheerleading in Redruth and met with Rhea, the owner. After a brief chat, I was introduced to my classmates, who looked all made up and beautiful, while I was sporting a pale, post-illness complexion and lank hair. Damn it, I should have made more of an effort and put a bit of slap on.

We entered the gym and I was delighted that they had a sprung floor. I see these all the time, as my girls do gymnastics and I've always wanted to have a bounce. The class started and straight away my naive illusions began to shatter as we got on with a SAS style warm-up around an assault course. We had to climb over something, then under, then over. Roly-poly next and a walk over a beam, run over the inflatable mat, then a burpee, a sit-up, a burpee, a press-up and a burpee - five times!

I was heaving and blowing like a distressed elephant already. Next up was gymnastics, as I yearned for a sparkly pompom to appear. This is challenge number 55 and I feel I have become a little immune to indignities. I leave my dignity in the car on the way in and on the journey home I have a rummage about for it again. This mind-set has enabled me to cope with most situations which I'm presented with but I'm delighted to report that the bar has been raised again, as I attempted to tackle gymnastics.

Firstly, some roly-poly's into straddle and tuck, which was OK. Then, we moved onto forward and backward handstands - yes, handstands! I haven't attempted one of these since primary school. To say my attempts were rusty would be a massive understatement. My T-shirt kept flapping up to reveal my attractive wobbly bits. The Gods who control dignity rolled the dice again for further entertainment, as I attempted to bunny hop across the floor and then for more amusement, reverse bunny hop back, with my fat arse waggling around in the air and my T-Shirt eagerly trying to escape the humiliation of the situation. I did manage a few cartwheels, though, which is quite a feat to accomplish sober.

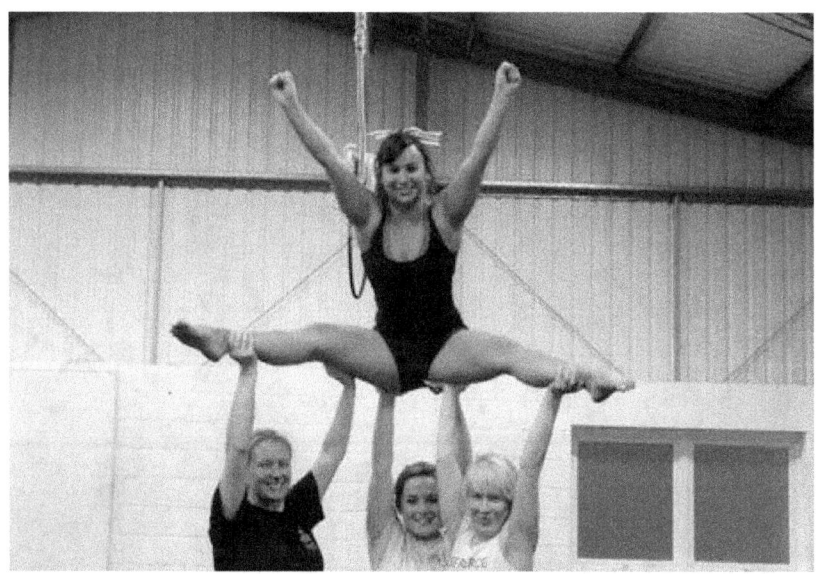

Supporting the flyer

Next up, we practised a few stunts. The person who is flung about and caught by the rest of the squad is known as the flyer. The usual flyer wasn't there this evening, so the girls looked for a replacement. As I have the physique of a small bungalow, this was not a position I was going to put myself up for. Instead, I acted as a "limb holder" as our flyer was launched in different positions into the air. I then stepped back to watch as they progressed to full swinging in the air, rolling about and catching. The girls described all the injuries that had been sustained when this has gone wrong – it turns out cheerleading is quite a dangerous sport after all.

Finally, and I think purely for my benefit, the glittery pompoms were brought out. We were taught a "simple" routine, which I tried my best to follow but I ended up looking like the Gary Barlow (circa 1994) of the group, as I tried forlornly to keep up. It was good fun, though, as we all tried to perfect our routine.

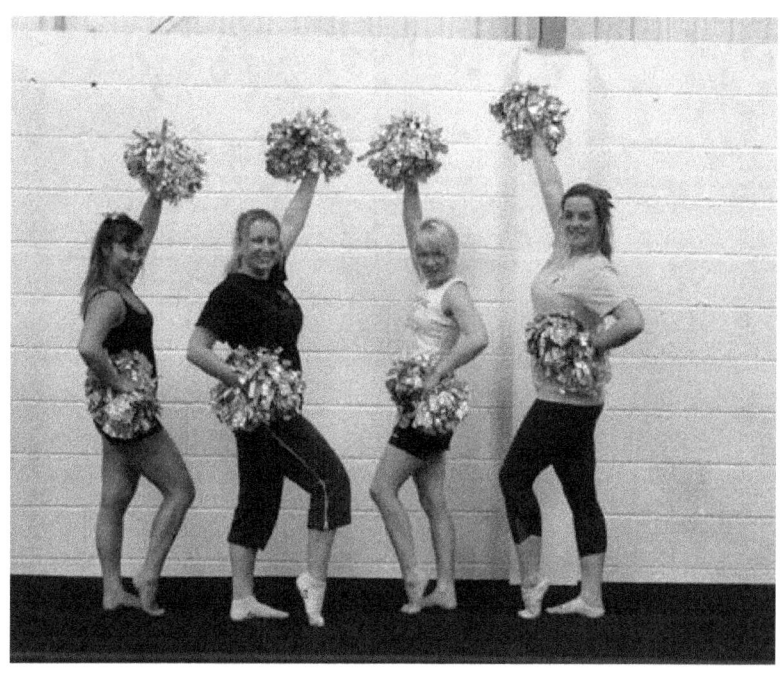

Yay! Glittery pompoms!

We finished up and my body really felt like it has been through its paces. It was as physically demanding as any fitness class I have taken. If I'm honest, I would have to admit that my body isn't as flexible as required but it was a lot of fun and very enlightening to see that cheerleading is a mixture of dance, gymnastics, acrobatics and weightlifting; certainly something my daughters would absolutely adore. I will hand my pompoms over to them, I think, as I get back in the car for the journey home. Now, where did I put my dignity again?

Golf – Number 56

There are two sports which I play and am competent at: hockey and tennis. The common thread with both is that I get to smack the hell out of a ball. Smacking the hell of the ball is my release and substitute for feeling the need to smack the hell out of something else in my day-to-day frustrations, whether that be a computer playing up, a human being on the end of an exasperating customer service call – the list could go on.

On the surface, golf has the potential to be a sport I really like. It seems to fit nicely within my preferred sporting criteria i.e. the ability to legally hit something. I was invited to bring a group of novices along with me for some expert tuition at my local golf club, Lanhydrock. Paul came along, with my friends Sarah, Harry and Chris, who seemed happy to pop their golfing cherry with me.

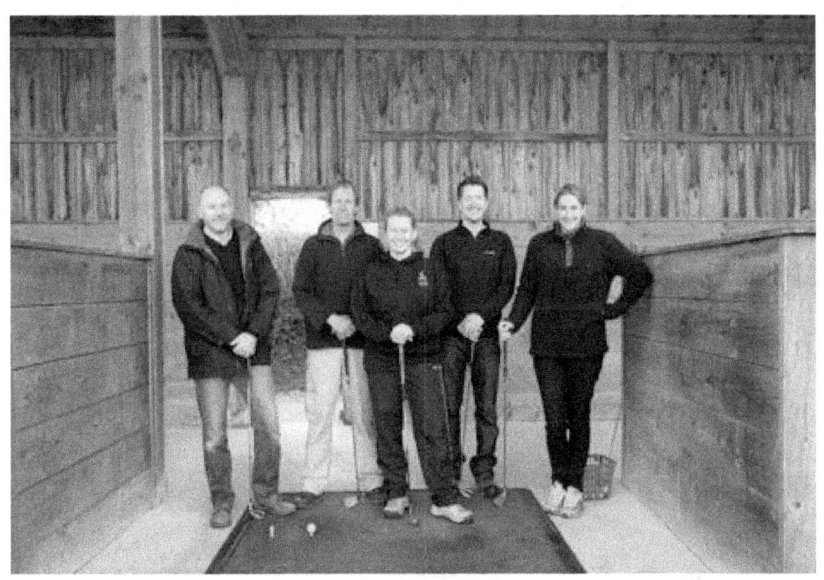

Swingers Party

I have to confess that I'm not a complete novice at golf. My father, a keen golfer, used to teach me as a child. Home video footage shows little me, swinging clubs about on the beach or on walks, or in the park. On more than one video, Dad can be heard to indulgently remark to my mum in his Cornish twang "Ann, she's got a good swing!" The trouble was that I wasn't a very compliant student and didn't want to hone my technique. I wanted to bounce about and build sandcastles. Dad finally gave up when I was 8, when he dragged me around a course and in trying to avoid the long route, I instead climbed over a fence, fell and face-planted straight into a muddy bog. I ended up in a flood of tears and Dad gave up on his golfing ambitions for me.

I didn't mention any of this to Alister, our instructor, but inwardly I felt confident with this one. We went down to the driving range and selected our little holding pens, as Alister went through the stance required and how to set ourselves. I was eager to start clubbing some balls about and once he was satisfied we were holding the club correctly, off we went. I popped my ball on the tee and looked out to the 100 -150 yard markers, with confident expectation. I focused on the back of the ball, with my head still, as I raised my club and violently swung through. The ball smashed loudly to the wooden side of the area and dribbled pathetically onto the grass about a foot in front of me. Everybody laughed.

I brushed off my own humiliation and I tried again. This time, it went high and far. I carried on, attempting to recapture my childhood natural ability, which my father reminisces about to this day. As the session went on, I started to think of myself as Tigress Woods. I battered the ball about, lashing it here, there and everywhere. Some went straight, some sliced off in different directions but either way, I recaptured that lovely feeling of smacking a ball about and the release of tension which goes with it.

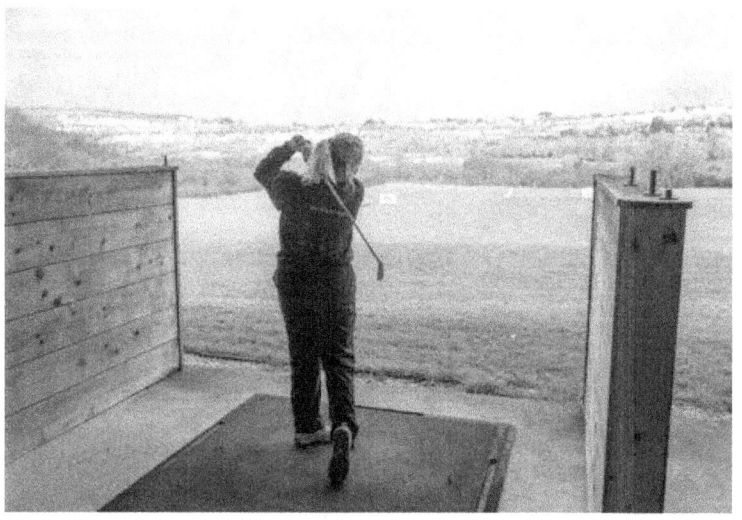

Battering the ball

As my hockey career winds up, this may be the next sport of choice, although I am rubbish at crazy golf and I am not sure I would be able to do the pitching part very well either. I start to consider a new variation to golf, which would be perfect for me: relay golf. You play in a team, one person or the "Smacker" hits the first shot (that would be me), the next ball is hit by the "Pitcher" and the final shots are played by the "Putter." I look around at the efforts of Paul and my friends and decide I would need to find a different team to compete with, as they clearly wouldn't grace my new variation of the Ryder Cup.

Yes, I like golf. Alister encouraged me to take some lessons and maybe I will. If my relay golf idea doesn't take off nationally, I will have to learn the other strokes required. We left the course after a cup of hot chocolate. I went to report back to Dad and whined at him that he should have made me continue with golf. In return, Dad smugly sat back with the unspoken words "I told you so" written all over his face.

Rugby – Number 57

For the first time in my challenge, I was late. The margin of error with carting 3 children around to their various pursuits is very fine and the coordinated drop off/pick up with my father went wrong, which meant I turned up 15 minutes late to rugby. The girls were already warmed up and performing a drill, so I made a quick introduction to Ann, who I had spoken to on email and joined straight in.

This flurry of panic and urgency had ensured that I didn't have the time to consider the potential pitfalls of the sport I was just about to try. If I had allowed myself the time to reflect on rugby, I would have felt pure apprehension and dread of being potentially tackled and thrown into a muddy bog. So, all in all, it was probably a good thing.

I was delighted to find there were a few newbies joining the session. I am always comforted to find fellow clueless people, as I don't stick out as much. After a fairly taxing routine of running in circles, changing direction at speed and picking up the ball and repeating, we moved on to a game of touch rugby. The coach told us we could pass in any direction, forward or back but we would have had to have passed the ball at least three times to score a try.

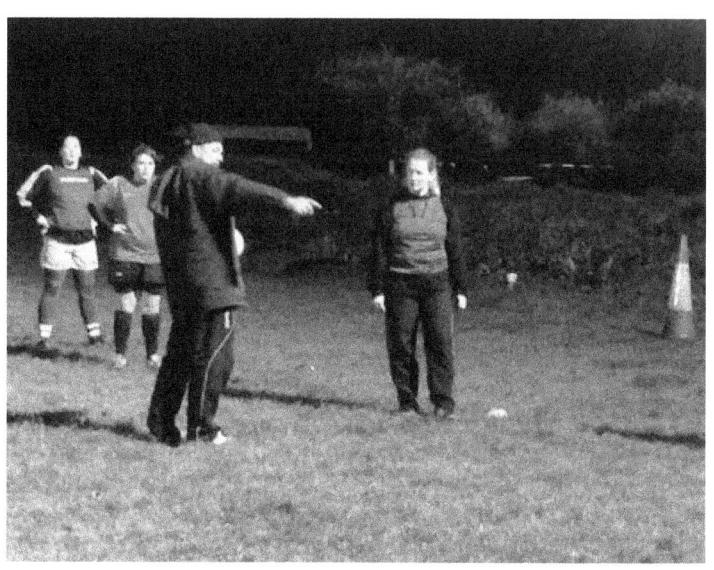

Getting some direction from the coach

It was four v four as we lined up against each other. I knew what my strategy would be, as it has served me well in previous sports such as handball and football: the old hot potato (HP) technique. In these situations, I like to be in charge of a ball for no longer than 2 seconds; anything more and a defender is all over you. This then incites me to panic, which is usually accompanied by my pterodactyl scream but ultimately it ends with me losing the ball. Not great for team sports.

The game began and my HP technique was deployed. I must try to develop this technique to ensure somebody is actually there when I throw the ball, as I repeatedly offloaded into thin air. Another problem I found was that when I got the ball, it felt like netball, so I stayed rooted to the spot and looked to immediately pass. What I needed to do was run with the ball. This was harder than it sounded as I kept getting tagged by the opposition.

One girl, who seemed very good, would receive the ball and dodging outstretched limbs, darted to the other side. I decided to try it. After several aborted efforts, I caught the ball and made my way through a slither of space and triumphantly put the ball on the ground. That felt really exhilarating, if not unnatural. We then progressed the game to passing only backwards and this is where it kind of fell apart for me, as I found it very confusing to not run to a space for a pass. When I did receive a ball, I would run as far as I could and then pass behind, then carry on running ahead, before I checked myself and ran backwards. I think that would take a while to actually master.

Training ended with another passing drill, and I was relieved to get through the session without ending up face first into the quagmire we had made. Although, thankfully, we hadn't practised tackling, I found the session physically demanding, as we barely stopped running. I must have enjoyed it as I wasn't even bitter about running around in the mud in the pouring rain on a Friday night and not being in the warm, having a glass of end of week wine.

As we stood for photos, the girls were quite shocked to hear about why I was there and that I wasn't coming back. That is the thing I love about team sports; you are automatically accepted into the group. Usually, I have time in the beginning to introduce myself, so I apologised if they felt deceived but no, I wouldn't be back next week - God knows what I will be doing in a week. Last Friday night I was cheerleading and this week I was playing the polar-opposite sport of rugby, so who knows what next week will bring?

TRX – Number 58

Twas the night of the school Christmas play, as I sat in eager anticipation to watch the panto unfold. I made small talk with one of the dads sat next to me, as he enquired about my challenge and how I was getting on. "How nice of you to ask," I replied. I gave a brief account of where I was up to and that my next class would be TRX. A sharp intake of breath was the response - in my experience, this is not a good sign. It turned out that he took the class as well and jokingly warned me I could kiss goodbye to walking up or down stairs the day after.

With this knowledge, I was filled with trepidation as I entered the class. I knew Chris the instructor already and was pleased to see him, knowing that he was already aware of my limitations in the areas of balance, strength and stamina.

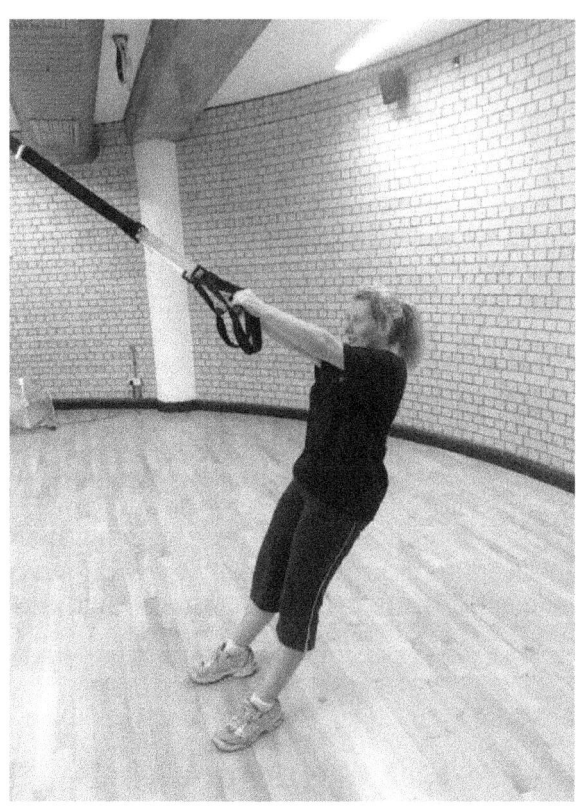

and pull....

TRX is a suspension based workout, where you work each part of your body against the tension of a pair of straps dangling from the ceiling. They looked a bit suspicious to me, as it had a passing resemblance to a sex swing and I certainly didn't feel confident putting my full weight on them. What if I pulled the ceiling down? I haven't done a challenge for a week now and I have been indulging in pre-Christmas wine and nibbles.

We started the warm-up with a few lunges and squats. Usually, I am falling all over the place but the straps were keeping me steady, like a wobbly toddler on a pair of reins and I felt more confident using them as a support.

With all of the exercises, you could go at your own pace. If you took a step forward or back depending on what you were doing, it would provide more resistance. Chris seemed to enjoy watching me wince and then encouraging me to move and make it harder.

We went through curls, crunches, a variety of lunges and numerous other movements. So far, so good and I was certainly feeling the burn, as different muscles shook off the hibernation mode I had put them in for over a week. However, I should know by now that I am not going to get through a class without at least one experience of mortification; this time, it was when we had to put our feet through the handles and with legs akimbo in the air, work on our core. It looked like we were strapped into stirrups and about to give birth.

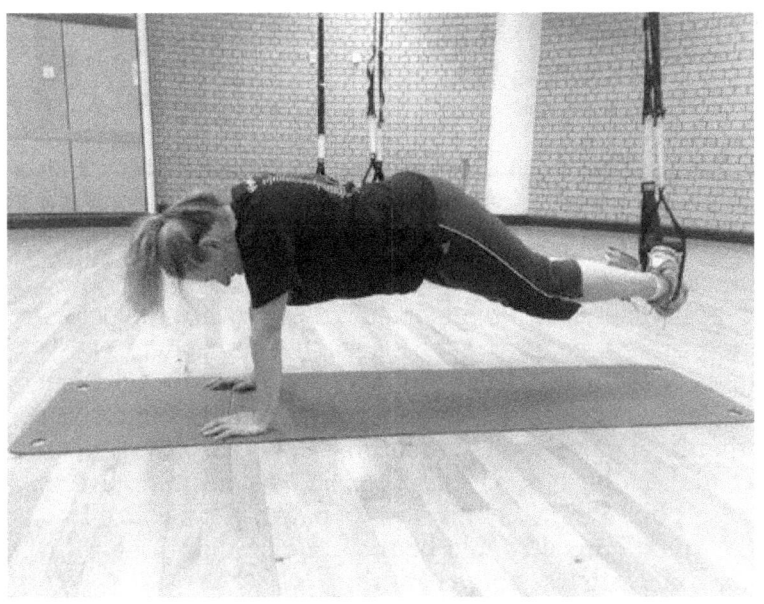

Looking like a right planker!

Having failed on an epic level to bring my arse off the floor as I pushed down on my hands, we moved onto my nemesis: the plank. I hate planking and planking hates me. I assumed the position with my legs behind me, strapped into my stirrups, my arse forlornly waggling in the air, as I attempted a full plank and when that seemed impossible, a half plank (elbows on the floor). This progressed into bringing our legs up, whilst in the same position and then for extra fun, we had to do a running man plank. I looked around to ensure everybody was making a meal of it like me, but my classmates were able to follow and assured me that it took a couple of classes before you properly picked up the technique. Although this was the beginners' class, one lady had been doing it for 18 months and looked great for it. This is the problem with my challenge; I only do things once and then I am off doing something completely different, which means I seem to find everything hard to start with but if I kept up with TRX, I'm sure I'd see a lot of benefit.

For now, my next challenge was a steep flight of steps to conquer, which looked and felt almost Himalayan. I almost planted a flag at reception when I got to the top. I can only imagine what tomorrow will bring and I'm considering whether I can put a Stannah Stairlift on my receipts for this challenge. If I can have toddler reins, surely I can have a stairlift as well?

Cardio Tennis – Number 59

I have high hopes for cardio tennis. Without even knowing what is specifically involved, it's in the running as a regular fitness class P.C. (post challenge). Mixing a sport I enjoy with the benefits of a cardio workout seems to make it a leading contender.

Usually, when I play tennis B.C. (before challenge), I occasionally made up a foursome with my neighbour and a couple of other local players, all in their 60s. Although very competitive, I don't find doubles too physically taxing, as you can have a natter between points and you only have to patrol half a court. I assumed with cardio tennis, it would be the same kind of thing, a bit more running but with less of the nattering.

I dusted down my tennis racquet, which had been left abandoned and neglected in the garage and joined Steve at my local leisure centre. Whilst waiting for the class to begin, I spoke to a lady who went regularly. My illusions started to shatter as she described the amount of running which was involved and advised me not to worry about where my ball lands, as it was just about getting to it before the second bounce. I felt slightly dejected at the thought that nobody would appreciate my one and only shot in tennis: my semi-powerful, two-handed backhand.

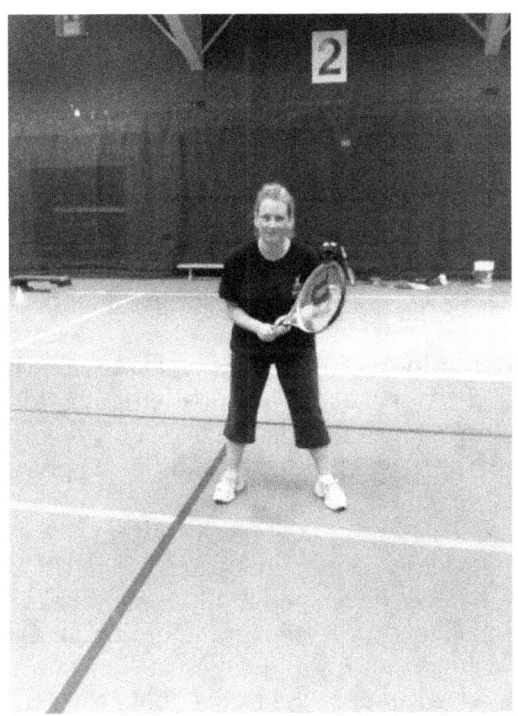

Ready for action...

Steve trotted over with a kind of shopping trolley full of colourful tennis balls and explained to us that due to lower numbers because of Christmas, we would have to work extra hard. He had a menacing glint in his eye.

We lined up for the warm-up, as Steve threw a ball to our forehand for us to run, hit, then back through the ladder and join the queue. We did this on the forehand and backhand side a number of times. So much for warming up, I was boiling already. The next drill involved starting from one side of the court and then running to reach the ball on the other side, then running and joining the back of the queue. It was continuous. We couldn't even have a slight chinwag.

Thankfully, Steve ran out of balls and we were ordered to retrieve them from the other side. Finally, a break and a chance for a breath. There were a few eager beavers quickly picking up the balls but I could see a strategic ploy by others to take a bit longer to pile the balls on their racquet. I followed suit.

Meanwhile, Steve was busy placing some step blocks either side of the court for pairs to use, whilst the others continuously repeated the drill and then swapped. Another few variations of this drill and then off to retrieve the balls. This time, I put myself in charge of the ones under the bench; I used the opportunity to sit for 10 seconds, whilst feeling for balls out of my reach.

Steve announced that the next drill would be hitting balls on both sides of the court; firstly a forehand, then immediately a backhand and run around the whole court and do it again, until the balls in the trolley were gone. I abandoned my lovely two-handed backhand, as I was finding it impossible to stretch to get to the ball.

We were forty minutes in and finally, I was over the shock of all the running and I was starting to hit the ball better and running didn't feel quite as exhausting. Was I enjoying myself? Steve carried on feeding from his never-ending supply of balls, until finally they were gone. We ended on some "winner stays on" doubles, where finally I could show off my one tennis shot. Unfortunately, the memory of this will be clouded by my horrific forehand, which never developed in the same way as its sibling.

The class finished and I was completely spent. One of the girls said we would have run up to 4 miles in the class - no wonder I was so exhausted. Although I had my doubts early in the session, I do think it remains on the shortlist P.C. When I got home, I popped the racquet back in the corner, knowing that I won't be leaving it so long next time.

Snooker – Number 60

Unfortunately, my 100 quest had come up against some recent hurdles, what with Christmas, kids' stuff and generally getting involved with a lot of over-indulgence over the festive period. Calling myself a Sofadodger has never been more ironic, as I squeezed myself into my jumper. So, to gradually ease myself back into things, myself and Father went off to the snooker club for a frame of snooker.

Our local snooker club is, without doubt, going to be my most favourite venue. It is one up from a tin shack and when I drive past it nearly everyday, it always makes me smile. Although very familiar with the location of the club, I had never actually been in, let alone played snooker. Once we had the OK from Gilbert, we let ourselves in.

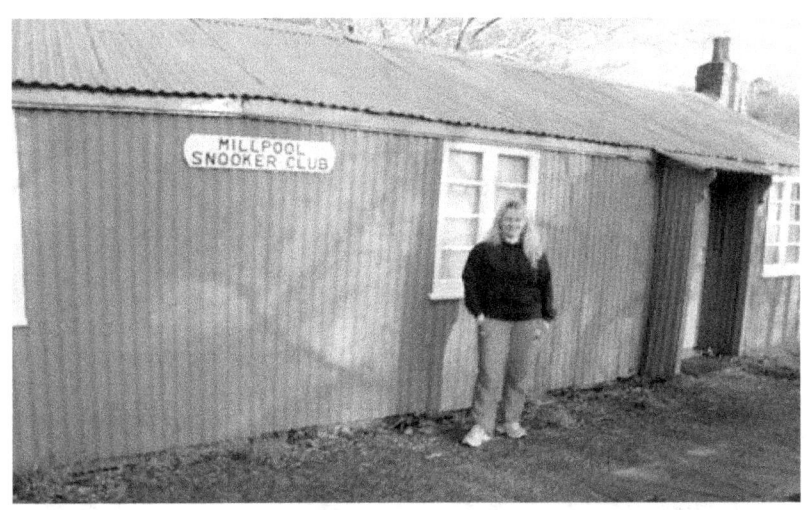

Not quite the Crucible!

Dad and I are very similar beings; we are competitive and we like a bit of banter. The banter immediately kicked off with the cue selection and then who was going to break. Although unacquainted with snooker, I used to watch it on the telly a lot and I occasionally play the odd game of pool, so I was confident I would be at least able to hit the things.

Neither of us got off to a flying start, as I quickly realised that this was nothing like pool. With my hitting and hoping and Dad's "just missed" pots, I glanced at the clock and wondered how long it would take to get through one frame. Apparently in 2001 when Ronnie O'Sullivan played Joe Swail, the frame latest only seven minutes - it took us that long to actually pot a ball. Dad finally opened the scoring and we were off!

I was having an absolute mare, with everything going wrong. Eventually, when Father was 20 points up, he made a foul shot, thus conceding me 4 points! I was cock-a-hoot with that. I had essentially scored the equivalent of four reds! I stopped moaning about the lack of chalk on my cue and started to concentrate. My technique was the problem here and Dad kept advising that I kept raising my head after a shot. I focused and hit another red, it missed. Whilst we were busy arguing about how quickly my head had moved, I noticed out of the corner of my eye, that the ricocheted ball had slowly plopped into the corner pocket. I celebrated like I had won the World Championship against Ronnie O'Sullivan himself, as I triumphantly moved my counter a few centimetres to the right.

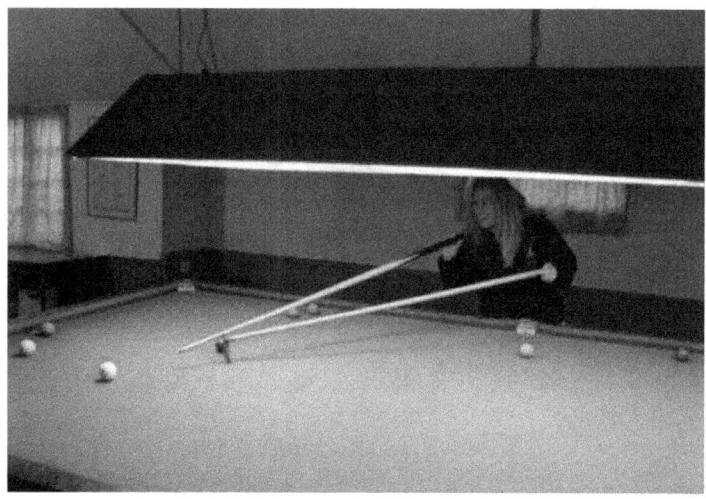

Just told Dad to give it a rest! Classic...

Suddenly, Dad got into gear and started potting balls from all angles and then unfairly, put me in "snookers". Apart from my foul and my fluke, I was still not potting anything. I struggled with the length of the table, using a rest, using a spider, using a long cue and finally angles. All of which were critical to my success. Forty minutes in and we finally got down to the colours – I was determined to pot one of these spherical foes.

Dad, whose highest break was standing at nine, potted the yellow and went for the green but missed. It sat tantalisingly over the pocket. I chalked my cue as I tried to control my adrenaline. I was aware that a poor sighted, one armed, octogenarian could probably pot this ball but as Dad kept murmuring, "there are no easy pots". I took aim and feebly managed to kiss it into the pocket. Sheer joy!

The frame ended after an hour, with Dad scoring 60 odd and me a measly 10. I enjoyed the game and was glad I had experienced the mysterious activities of the fabled "green shack". As Dad crowed all the way home, it felt that my game was more You've Been Framed than a frame of snooker but that didn't matter. It also reminded me why I never asked Dad to teach me to drive.

The Challenge So Far - Number 51 to 60

The journey between challenge number 50 and number 60 has been fairly long and arduous. I knew that it wouldn't be plain sailing but it has taken me nearly two months to complete only 10 challenges. This is way away from my target of two a week and has really put me behind schedule. December, in particular, seems to have presented endless hurdles; from illnesses, to car troubles, to the obligatory festive school activities, to the celebrating of the birth of baby Jesus himself. It all seems to have happened together and put me completely off track.

Historically, as soon as I feel off track, I talk myself out of what I am doing and promise to myself that I will "start again" at a better time; whether that it is a diet or an exercise plan. Had I not publically set myself this challenge and imposed a deadline, I would have used every excuse under the sun to give up and try at a more convenient time. This says a lot to me; firstly, I need an objective and a deadline and secondly, I need to stop making up excuses and understand that it is OK to take a pit-stop but that the journey must continue. I can't keep going back to the start each time.

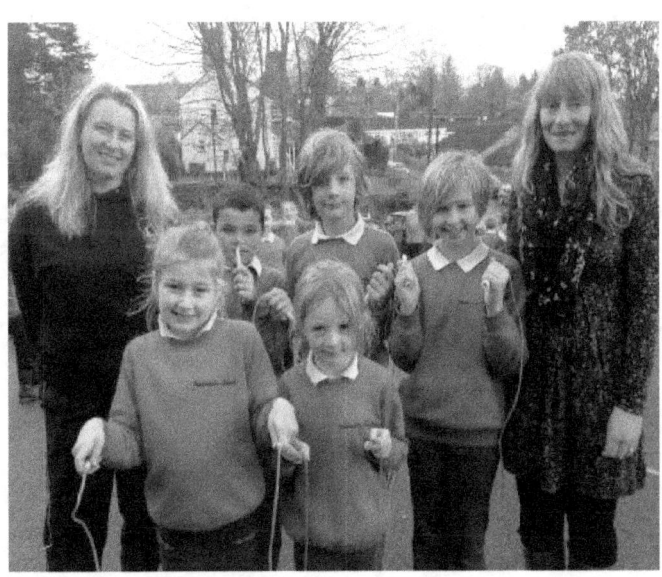

Mini SofaDodgers!

There have been other positive things to happen recently; as a by-product of this madness, the local primary school have given the go ahead to pilot the idea of a "mini SofaDodger challenge", whereby the children will take on the challenge of trying 20 different sports over the course of two terms. The sports included are: ice-skating, surfing, climbing, archery, squash, bowls, aikido, yoga, dance, American football, trampolining, mountain biking, golf, Zumba, judo, orienteering, table tennis, badminton and handball. The local Rotary Club have sponsored the printing of T-Shirts and after announcing the idea on BBC Radio Cornwall, we are all set to go in the New Year.

The obvious benefits of getting the kids involved is that they get to try a range of sports which they might not have come across, the clubs get to link with the schools and give the kids a taste of the sport and for the school, it works towards their objectives in this part of the curriculum. We are hoping that parents may also get involved but that might be more of an uphill struggle!

Another bit of news and this is purely a headline for the old ego but my blog has made it to the finals of the National Blog Awards, taking place in London in April. The competition looks stiff but it will be nice to get a new frock and mingle with the crème de la crème of the blogging world...I won't be preparing a speech, though!

So, as the New Year starts and I reflect on 2014, I have to concede (in a cheesy X-Factor style sound bite), that it has been a truly life-changing year for me, as I have pushed myself far beyond my comfort zone. I have also had the privilege to have met lots of truly inspirational people along the way. It hasn't been easy juggling the demands of work, deadlines, motherhood, after school clubs and life in general but my family have been incredibly supportive and I just ask that they hang in there for a few more months, as I drag myself, by hook or by crook, over the finish line - no more excuses!

Chapter 8 - Challenge 61 – 70

Online Exercise Class – Number 61

The festive period has certainly taken its ritual toll, as I attempt to squeeze myself back into my gym leggings. My tummy resists any type of confinement after weeks of freedom, as I opted for looser fitting waists. 2015 sees me more of a Jammy Dodger than a SofaDodger!

Not 10ft from my sofa resides my TV and on the sofa itself lodges my laptop. Between the two of them, their sole aim seems to be to corrupt my attempts to live a non-sedentary lifestyle. Along with their secret weapon, Sauvignon Blanc, they work together to derail the attempts of Will Power to change my habits. Will and I fluctuate between friend and foe but Will's powers are in the ascendancy, as today we turn the tables on laptop and TV. We use their powers for good and sign up for an online fitness class.

I kick the family out of the sitting room (ironically into the fresh air), as I signup to Gymcube - which is the first Non-American website I came across - no offence to my transatlantic friends! I sign up for a free membership but can't access the on-demand videos unless I give the monthly subscription a free trial, so I pop in my details and I am good to go.

There seems to be a fair amount of choice, so I filter by most viewed and click on the Little Black Dress challenge and was surprised to see the gym lady from the Apprentice (Katie Bulmer-Cooke) taking the class. The class is for half an hour and we kick off with the normal warm-up and then work through a variety of squats, lunges, high kicking cardio moves and planking. The only problem with the way I have set it up is that I can't get the browser footer away from the bottom of the screen, so when they're doing something on the mat, I am not sure what is happening. I have to freestyle. Maybe this is the TV's way of retaliating?

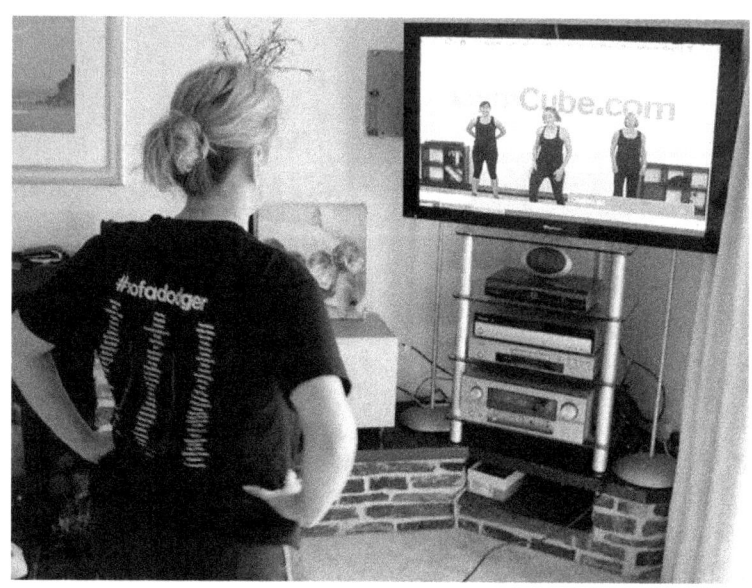

Following the instructions

One of my usual strategies for getting through a real life gym class is to "cheat a little" and when the instructor's back is turned, I tend to slow right down before I am back in full view. Online exercise classes present a massive opportunity to do this throughout, so I have to fight my urges on the basis that I am only cheating myself. The class lasts for 30 minutes and at the end, I am genuinely out of puff.

I can see lots of advantages with exercising online: it is easily accessible, cheaper than a gym membership, it doesn't matter if you haven't shaved your legs or painted your toenails and you can use your TV for good not evil (sofa dwelling). It also trumps fitness DVDs hands down, as it has the variety to keep it from going stale. On the flip side, I did have to put up with various family members peaking in to see what was going on and ask, "what time is dinner?" and "can I go on the computer?" but that's just about timing. There are also the advantages of training with an actual instructor to consider; they are able to correct technique and get that little bit more out of you and obviously have a variety of equipment on hand. When you also take into account the social aspect of going to a class, there are a number of different pros and cons to ponder.

However, I think it's something that would work for me, being a busy working mother who lives a thirty minute round trip to a gym. It is all about timing and flexibility and if I can't find a gym class to fit in with my schedule, this is definitely a good alternative.

Me and Will high five, as we triumph over the laptop and TV. I would celebrate with a drink but Sauvignon Blanc has taken a New Year's holiday, as I aim to cling on to the wagon for as long as possible.

Clubbercise – Number 62

Next up on my New Year's list is Clubbercise, which I found out about whilst cruising Twitter looking to pick up hot new classes. Clubbercise is apparently taught to dance/club music, in low lighting with flashy lights and with the provided glow sticks, it seemed more reminiscent of attending a rave than a fitness class. Combining darkness with my well-rehearsed strategic placement at the back of a room, it sounded like a winner to me.

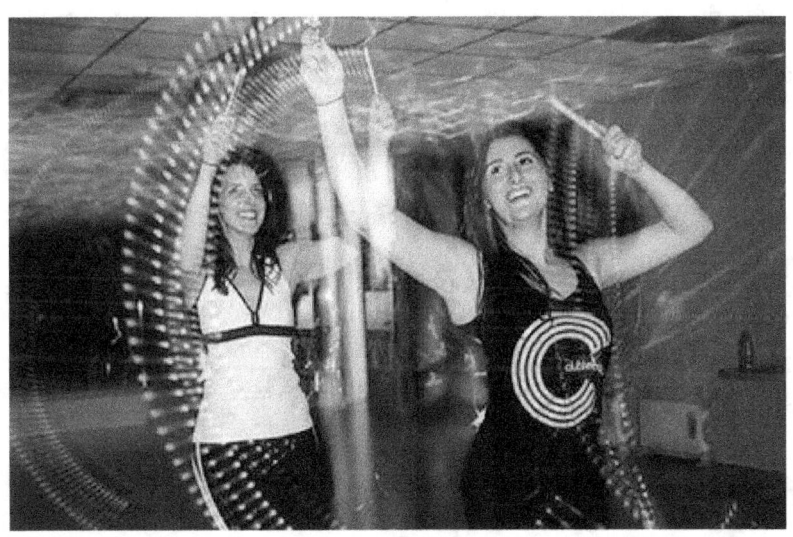

Spangly lights!

I arrived in Plymouth to meet Laura and Sara; twin sisters who actually founded Clubbercise with their sister-in-law just over a year ago. I was swept along with their enthusiasm as they told me the story of how they started up and how it is growing nationwide. I was completely in their thrall, as they told me their tales, whilst finishing each other's sentences and barely pausing for oxygen!

I was handed my glow sticks as I entered the hall. This was the first fitness class of 2015 and it looked more like Noah's Ark than a school hall, as friends of all shapes and sizes huddled two by two around the parameter of the hall. I shuffled to the back, marking out my territory, as the lights went off and the disco lights cranked up. I switched on my glow sticks as the music started.

The first track was slower, so we could warm-up and then boom, into some proper tunes. I didn't get all of the moves but being in the back, alongside the other newbies (who had also staked their area) and being in the dark, it really didn't matter. It seemed like the people in front were at a proper rave and knew all the moves and I had the sneaking feeling that I looked more like the person who waved in landing aircraft.

That all changed when "Rhythm is a Dancer" by Snap came on. I busted my moves to that tune. Those moves were tried and tested and have been in the locker for over two decades now. They weren't actually coordinated with the moves everybody else was doing but I couldn't help myself. When I finally abandoned my rusty teenage dance routine and synchronised myself with the rest of the class, it was quite a sight to behold as the glow sticks waved in unison and the lights danced around the room. Then N-Trance's "Set You Free" came on. I was in musical heaven.

If I'm honest, I would have preferred to continue in that genre of music but I'm aware that the class cannot be solely catered for selfish ravers in their late 30s, as the class was attended by people in their teens, right up to people in their 50s. The subsequent music were all floor filling dance tunes, so I was more than happy going through the 90s to the present day.

The class was a lot of fun and I was sad to relinquish my glow sticks back to the girls. I felt like a dancing Darth Vadar toward the end, as I waved my mini light sabres about. The obligatory photo was taken and a few of the other class goers came up to me to ask about my challenge. The people I talked to absolutely love the class and were campaigning Laura and Sarah to offer more dates.

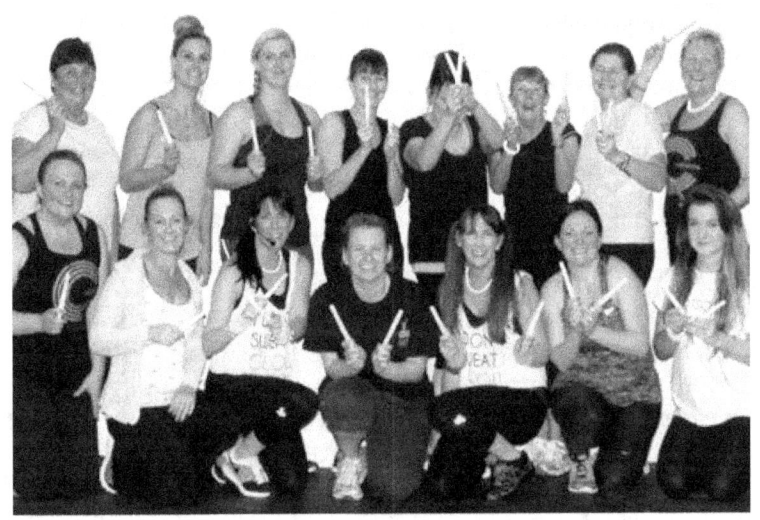

Some of the lovely class

I really recommend the class if you are looking for something which is fun and doesn't feel like a fitness class. If you feel conscious about exercising, the darkness really does give you that anonymity and if you worry you can't dance, don't because there were plenty of people shuffling along at their own pace and completely out of time – including me!

After a further chat with the sisters, I made my way home. The business woman in me really respected these two accidental entrepreneurs, who have a really inspiring story behind their business. I wish them all the luck in the world, as I really believe they are on to something.

Kettlercise – Number 63

Kettlercise is the next "something-cise" fitness classes on my agenda, with Mike Charlwood from Priority One Fitness. You may remember Mike from the Insanity challenge, as I fondly referred to him as "Tigger on Smarties." This time, I think he'll be less bouncy, on account of the fact we'll be swinging clumps of metal about. There are various weights to choose from but I immediately bonded with the runt of the litter - the little 4kg kettle.

Mike explained that we'll be working through sets of exercises to a tempo and we must concentrate on our technique where possible. I said I was a little concerned about my lower back but he explained that if my posture was correct, I would be fine. This included ensuring the shoulders were back, with knees slightly bent, looking up and to clench the buttocks. To help with this, he told us to imagine that we were clenching a £20 note between our cheeks. £20? After the indulgences of the past few months, I could probably clench a whole ATM machine.

We grabbed a mat and found a space; to my horror, the back was already taken, which meant I was in prime eye-line position. Not good. I placed my kettlebell next to me as the music started and we commenced the warm-up, with me under Mike's watchful eye. The warm-up was very straightforward but then came the start of the workout and the relationship with my new metal friend. Kettlebell was so informal that I vowed to think up a new name for it by the end of the session.

Kettlercise is essentially a fat burning class, where the kettlebell exercises are designed to strengthen and tone. Mike is Mr Kettlercise and as an instructor, I know he is a massive fan, so I was happy to place my trust in him and follow his instructions, even though I was starting to wince. As the class went on, we tackled different areas and awoke different muscles, I was starting to find it really challenging but because the exercises moved on so quickly, it was manageable. Although the kettlebell felt like it doubled in weight every 10 minutes, and it was starting to test our relationship.

I was pleased I was following fairly well and hadn't managed to bang myself with my weight, even when it had to be swung around our head. As I gritted my teeth for a 30-second countdown, I distracted myself by renaming my kettlebell, Bella. I transported my mind to me and Bella on a beach, working out. Mike interrupted my day dream by adjusting my stance, as I don't seem to understand that shoulder width apart and hip width apart are different.

Next to the floor, as we momentarily collapsed on our mats before Mike showed us the next drill. We had to lie down flat and lift the kettlebell above our heads and back and repeat. I slowly lifted Bella behind my head to the count of three and lowered her to the count of three then for some reason dropped her on the floor and lifted my head up, not realising that I had dumped a 4kg weight on my ponytail. As I came up, I was yanked back down like an elastic band. This would be bad enough on its own and I checked to see if anybody had noticed but on the next one, I did the same thing again. How?

It was there that my relationship with Bella ended. I resentfully renamed it "Kev" the kettlebell - apologies to all Kev's out there - but Bella was too pretty a name for it now. I wonder if anybody else was having the same kind of internal discussions as I seemed to be having with this inanimate object. Possibly not...

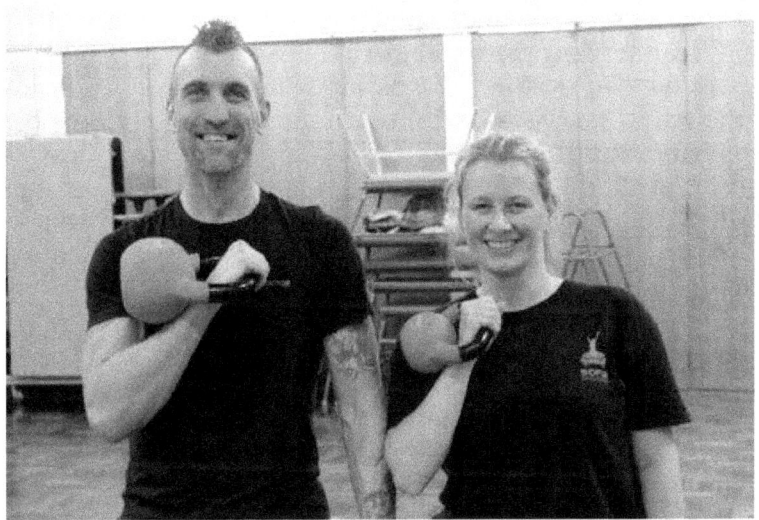

Big kettlebell and little kettlebell/baby bell...

Anyway, apart from the fact I probably won't be able to move the next day, as I feel the grey cloud of aches already descending upon me, I enjoyed the class and it makes the shortlist for classes enjoyed and to do post challenge. I have decided that as long as it doesn't have a burpee in it, I will be taking up some kind of fitness class after the challenge...but not with Kev - Bella maybe but not Kev!

Table Tennis – Number 64

As I arrived at my next challenge in the pouring rain, I walked past a dozen sodden rugby players training and was relieved to be heading for the warm, dry bosom of St Austell Table Tennis Club. I was five minutes early, as I had to do the customary children's club drop offs.

Di, the club secretary, pulled up two minutes later and chastened me for being early. We entered the large expanse of the club, which can fit up to 16 tables. I introduced myself and explained about my challenge. Di looked suspiciously at me. As a 75-years-old, veteran table tennis player of 45 years, she had seen rookies like me come and go but I vowed to win her over with my engaging personality and willingness to learn. Alternatively, I would wear her down into submission.

I was handed a bat as Di took me under her wing and showed me the ropes. I have played the odd game of table tennis before but not for over 15 years and the last time was more tipsy table tennis than anything competitive. It appears that with my limited knowledge of the game, I had been holding the bat the wrong way. Di encouraged me to put my finger behind and move my hand up for more control.

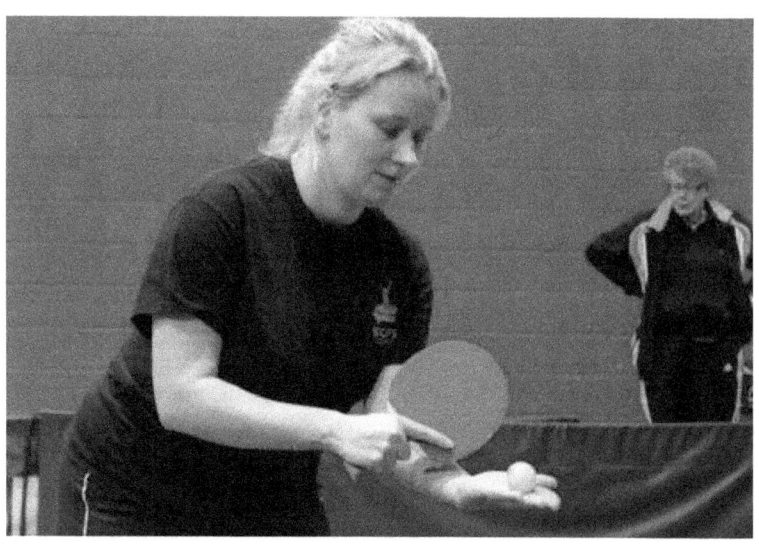

Di keeps an eye on me, as I try to serve

We then practised simple returns, which involved me not flapping about my arm but a smooth motion. Once conquered, we moved on to the forehand, which I found more challenging and became increasingly apologetic as my wayward shots meant Di had to be continually picking up my stray efforts. I suggested that the sport clearly required a hand-held hoover device, reminiscent of a straw and a Malteser.

We moved on to some rallies. In one rally, I counted 23 strokes and remarked that it felt very Forrest Gump-esque. I remembered to hold my tongue and focus on being a model student but I was really, really enjoying myself and I tend to get over-excited in these situations. Di handed over babysitting duties to Mike, a player in league one, who spotted immediately that my knuckles were white as I was gripping the bat too hard. As he was telling me to relax, I could hear Di in the background telling off some errant teenagers for messing about.

Mike and I went into some rallies and I took the audacity of smashing the ball hard into the corner. That felt really good! I tried to continue in that vein but I had no consistency, as the three subsequent shots fell into the net or launched past the table. I felt I was giving Mike a bit of a run for his money but then felt a little perturbed when he started kneeling down for a couple of shots. Maybe I wasn't providing the stiff competition I had imagined?

After the obligatory photo, I chatted some more to Di, who had finished her admin duties. Mike went off for a match with another player. I mentioned how impressed I was by the venue and asked some questions about the club. I looked up to see Mike was actually sweating against his new opponent and felt a little disheartened, as he failed to produce even a drop of perspiration when I had him on the ropes.

Then whilst Di was writing down her email address for me, some of the "always misbehaving" youths fired a half-squashed ball, which landed on her head. I left the club as she went marching over to give them an earful.

I skipped out of the building and into a large puddle/small lake, which I had failed to see in the dark but there were no expletives – wet feet was a small price to pay for such an enjoyable evening. I will definitely be playing table tennis again. I just need to invent that hoover idea to take on to Dragon's Den and I will be quids in!

CrossFit – Number 65

I wasn't sure what exactly CrossFit was and because of a few people's good luck messages, I was reluctant to research it before I turned up at Newquay CrossFit. When I walked in the door, it was wall to wall beefcake (with one beefcake-ess). Before my challenge started, this would have been the stuff of nightmares for me, as I'm more fudge cake than beefcake. Even after all I've experienced since I started, I still felt really daunted.

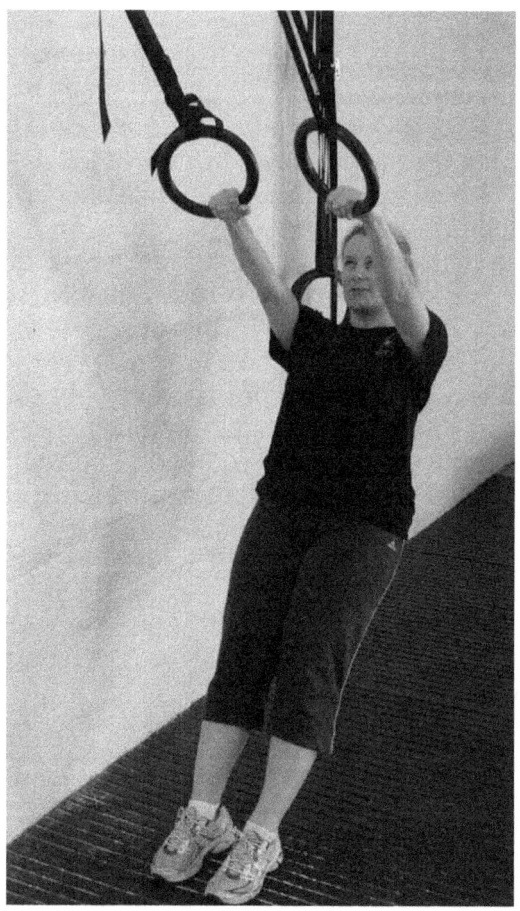

Trying out the equipment

Dan the owner came up and introduced himself and tried to allay my fears and said that I would be going at my own pace and finding my own limits. In response, I hurled a number of excuses about my back hurting and that I have self-diagnosed burpee-itis (fear of burpees). Dan took my whining on board and then in one fell swoop cast it aside, as it was time to warm-up. Thankfully, a few more ladies joined us to balance out the testosterone.

The idea of CrossFit is to build strength and conditioning through a set programme, with workouts of the day or WODs.

There is a competitive element to this, as you earn points for the reps you do in whatever is assigned for that session. The afternoon crew will then come in and try and beat those scores. Essentially, I was in a room full of bad-asses.

The first element was named "Thruster" and Dan told us to pick up a bar and with your partner alternate squatting and then lifting your preferred weight above your head. Your score would be the weight, times how many reps in 5 minutes. I was handed a bar but this was heavy enough, so I declined any additional weight. My jaw dropped to the floor as we lined up and I looked around at what everybody else was attempting. I managed 50 in two and a half minutes and although I wasn't lifting an actual weight, the 15kg weight of the bar was hard enough. I properly grimaced through the last reps.

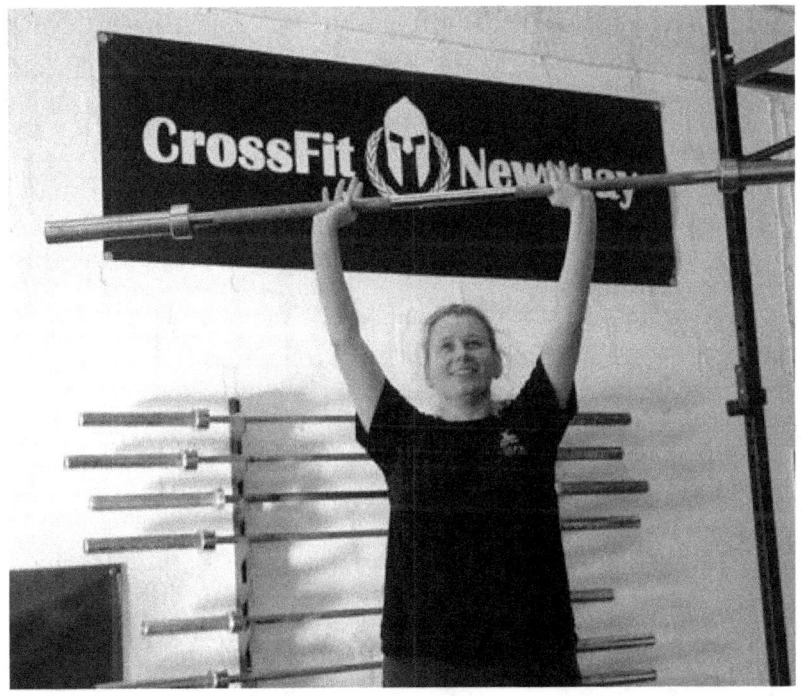

Weightlifting but without the weights

Next up, Dan instructed us to get onto a bar and then we had to swing our feet up to touch the bar and repeat like before. The exercise was simplified to hang from the bar and bring up your knees, or for me, who could only manage 6 before falling off, lie down and then lift up my legs – which was hard enough. I was completely letting my partner down but she was very sweet and understanding.

What followed in the next 10 minutes is a place where I have never seen people go in this challenge so far, in terms of pushing themselves. As I did the toddler version of this exercise, some of the guys were alternating pull-ups and getting their chest on the bar with handstand push ups. I'll explain this in the hopes of giving you the full visual effect. The beefcakes were getting into a headstand against the wall and then lowering themselves up and down, for a total of 60 reps. This was a different level altogether.

I just about managed to complete my version of what they were up to and I found it really tough but I was full of admiration watching everybody.

The hour was up, and I fist bumped with a few of the guys – thankfully there was no high-fiving, as my bingo wings probably couldn't have managed that, after what they'd just been through! Although this is definitely the toughest thing I have done, I was full of the old endorphins once it had finished.

CrossFit is definitely not for everyone and although it's on the far end of the spectrum in terms of strength and fitness, I'm glad I experienced it. These guys told me how much they absolutely loved it and how they got so much out of it. There's something out there for everybody and if you want to go to that next level, this is definitely for you.

I said goodbye and as I get to the two-thirds mark of the challenge, I look at what is left and feel relief that I am through the hardest but actually I still haven't tackled the likes of wrestling, gymnastics, water polo, wheelchair rugby and snowboarding. Maybe I will wait until I have completed those before I declare this the toughest.

Gymnastics – Number 66

Both of my daughters are keen gymnasts and sank to new depths of mortification when I mentioned that I was going to the adult gym class immediately after Izzy's session. As I watched my little daughter warm down by doing the splits and placing her nose on her leg, I had to wonder where this flexibility has come from. I certainly don't possess such powers, although Paul can proudly touch the floor with his hands whilst keeping his legs straight.

Once Izzy was safely deposited with Daddy in the car, I joined the rest of the adult gymnastics class. The class had only been going for 2 weeks and I was surprised to see so many people there. I was a bit apprehensive, as I assumed they were all going to be ex-gymnasts but it turned out that nobody had any particular gymnastic heritage. Both men and women were there, either because they were parents of some of the gymnasts or just randomly fancied giving it a go. I found this very comforting.

We lined up at one end of the springy floor and alternated forward rolls, forward rolls to straddle, backward rolls, cartwheels and round offs. My rolls were not pleasant to behold but I am really pleased with my cartwheels. Looking around, it was quite amusing to watch 25 adults, all veering off in various directions, landing in different heaps around the floor. It was certainly performed in a good spirit.

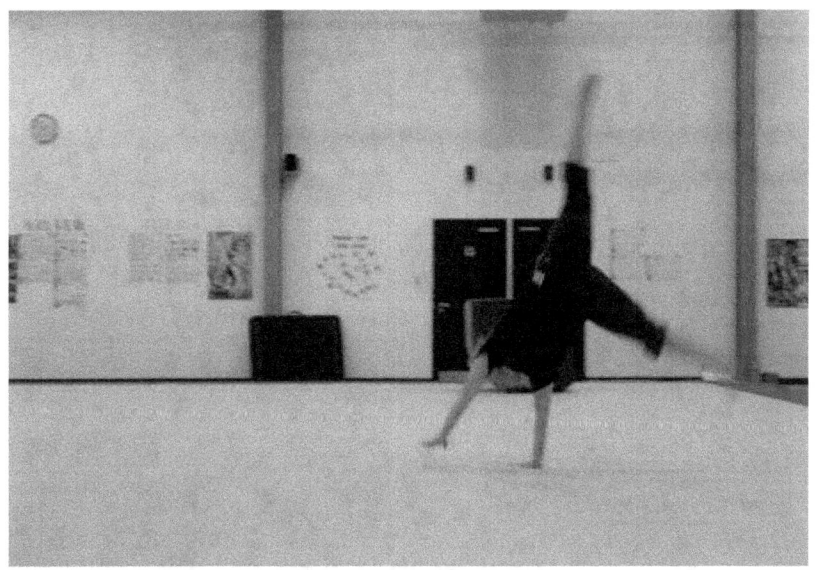

I am head over heels in love with cartwheeling...

Once we had conquered the floor with our misshapen moves, we were free to sample any apparatus we wanted, with the help of some of the coaches dotted about. For me, this was reminiscent of a chapter out of Charlie and the Chocolate Factory as this normally forbidden apparatus, usually reserved for children, suddenly became ours. No more standing behind a cordoned off fence, watching enviously from afar. Our faces lit up as we charged toward our most desired apparatus. For me, it was the vault.

As I come to the final third of my challenge and the finish line comes in sight, I feel like I need to make the most of every opportunity presented to me because in reality, a large number of things I am trying, I probably won't do again. I mean to make the most of it and for the vault; it meant that I was going to charge at it like I was an Olympic contender!

After a quick lesson in technique, we formed a queue. I strategically placed myself at the back and watched the people in front nervously canter up to the springboard, vault and then land on the mat. I decided to charge, like I've seen on TV and launch myself as best I could. The result was the best I could have hoped for but it felt really good. No wonder my kids love spending so much time here!

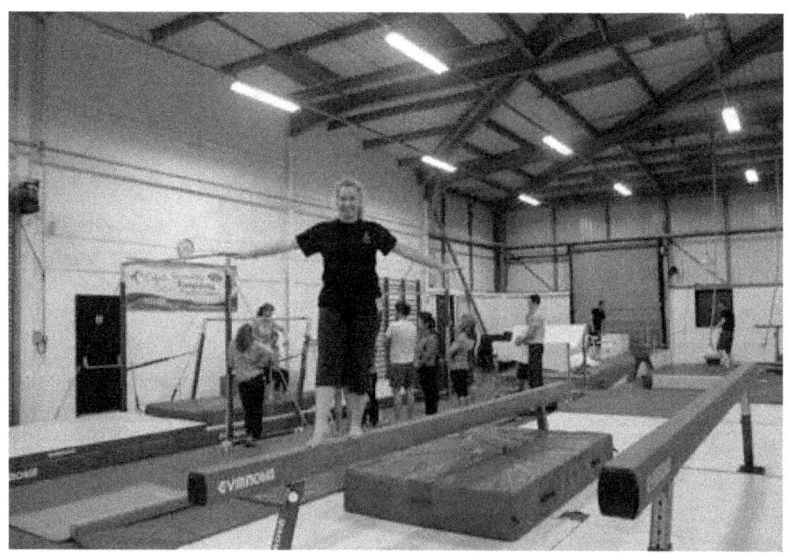

Beaming on the beam

Next was the beam, which really tested my issues with balance. I was encouraged to keep looking up but even on the baby beam, I was like a newborn foal. I moved on to the bars and again, there did seem to be some physical limitations to even reaching up to the bar. For one, I am a short-arse and secondly, I have big boobs. I had a few attempts to get up but for once, I decided to preserve my dignity, as I shrugged off my attempts with my self-deprecating barbs and moved back to the floor where I tried to perfect my cartwheels. We ended with some conditioning, which meant more planking. I am not going to miss planking or burpees after this challenge.

I really enjoyed gymnastics and I actually didn't need to feel daunted at all. The class was completely inclusive of all ages and all abilities. I don't think I will be challenging my daughters anytime soon for room on the podium but it was great to enter into a bit of their world. At the rate I am going, I will be attempting to shoe horn myself into their relay race at sports day or turn up on a Duke of Edinburgh excursion. Now that would really crank up the Shame-O-Meter for them!

Volleyball – Number 67

Volleyball is my next pursuit and from my distant school memories, I remember that I wasn't too shabby with my dig and serve, so all I needed to do was dust off my skills and I'd be sure to impress them. Maybe they would ask me to sign up. It is not unheard of in this challenge for a club to invite me to sign up with them after. I usually shrug off my nagging doubts and suspicions of their desperation in putting together a team or their financial survival, or dwell on the fact at hockey, we will have any old person who can hold a stick. Instead, I focus on revelling in their invitation and accept their praise as truly sincere.

I met Dave from Kernow Volleyball, who plays in Truro. Issue number one became apparent, as I stared up at Dave, who was over a foot taller than me. A foggy recollection came to me, as to why I didn't progress with volleyball. Ah, yes – I stopped growing at thirteen and remain to this day, a short-arse. I filed this away and continued to discuss the club and the sport in general. Apparently, volleyball is the second largest participation sport in the world. I imagined a beach volleyball court, on an exotic beach. I sniggered at the thought of turning up today, in a bikini, introducing myself normally and maintaining a straight face. I remembered that I didn't own a bikini and that I must not be odd in front of new people.

I was introduced to Rachel, who was assigned as my babysitter and I was delighted to see that she was no taller than me. We practised setting the ball and I really struggled to get the technique. I practised it about a dozen times and it just wasn't sinking in at all. I joined in with the main training and lined up against three people, who in turn threw a ball at me. My job was to run to receive the ball, use that stroke to give it back to them, run back and then run to the next person and continue on a loop. Everybody was really helpful with their words of advice but I just couldn't get it.

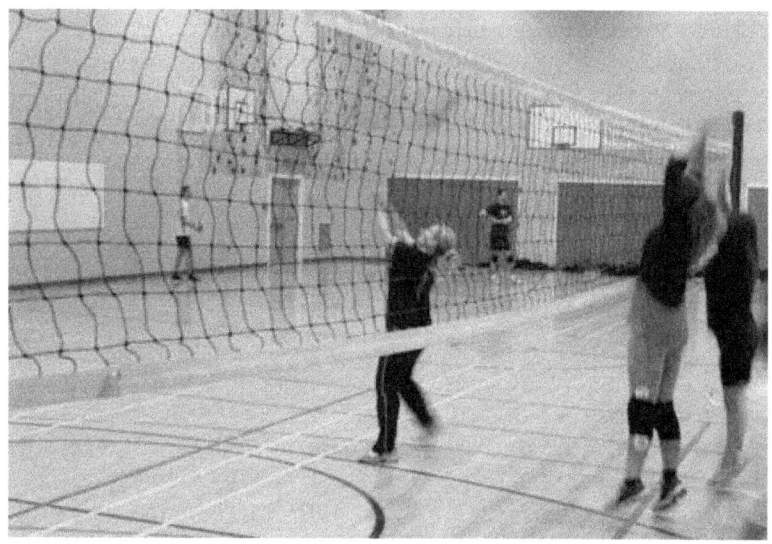

Playing the ball, whilst looking in the opposite direction from the net, is in no coaching manual

I was relieved to move on to digging the ball. This is where you grip your hands together to present the ball with your forearms. To receive the ball, you kind of need to squat and then use your arms to power the ball up to your teammate. We stood facing our three feeders again and as I received my first ball, it went careering off my arm into a different direction and it kind of hurt. More advice on technique was provided by a number of people.

I carried on but it was really stinging my arms! I watched as they started to glow red and my veins began to pop up. Then the whining started as I winced and screamed every time I hit the ball. I asked my teammates why I was being so pathetic and the general consensus was that it took a few goes for that to wear off. I kept taking "water breaks" as I caressed my throbbing arms.

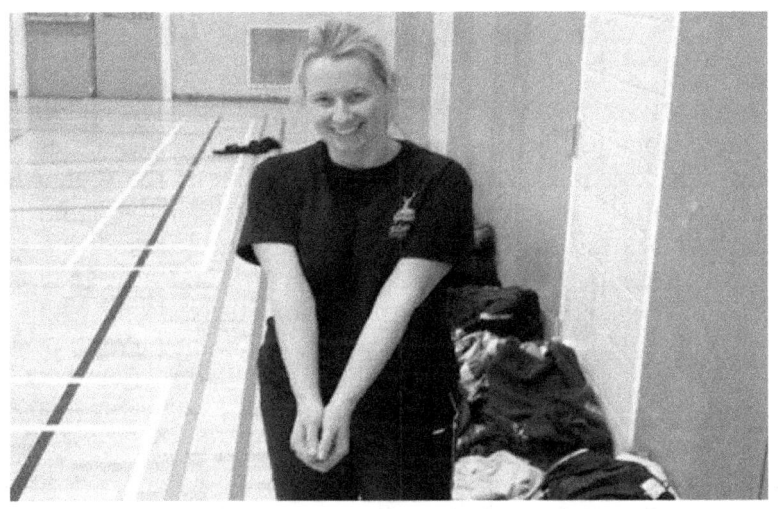

Not sure why exactly I am smiling!

I was delighted to move on to serving, which required the palm of my hand and not my arms. This went very well, as I managed a high percentage of serves in. It felt a bit odd using my limb as a racquet but my underarm serve was certainly doing the business. We moved on to a game, whereby the two "stars" of the team were pitched against six on the other side of the net. After yet another pit stop, I went to join the herd on the latter part of the court but they shooed me over with the stars. Oh no – I had nowhere to hide.

I managed to scupper a number of the points which they would have won, had I not intervened with my flailing arms but towards the end of the game, I managed to hit a fluke shot over the net to score a point. The girls high-fived me. I winced as our skins touched.

The All-Stars (and me) won the match and I took myself home. I heard that all athletes can benefit from an ice bath after a hard session, so being mindful of that, I adapted it, by putting half a dozen ice cubes in a glass and then poured Baileys all over them. Between sips, I rested the glass on my poor arms and reflected on how rubbish I was and that I probably shouldn't look out for an invitation back anytime soon, bikini or no bikini.

Kickboxing – Number 68

With my attractively bruised upper torso, I decided to make a last minute change to my schedule and focus on a lower limb activity instead: kickboxing. James, the instructor from the Krav Maga challenge offered me a class at his newly refurbished, swanky gym at Kernow Martial Arts in St Austell. Last time I was at this gym, James had me pinned against the wall with a mock weapon, so I wasn't entirely sure what to expect this time. It very quickly became apparent when chatting to his wife, Elaine before the class that I had focused on the word "kick" and failed to give the same priority to the word "boxing." My face fell as I realised I might be bruising my bruises. I looked up from my moping to see an angel staring back at me, in the form of Trina, who once worked for my good friend a few years ago. We recognised each other immediately and had a quick catch up while walking into the class.

I was over the moon; Trina would be my salvation. Trina is a lovely, sweet girl, who I could partner with and at most, I could expect just a light skirmish, with a few marshmallow soft taps around the torso. Josh, our instructor, set about warming us up, with a variation of push ups, crunches, star jumps and running. Trina and I whispered a few headlines to each other about what had been happening in our lives since we last saw each other...this was brilliant, we were having a good old chin-wag.

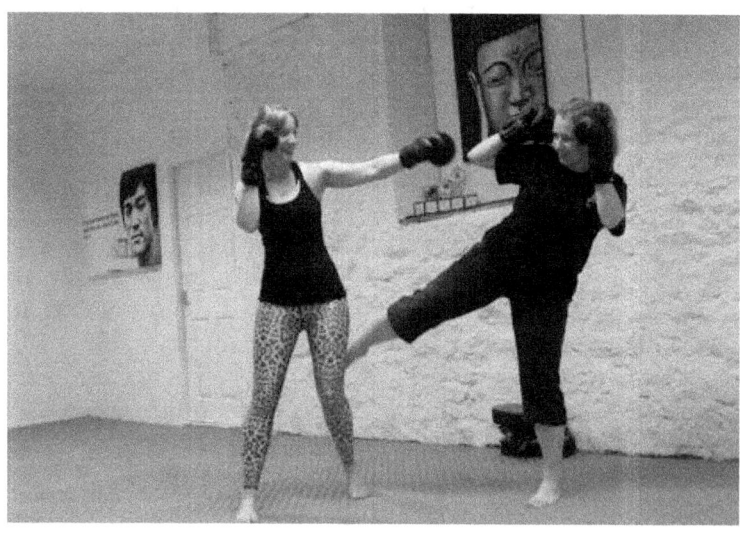

Having a laugh

Josh instructed us to get our gloves on and with our partner, practise a few blocks, parries and punches. Trina and I giggled through our attempts as we struggled to follow the instructions. We kept breaking off to see how other people were doing it. As previously noted, I have learnt so many other methods of blocking and defending that I just end up confusing myself and in a real life fight, I would be out for the count within 30 seconds as I attempted to figure out where best to put my hands.

We moved on to incorporating some roundhouse kicking. I was really looking forward to kickboxing, for specifically this reason, as I've found that I enjoy kicking. I seem to have far more strength in my lower body than my upper body. Although my left side is far weaker than my right side, which essentially leaves me with one quadrant of my body that's of any use and this is my right leg. I am fully prepared to weaponise this limb to best effect but not today, not with Trina. It wouldn't be fair.

We faced each other and Trina casually mentioned that she had some experience with this part of kickboxing and knew a little about roundhouse kicking. I furtively kicked her in the thigh as she turned away from the blow; she threw a couple of punches which were a little harder than our practise blows. Trina was starting to change, turning into Trina the Warrior Princess, as she demanded that I "kick her then punch her!" I followed the demand, while still apologising for any blows I landed.

My turn and I began to take a bit of a pummelling as I was kicked in rotation, firstly in my thigh, then my midriff, a glancing blow to the boob and finally, her leg swung up to hit me on the side of the head. I am sure she left my friend on good terms! Why is she beating me? I tried to follow suit but it still feels very alien to me to hit somebody with any great force. We parried and added new moves and I enjoyed being the kicker but not so much being the kickee.

The session ended and we all bowed. It was a very unexpected type of session for me and although I really enjoy kicking, I think I prefer kicking a pad rather than a human. I thought I had enough padding of my own to not feel the blows as I did. What is the point in having flabby thighs if it doesn't get you through a bout of kickboxing? At least, I will look symmetrically proportionate tomorrow with bruises on both my lower and upper limbs, kind of like a battered, old butterfly.

Squash – Number 69

If it hasn't come across already on my challenge, I am a big fan of racquet based activities. My father was a league playing, squash player back in the day, which meant I spent a lot of childhood weekends twiddling my thumbs at local leisure centres whilst he played his matches. So coupled with my predisposition to hitting a ball about and a possible genetic connection, I have high hopes of nailing this sport.

I badgered Tom, who works at my children's primary school and who also coaches squash in his spare time, to give me a training session. I have heard rumours that Tom includes 3-year-olds in the punishment lap at school football practise on Saturdays, so I knew he wasn't going to take any kind of pathetic behaviour from me.

Tom handed me a racquet as I excitedly reeled off my tennis pedigree. He sniggered at my reference to my prized two-handed backhand. Something told me that it wasn't going to make a showing today. Tom also introduced me to Aidan; he would also be joining us as his "assistant."

Firstly, we kicked off with some simple forehands and again I was discouraged out of my typical tennis stroke. All was going well, until the ball veered too close to the wall. There seemed no feasible way to get to the ball without smashing the racquet against the wall. Tom went up to the wall and gave it a bit of a smack and explained that it happened and was part of the game. I accepted it and the next time it veered near the wall, I followed suit, whilst wincing at the noise.

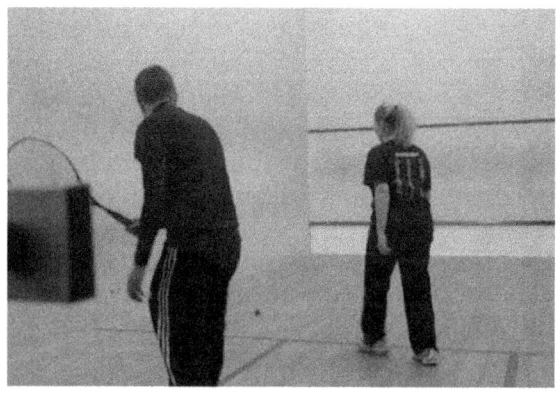

Tom showing me the backhand technique

Next, we moved on to the backhand, which is usually my strongest side but my powers would be halved with the use of only one hand. To reiterate the point, Tom told me to put my redundant hand in my pocket. I was really enjoying hitting these balls about, even if I couldn't always judge the bounce. I managed to perfect three methods of returning; firstly, running to the ball and then watching it bounce lower than I had judged, which left me swinging into the air, secondly, I would majestically return the ball and then just stand rooted to the spot as I admired the shot or thirdly and most annoyingly, I would hit it right back at myself and thus foul my competitor.

Tom felt that it was time to step it up a notch, as he told me he would be feeding in a forehand drive on one side of the court and Aidan would be feeding in a drop shot into the other corner of the court. My job was to get to both, 10 times each. This was obviously exhausting, so I had to play tactically and try and hold them up by returning the ball away from them, thus buying me a bit of time while they retrieved the ball.

A young lad called Owen made an appearance just in time for "winner stays on." I sized him up and felt I could take him on. I cobbled together my own version of a serve and the four of us rotated the points. I really appreciated how fit you would have to be to be a good squash player, as I got to play a point and then watched the pros play – it looked pretty brutal. I felt like I held my own, apart from when the ball was played behind me towards the back of the court. I was completely flummoxed as to how I would be able to play that ball. Owen, sensing a full on weakness, persisted in playing it there.

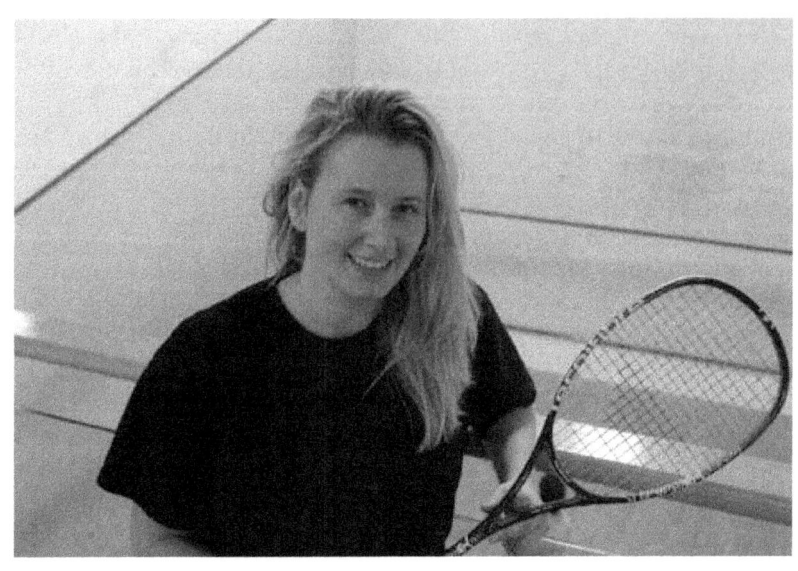

My new love interest

We finished up the session and I was completely puffed out and also confused. Squash seemed to pull on my heart strings. Was I cheating on tennis by flirting with squash? I have been loyal to tennis for so long and we have a lot of history together but squash has come along with its ball which almost winks at you. Add badminton in the mix and I seem to be turning into a racquet based floozy! Maybe that is the point about sport – you don't have to be monogamous. Maybe it is a relationship where you still have to be committed, yet not fully loyal but if you don't keep your eye on the ball, you can get hurt. That's enough pondering; I feel like Carrie Bradshaw in an episode of Sex and the City.

Kickboxing Aerobics – Number 70

With my love of kicking confirmed, I was invited by Tara of Versatile Fitness Choice to try her spangly new Kickboxing Aerobics class. The last time I met Tara was in her Piloxing class, where I fell ill mid-jump. I went on to spend the next three days in bed, which is completely unheard of for me. I was keen to go back to show that my complexion isn't usually green and Tara was keen to show me the only thing usually infectious in her classes is her enthusiasm.

The evening didn't start well, as I got out of the car and dropped my iPhone on the ground, thus smashing the screen. I had to pull myself together, or Tara would think I'm a complete liability. As I entered the class, I could see that it was packed, with everybody in high expectation as to what kickboxing aerobics was all about. Clever Tara had choreographed the whole class herself, taking influences from pilloxing, aerobics and well...kicking.

You can tell when there is a class full of newbies who are just getting into fitness, as they are usually lined up in this type of formation: 3 in the front, 5 in the middle and 20 in the back row. I had already spoken briefly to a couple of ladies, who were keen to show off the post-baby bellies they were trying to shift. I empathised with them but didn't mention that my youngest was coming up to seven and I still had that belly to lose! Tara encouraged everybody to space out for health and safety reasons, so there followed a reluctant manoeuvring around. The music started up and off we went.

The pace was bouncy but manageable as Tara built up the sequence. As there is the hierarchy of confidence and perceived ability in the front, middle and back of the class, I had situated myself in the middle, which meant that I had a girl in front of me, who I could follow as she seemed to have the moves off pat. What it meant for the poor person behind me is that they had my uncoordinated self in front of them, swinging in the opposite way to everybody else and always that one beat out of time.

At the start of the challenge, my timings and coordination issues would make me really self-aware but now, I just enjoy the music and follow as best I can. In that sense, I do feel I have come a long way since I started. I also have a new admiration for fitness instructors. I would compare it almost to being a stand-up comic and tonight, Tara was performing her own material. Having met a number of instructors over this challenge, I have been surprised that some do suffer a bit from their version of "stage fright." It takes a lot for somebody to stand up in front of a room and then perform and try and get it right for so many different abilities. As the crowd, you pay your money, but you must be open and enthusiastic and if you don't get every movement – or joke in this analogy - hang in there because the jokes change and you are bound to find something you enjoy.

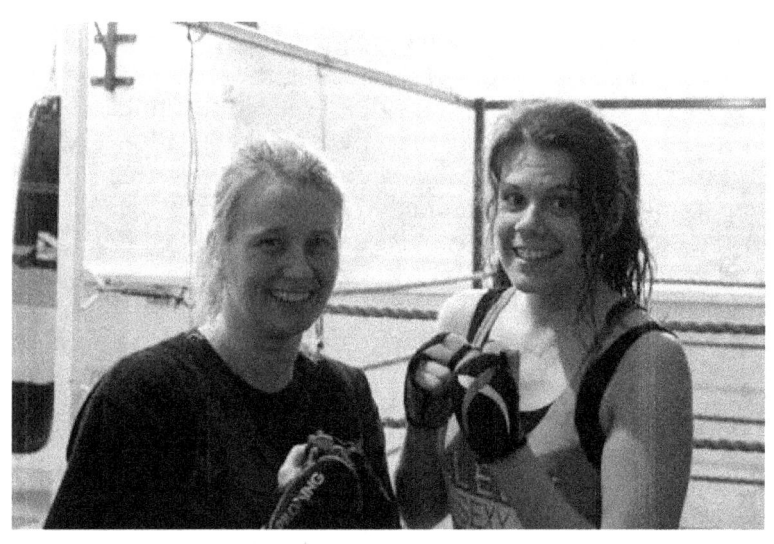

Tara and my sweaty selfie or "swelfie"

Tara ended her class by incorporating the "funky chicken" into a sequence, which everybody had fun with. If you choreograph your own class, you hold such extraordinary power...power which I should never hold. I don't think I could resist including a bit of an arse-dance or a baboon inspired element. This is why the power I wield over people should be limited. My children only realised that baboon arse-dancing was not cool when they hit school age.

The class was a great aerobic workout and I was full of praise after the class for Tara. There was an influx of people for the next class, so the goodbyes were swift. It was nice to finish one of Tara's classes with a smile on my face. I just had to break it to Paul about the phone. I decided to go home and ask whether he would prefer it if I had smashed the car, the camera, had the wallet stolen or smashed the phone...I was banking on one answer to turn it into a positive story.

The Challenge So Far - Number 61 to 70

My last ten challenges have encompassed the start of 2015, to the second week of February. Along with over 16 million people in the UK who have vowed to do more exercise at the start of year, I joined a host of newbies in a range of fitness classes, including a home exercise class, Clubbercise, Kettlercise, CrossFit, Kickboxing and Kickboxing aerobics and I also tried table tennis, gymnastics, volleyball and squash. Yet, unlike over 60% of people who would have abandoned their new year's resolution by now, I am still going and if anything enjoying it more and more.

I seem to have got through the pain barrier of December, when getting out of the house was a struggle and the end goal seemed a long way away. I have now adopted an attitude which makes me remember that I might not ever do most of what I am trying again, so I must go in with a mind-set of complete and utter enthusiasm and wonder. In gymnastics, this saw me motor at full pelt to the vault, like an Olympic medal hopeful. I have found that what I lack in natural ability and skill must be plastered over with a whole-hearted commitment to the activity in hand.

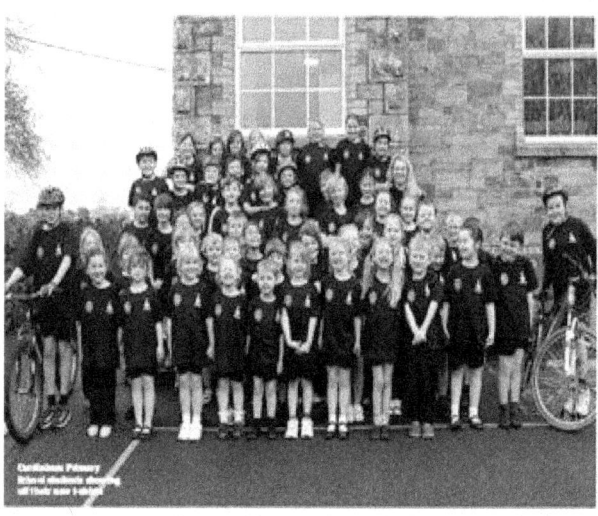

School does mini challenge

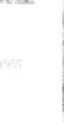

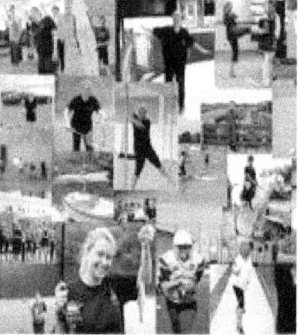

Coverage from the Western Morning News

January also saw the launch of the Mini SofaDodger Challenge, which has been covered in the local press. We even had the local BBC TV station come down and feature the school. Essentially, the kids are encouraged through school and outside of school to try up to 25 different sports until the end of the academic year. They've already tried street dance, yoga, squash, orienteering, mountain biking, gymnastics, trampolining and as I type, they are boarding a coach to The Eden Project to try ice skating.

It is lovely to see the kids sample the range of sports which are being offered to them by the school and I am so pleased that my children go to a school which encourages healthy living and learning. To achieve their 25 sports certificate, my own kids are desperate for me to take them to different venues and try different sports, so I am essentially running three SofaDodger challenges. This wasn't exactly the plan!

I've put the Mini SofaDodger Challenge concept to the website MindOpen to seek further thoughts and ideas of possibly extending this to other schools. Clubs are keen to increase the number of children "sampling" their sport and the kids seem excited to give new things a go, so maybe this is something which schools might be interested in taking on.

Finally, in this pit-stop of progress, I have signed up to a 6-hour danceathon at Wembley, for Comic Relief - whilst tipsy on Twitter, which seemed a great idea at the time. This promises to be a gruelling challenge for me, as I have to work out how many "toilet breaks" I can feasibly take, without showing myself up as a cheat!

The next 10 challenges are firmly in my sights and so far include Walk Football, Wrestling, Wheelchair Rugby, Basketball, Hockey, TyreFit, Snowboarding, Skiing, Bootcamp and BuggyFit - over half of these I am deeply apprehensive about and I will leave you to guess which ones.

Chapter 9 - Challenge 71 – 80

Zumba – Number 71

I started with a number of phobias before this challenge started: gym phobia - the thought of hauling my Lycra-clad arse into a hot and sweaty room, with a bunch of different machines I didn't understand, was and still is a relatively distressing thought. My other phobia was being part of a fitness class which involved any kind of requirement for rhythm. There are numerous other phobias: fear of heights, fear of wetting myself in public, fear of death but I put them in the normal/can't change category. I have retained all of those phobias but I have smashed my fitness class phobia out of the park. After Fitsteps and Clubbercise, I've realised the only thing you need for such classes is a positive attitude and a bit of sass.

I was invited by FunFit Dianne of Pilates and Powerhoop fame, to join her at a Zumba Master Class, with Hender Corredor-Escalante (apparently a veritable Zumba Overlord, as he is an International Zumba Jam Specialist). Unfortunately, I had left a little bit of sass at the bottom of a bottle of Prosecco the night before, so would need to muster extra swagger for what was about to hit me.

The event in Plymouth was sold out. Dianne introduced me to a number of ladies from her Zumba class and then took me off to meet Hender himself, who was very welcoming and fantastically effervescent. I bagged myself a prime position at the back, whilst taking in the variety of ages and shapes and sizes in the room. I wasn't quite sure what to expect but from the minute the music started, I was swept along with the Latin vibe and the energy in the room.

I've heard a lot of my friends talk about Zumba before but because of the aforementioned phobia, I had never gone along but wow, I can now see what all the fuss is about. I was loving it. The tempo was high and although I didn't get a lot of the moves to start with, it didn't matter. Just because I've had a change of attitude doesn't mean I have suddenly located rhythm but for that hour, I was shaking my booty like J-Lo herself.

Adham Abou-Shehada (the host for the event and a Plymouth based Zumba instructor) and Hender must have gone through about a dozen songs but there was none of my usual clock-watching. When the hour was up, I felt like I could have gone on for another hour, good news considering that six-hour danceathon I mentioned earlier. I definitely felt the benefits of a cardio workout but more than anything, I felt my mood completely lift and any remnant grogginess from the night before was gone. This stuff should be prescribed! By the look of the room, everybody felt the same.

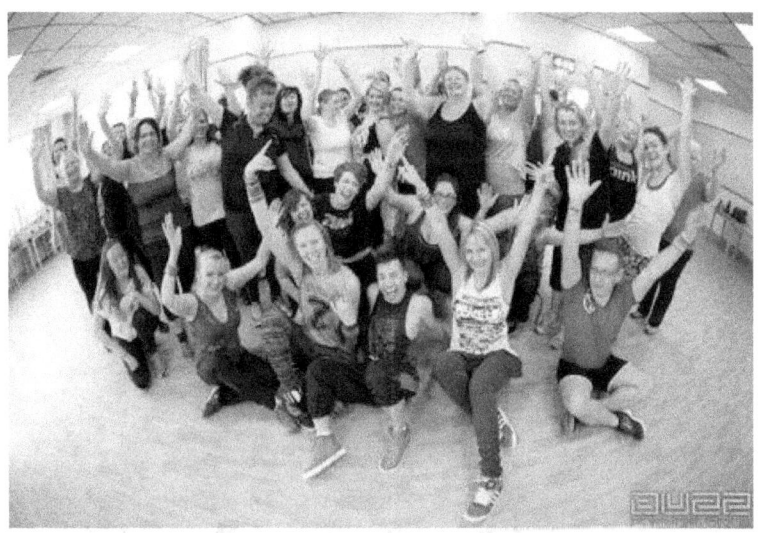

Put your hands up if you feel good!

I will definitely be combining a dance fitness class into my post challenge timetable. Yes, I do have a Wii and yes, I could stand in front of that but to be honest, I don't have a lot of willpower (or Wii-power) and if left to my own devices, I'll find an excuse, whether it be work related, child related or housework related. I, therefore, need to book a class and commit to it. Plus, it is good to feed off the energy of the instructor and the class itself - in my experience, an instructor will get at least 25% more out of you. So yes, I am one phobia down in this challenge, which is a fantastic feeling in itself. I'm definitely feeling "Sammy from The Block!"

Walk Football – Number 72

Some of the sports I have left on my list are at best daunting, at worst scary; one of them is even called MurderBall for God's sake! It's my own fault for not spreading them out across the year properly, so my next challenge of Walk Football should be literally a walk in the park.

Walk Football is a relatively new sport and has been featured on various adverts on TV. On the advert, there is a bunch of older gentleman popping the ball about. I was, therefore, a little baffled when I turned up at Newquay Sports Centre to see that the age range went from guys in their 20s right through to the more established gentleman. Annie, who ran the session, said that they were laid on for free and some of the guys were recovering from injury and found this sport works really well for them.

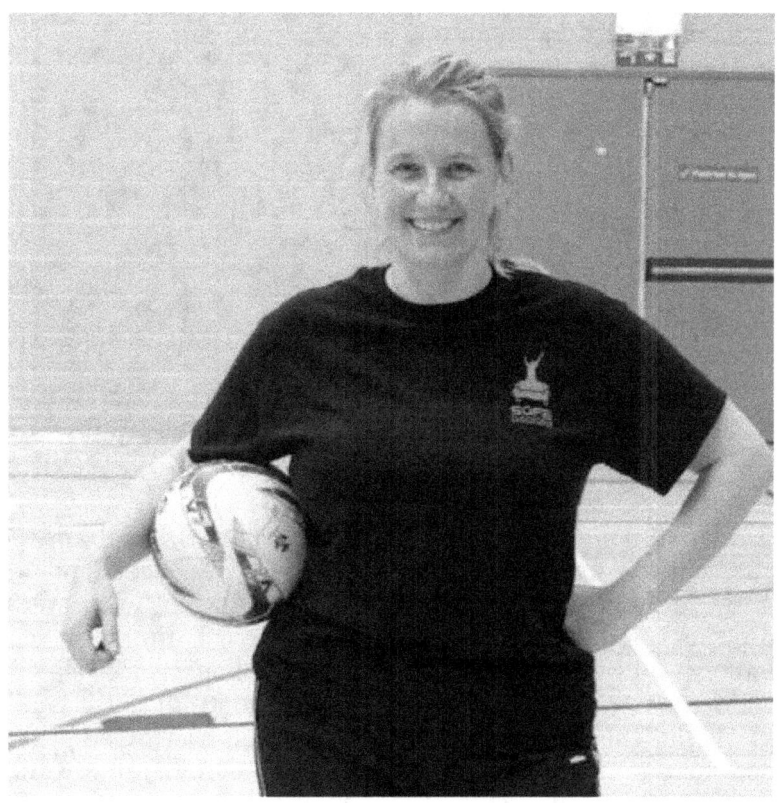

Ready to kick off

We went straight into a 4 a-side match, with me making up 4 and a half on one team, which would either turn into a help or a hindrance to them. How hard could this be? No running and just a bit of passing... Within the first 2 minutes, balls went whistling by at speed and just because there was no running, there was nothing saying the ball couldn't be hit at full pelt. I quickly learnt that as well as no running, you could only shoot in a certain area, only the goalkeeper was allowed in the circle and that the ball wasn't allowed to go over waist height. You could also pass off the wall, which meant that, along with no side-lines or backlines, the play was continuous for the whole hour.

It felt very strange to see a ball and not run to get it. I felt like a penguin waddling towards an egg. It took me a good few minutes to adjust. Whilst my brain was adapting to this new method, I clicked into the familiar and went off to waddle into space. My teammates passed me the ball, as I got myself into glaringly good positions, which they couldn't fail to look up and pass but they soon realised I was pretty awful at controlling the ball and the passes became less frequent. This was fine; I adopted a "making space" and "taking a player" out tactic.

As I was finding my confidence, the only efforts toward a goal I could get were accidental ricochets off the wall. One landed at my feet and I had a shot on an empty goal. It was more difficult to miss it, but miss it I did. Around my car crash efforts, goals were being thumped in left, right and centre and the game was getting competitive. Mid-way through the first half, the ball came to me again and instead of passing it, I went for the corner and it went in! I was still celebrating when the ball was saved up the other end. I had to remember that there was no stopping.

I was absolutely sweating at half time. One of my teammates came over to me with new team orders; I was to defend and mark a player – essentially, stop arsing up all of the chances up front. I'm not too keen on defending but I shadowed my player without diving in and tried to hold them up. Annie then unleashed a shot and I tried to block it and got a stinger on my thigh. Ouch! With me in defence, suddenly our team's fortunes turned around as the match got to 11-11, with 2 minutes to play. Bob, one of the senior members of the team, who remained competitive throughout the match, cranked it up a notch and started berating any bad passes.

I hear you, Bob, I thought and when the ball (accidently) came to me, I saw my player on the wing and I attempted to bounce the ball off the wall to him, as he was in acres of free space. He could then turn and shoot and we would all run towards each other embracing the last minute winner, and I would be credited with the assist. What actually transpired was that my feeble pass was intercepted and what I planned for my team happened to the opposition. Could I still claim the assist? I held my head in shame and couldn't meet Bob's eyes. Time was up and through my glory hunting, we had lost. I apologised profusely but the moment the game finished everybody shook hands and all had a laugh. Bob even congratulated me on my debut.

Walk Football was a real workout and I would thoroughly recommend it to anybody who enjoys team sports, as it can be played at different intensities. I have learned that preconceptions are a dangerous occupation of mine and I really need to halt this habit and remain open-minded. I might start this new resolution after Murderball though.

Wrestling – Number 73

More than once that day, I did question whether Friday the 13th was the best day to actually try wrestling, given that it was in my Top 10 Most Fearful Challenges To Try list. I was trying Cornish Wrestling today, rather than the more standard types seen elsewhere.

When I arrived at the club, I introduced myself to Mike, who is a Cornish wrestling veteran and by all accounts, a bit of a legend. Looking around, I could see young kids right through to adults. First things first and I was given what looked like a strait jacket to put on and with everybody resembling a bunch of inmates in an asylum. We set to warming up and having a stretch. I was introduced to some of the club members, including Mike's son, Richard and also Laurie, both champion wrestlers. I made a mental note to avoid those two and try and wheedle my way in with the kids.

After our limbs were sufficiently stretched, we all went in a ring and holding the jacket of the person either side, we set about trying to get each person on the floor, just by using our legs. This was highly tactical and you could gang up on somebody to get them to the ground. I tried to follow suit and hook my foot around my neighbour's leg. The leg didn't budge an inch and within a micro-second, I felt a small brush on my leg and then I was looking up at the ceiling.

Thankfully for me, the crash mat was produced and in twos, we were told to practise various moves. I was paired with Laurie, who turned out to be a very patient teacher and as a bonus, she was very light, so when she landed on me, it didn't hurt too much. The ironic start to each tussle in Cornish Wrestling is a hand shake, which made me smile, given the relative violence which follows. The moves were reminiscent of judo but unlike my judo challenge, I had a wonderful crash mat to land on.

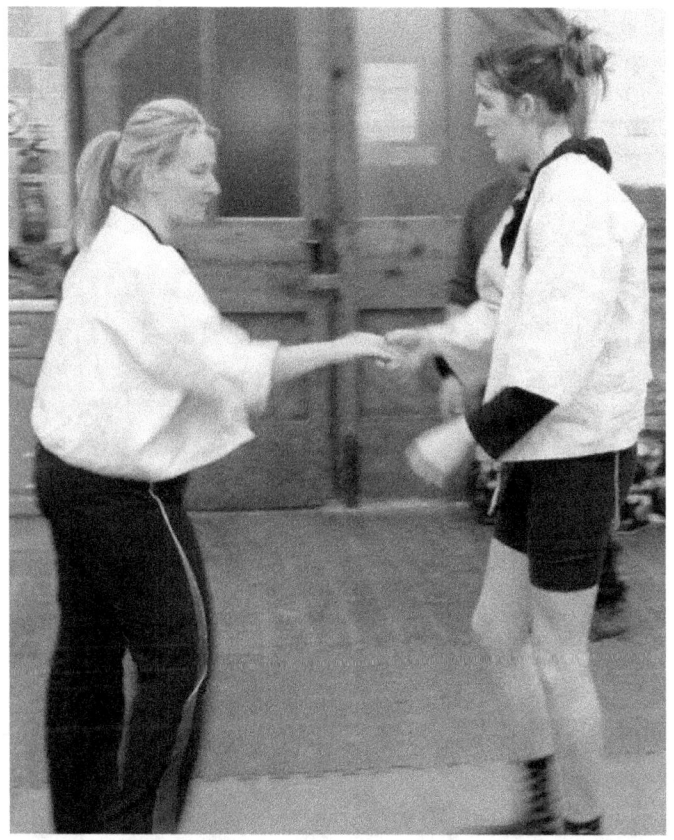

I shake thee hand, before I throw thee to the floor

Laurie was quick and nimble and when it was my turn to be thrown about, I would feel a slight tap and then be hoisted into the air before crash landing on the mat. We learnt four different moves and each time, when one was being demonstrated, Mike would animatedly describe the move and then regale us with stories of bouts yonder past, including in the 70s when they fought the Bretons and had to use doors when they ran out of stretchers!

After a cup of tea, I was horrified to see that my safety blanket (the crash mat) was perched up against the wall. My confidence drained away as I looked at the padded floor and considered all the ways I could injure myself. Similar sized opponents faced off against each other in a 3 minute round. It started with the younger kids and then moved up to the adults.

Laurie and I were up next. Whilst waiting, I considered fashioning a white flag out of my straight jacket but I didn't have time. We circled each other, with Laurie providing commentary on what to grab and how to attack. I made some half-baked attempts at crooking her leg, which she danced out of and compliantly waited for my next shambolic attack. Sensing that I was acting like a distressed animal, she swiftly took my feet and put me out of my misery, so I scurried off to the corner and hid behind Mike.

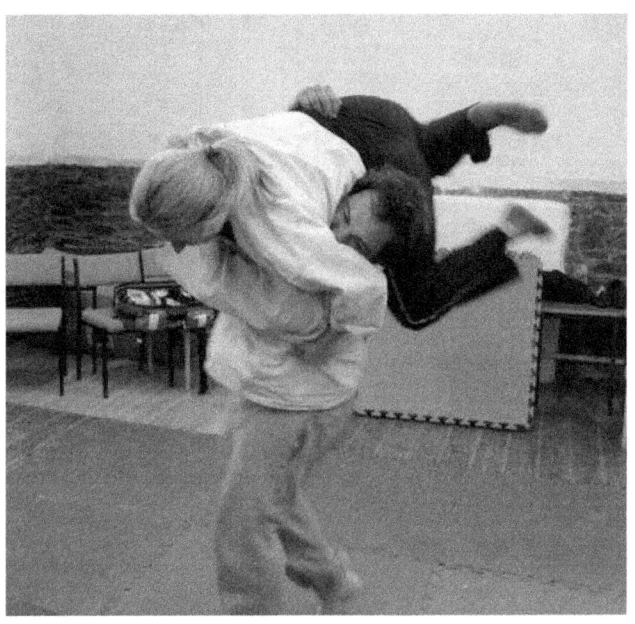

What goes up...

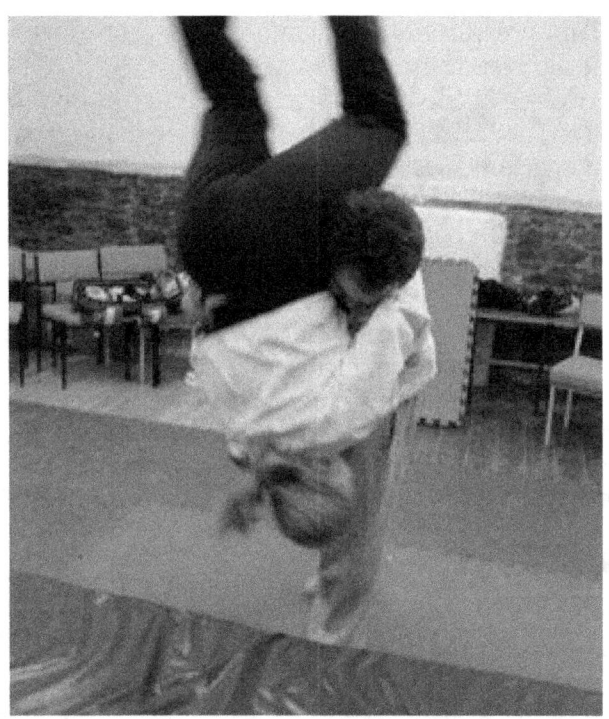

Must come down...

The session finished with another group tussle and then finally, Richard showed me a few the moves which hadn't been taught. Thankfully, the mat was brought back and I spent the next five minutes being hurled in the air and chucked about for the purposes of a good photo. Photos obviously do not convey my screams and shrieks.

I loved my time at the club. Everybody was very friendly and welcoming and I really enjoyed listening to the stories and learning the heritage of the sport but most of all, I loved that big, blue crash mat...I need to get me one of those!

Wheelchair Rugby – Number 74

If somebody said to you: "Come and have a game of Murderball"...that wouldn't sound very enticing. That is why when Caroline of The West Country Hawks presented it as Wheelchair Rugby, I readily accepted the invitation. It was only through my own YouTube research, and some ribbing on Twitter, that I realised the alter-ego name the sport went by.

I met Caroline at the impressive Life Centre in Plymouth. I was introduced to the team and coaches and they helped me strap into one of the specially designed wheelchairs, which had an almost shopping trolley vibe going at the front (which I later realised, would be helpful to barge opponents). Now, when I mean "being strapped in," I mean I was fully strapped in. I had a Velcro strap around my waist, attaching me to the chair. My feet were equally strapped at the bottom and once my gloves were on, I was approached by a strange man holding a roll of duct tape, which was very 50 Shades of Grey-esque! Not sure if this was the right time to say that I needed to go to the toilet.

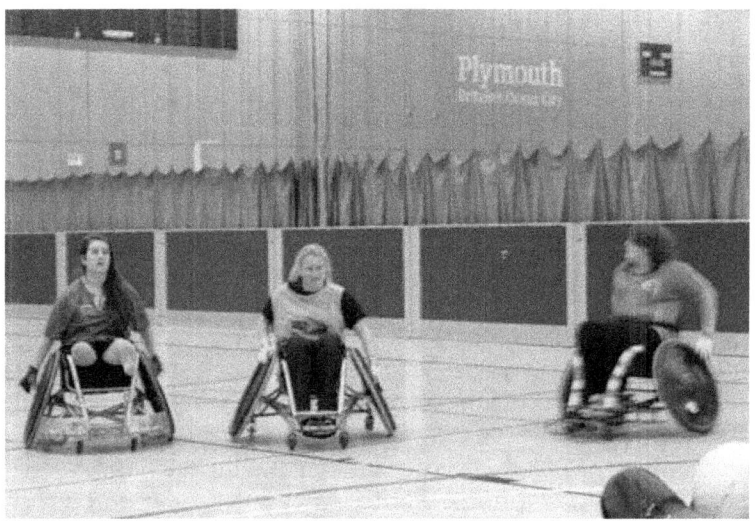

Getting used to the wheels

I set about rolling myself about and practising going forward and reversing. The key to this is to not think about it too much. Once I felt semi-confident, some of the team went through the rules with me. The aim of the game is to score by taking the ball over the line, whilst the defenders attempt to block you. There are four players per team, with subs able to literally roll on and off. Also if you hold the ball for more than 10 seconds, you have to bounce it - this wouldn't be a problem for me, as I will be deploying the old "hot potato" technique, which has served me well in the past.

As the head coach was away this week, the whole training session was to be a match. As soon as the whistle went, I set about getting myself into space, only to find that the space was immediately gobbled up by the opposition, who intercepted passes and then whizzed off in the other direction. The collisions were brutal and the game was punctuated with punctures, which required on court pit stops. The odd times I managed to catch the ball, I panicked, then reversed, then screamed, then winced as I expected to be crashed into and then offloaded the ball as quickly as possible, usually to an opposition player.

There was a lot of banter going on and some questionable tactics. My own ineptness just made me giggle, as I was really trying to go fast to catch people on the break and even with a 2 metre head start, I was like an old granny trundling along, in comparison. This effectively meant that my team were a man down. I decided, what the hell, I am going to try and start barging people. Apparently, you can block people who don't have the ball. I hunted down my prey as the opposition broke. With steely, wheely determination, I went hell for leather at one of their support players, rotating my wheels as quickly as possible. As I approached the inevitable collision, I shut my eyes and braced for the impact. When I opened them, I saw that I was careering toward the wall, as my player had managed to escape with a slight shimmy and went off to score. Rats!

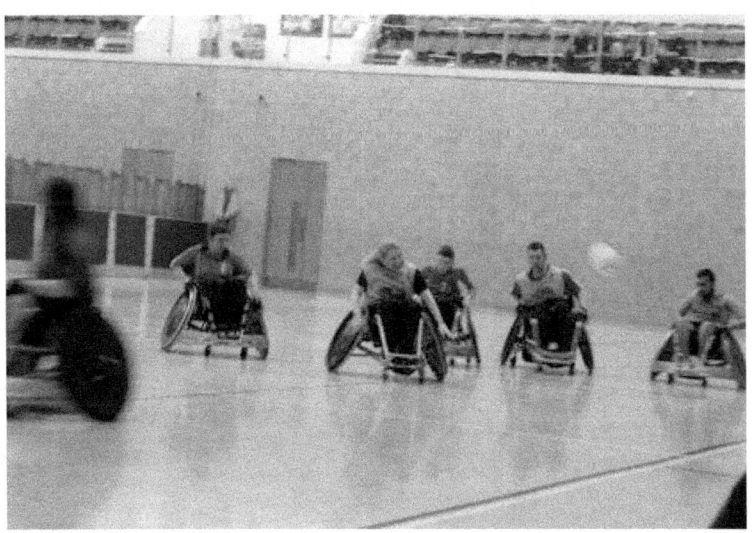

Can't quite get the ball....

The whistle went for the end of the game and everybody high-fived. I even missed a high-five and we had to roll back to try again. How embarrassing! When I was unpacked from my chair, my thumbs were sore and my arms felt heavy but it was a very enjoyable match and I was very thankful that the team went easy on me - so no whiplash, just an immense sense of pride that I survived MurderBall!

Basketball – Number 75

Basketball marks the end of my foray into American sports. As part of my challenge, I have dabbled in American Football, cheerleading, dodgeball and baseball, so I do feel like a bit of a pro when it comes to the preferred sports of our transatlantic cousins (I have ruled out ice hockey on the basis that I can't ice skate, so I probably won't be allowed on the ice with a stick). Turns out, I was a little too smug, as I was immediately told by one of the guys in the team that I had made a "rookie mistake" by not wearing basketball shorts. I never seem to learn; I remember forgetting the cap in baseball - these missing garments must surely detract from my powers.

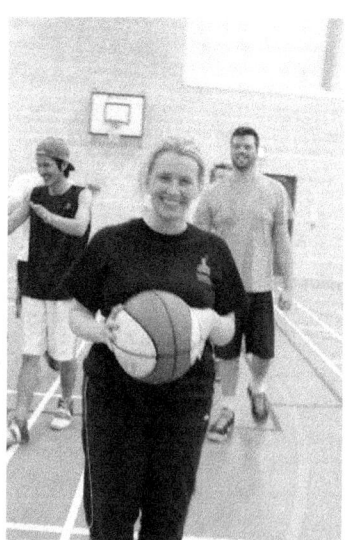

Tracky bottoms are for losers...

Other than that, I was set to go and met Dom the coach and the rest of the guys at the Ben Ainslie Centre in Truro. Before the full training started, we shot some hoops. I watched the lads shoot from a range of distances, with an impressive conversion rate. The ball bounced to me, so I lined up my shot and went for it. Immediately, I had an ETI (Emergency Technique Intervention) from one of the lads. I was quickly tutored that it wasn't like netball, as it required two hands and a knee bend to get the necessary technique. I learnt the backboard was my friend and to aim for that. I continued to practise my shooting before we were called in for the warm-up.

The warm-up involved "suicide runs" - I did not require a basketball manual to appreciate that this wasn't going to be fun. It basically requires you to run a quarter of the sports hall and back and then half way and back, then three-quarters and back and yes, you guessed it, to the end of the sports hall and back. After completing a few of them and a drink, we moved on to some drills and given the complexity of the first drill, I got to sit out and practise my cheerleading instead.

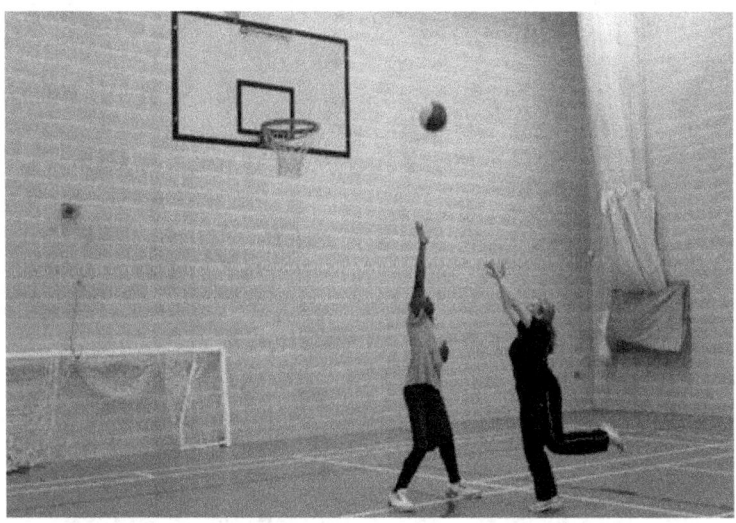

Needless to say, it didn't go in!

I was included in the next drill, as we split into two teams. The exercise was to shoot the ball from different sides. If you scored a basket, you got 2 points and if you caught the rebound, you could get an extra point. The first team to 21 won. I managed to score a couple of baskets, which I was chuffed with but our team still lost all six games and, therefore, started 6 down on the final game, which we lost. The reward for losing was more suicide running.

We ended with a match and luckily there was a sub on each team, so I embraced the side line and donned my imaginary pompoms. Basketball is pretty non-stop, which Dom confirmed by saying that playing a match was like doing one long bleep test. I was never a fan of bleep tests and always thought that it was named Bleep due to all the swearing that had to bleeped out whilst doing it.

My cheerleading was (I felt) inspirational and motivational and I thought if I did a good enough job, I wouldn't be subbed on but to my horror/terror, one of my team mates came off and I had to go on. I hauled all 5ft 3 of myself on to the court and my team gave me somebody to mark - was it me, or did I see my opponent smirk? I stuck to my man like glue and even called for the pass once or twice. I managed a few minutes of this high intensity match before subbing myself off again, as I didn't want to completely screw up my team's chances of winning.

I made one last appearance and I even felt confident enough to bounce the ball twice and have a shot. It was more Harlem Pig Trotter than Harlem Globe Trotter, but I managed to not completely make a fool of myself. As with everything I do in this challenge, I tread a very fine line between enthusiastically attempting everything which is thrown at me, with varying degrees of success and totally losing my dignity and making a right **bleep** of myself!

Hockey – Number 76

This challenge has certainly thrown me squarely out of my comfort zone but I do have a few sports which take me back to the familiar and back to my zone. The main one is hockey, as I've been playing since I was 11. This sweet little trump card has been hiding up my sleeve all this time and now, I am ready to play it, as I've organised a "badgers" tournament, hosted at my club.

Due to the time commitments of running around doing all of these sports, I've taken the season off playing but I have retained my behind the scenes roles at the club, which include being Club Secretary and helping with the juniors. I'm not going to detail about what happened at the tournament, but it did make me reflect on what "my" sport means to me.

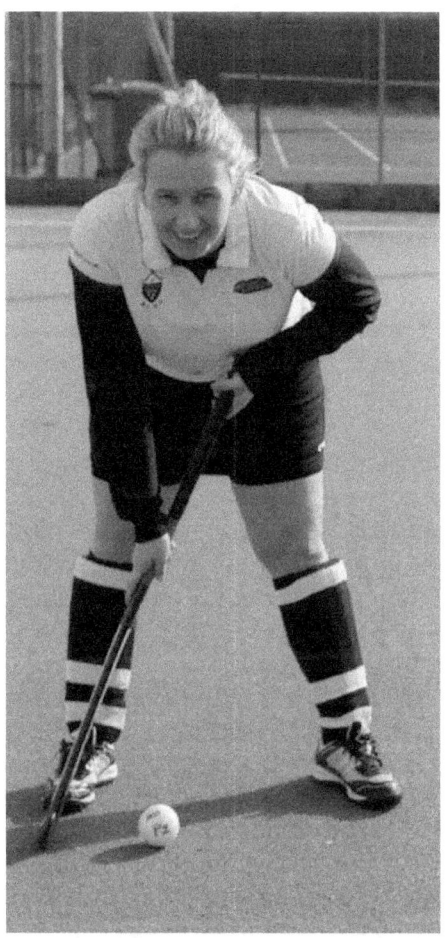

Finally, a sport I can play!

As a kid, I was quite sporty and one of the PE teachers, a keen hockey player, introduced me to the sport and over the next few years of secondary school, I developed into a club and county player. I am a massive advocate of children developing an interest in sport and if this challenge has shown me anything, it's that there is something out there for everybody. Maybe I should start a dating service for people to find their soul sport? Anyway, I digress - like 95% of teenage girls, I absolutely hated cross country running every PE lesson but I enjoyed team sports. The benefits of any kind of sport are obvious; it keeps you active and healthy but aside from the health benefits, I have always enjoyed the social side, the banter and my time with my "family away from my family."

When I moved to London as a 16-year-old, I didn't know anybody, so one of the first things I did was to join my local hockey club. Southgate Hockey Club happened to be one of the largest clubs in the country, so I got to meet lots of new people and every Saturday was taken up with playing a game and socialising after. I'm still very good friends with some of the girls I met, way back when.

As I have experienced so many other team sports to date, I can see common threads which I recognise from my own. Nobody really cares what job you do, how much you earn or what's going on in your life. For a couple of times a week, you are with your team as you train together, laugh together and encourage each other. There are obviously levels of performance depending on what standard you are at but you can tailor a sport to what you want to get out of it, whether it's the fitness or the social side or whether you want to train but not compete. With the team sports, I am welcomed wherever I go and even though it is usually my first time and am, more-often-than-not, rubbish at their sport, I am always enthusiastically invited back.

I'm not sure whether I'm ready to hang up my boots for good next season. Part of me isn't ready to let go of playing but part of me doesn't want to block the younger generation from breaking into the side either. I shall deliberate this over the summer to see what September brings. Whether I play or not, I know I will continue to be part of the club and help develop the youngsters, in the hope that they will get to experience what I have got out of the sport.

Oh, and just to give you the flip side: we lost all of our 3 games, none of our subs turned up, I had to play out of position and it was bloody freezing.

Skiing and Snowboarding – Number 77 & 78

Paul and I have been together for nearly 17 years and for 16 and a half of those years, he has been running a campaign for us to go on a skiing trip and more recently on a family skiing holiday. In my mind a ski holiday is one of those marmite things and to be honest, I would prefer to laze about in the sun, rather than be active in the cold - I do that enough in the UK. As my next challenges were skiing and snowboarding, Paul was extremely eager to advise me on technique. He even went rummaging in the loft for specific gloves and other garments. His efforts made me smile but I was pretty sure these next two challenges were to be endured not enjoyed.

I made my way to the Plymouth Ski Slope & Snowboard Centre. I was booked in for a Try-Ski session and then a Try-Board snowboarding session straight after. The first class was full and there were 14 newbies, all trudging up the hill to the nursery slope. I started chatting to a guy called Sam. This Sam was a much better Sam than me. His girlfriend was a skier and persuaded him to try a ski trip, so he was there getting in some practice before the big trip. The class started with a rundown of our equipment by our instructor, Dom.

Once we were in our skis, we had to shuffle our way across the nursery slope, like a winter wonderland conga. I placed myself in the customary position at the back of the queue and commenced shuffling. I was praying I wouldn't be the first person to fall over, so I made sure I concentrated. Once the conga was over, Dom showed us how to side step up to a gradient and holding on to the fence behind, to bend the knees, leaning slightly forward with our skis parallel, and then let go and ski down to the flat. This involved a journey of no more than three metres. Unfortunately, my back of the queue tactic had backfired, as the back became the front and I was first up.

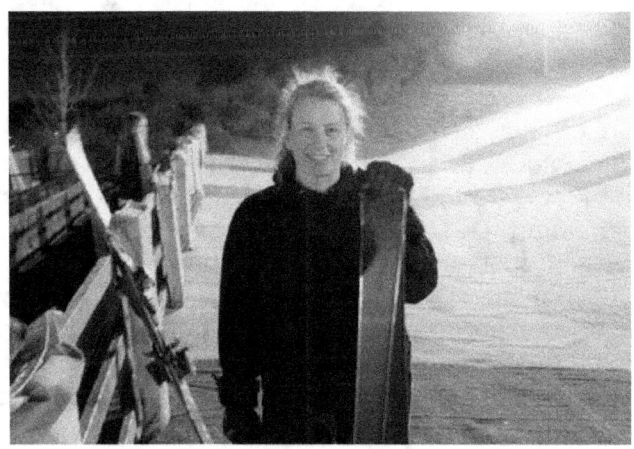

Me vs. Ski

I trudged up, clinging to the fence. Dom repeated the instructions. I looked up to see my classmates looking apprehensive but probably relieved they weren't first. I let go of the fence and leaned forward. A small snail would have probably overtaken me in a race but I made it down in one piece. Pride and relief washed over me, as I shuffled and sidestepped to my position, and we created the queue once more, to repeat and embellish on that exercise. This included lifting one leg up and also letting go of the fence. There were a few fallers and I am such a bad person for being thankful it wasn't me!

We progressed to higher up the slope but still it was only a third of the way up the nursery slope. Looking up to the top, skiing from there seemed unfeasible and must be lesson 3, at least. The lesson ended and I came out unscathed. I said goodbye to my class, as I waited in the bar with a hot chocolate, for the snowboarding lesson. Paul had regaled me with dark tales of the dreaded board as he hadn't got on with it, when he tried it. I started to think of Paddlesurfing, which didn't go too well at all with my legs shaking uncontrollably, meaning I couldn't even stand up on that board. I thought about going home under a false pretence.

Escape looked futile, so I gritted my teeth and went to get my boots and board. There were two other gentlemen joining me for the lesson and we all looked equally apprehensive. Dan, the instructor, was intrigued by my challenge and decided that he would take on the task of making snowboarding my favourite. *Good luck with that,* I thought, given my balance issues, fear of heights and lack of coordination.

We went through the equipment and we all got strapped ourselves in. Once clipped to the board, the only way to change direction is to bounce about, so we practised our bouncing. That went OK. Next, we had to get ourselves up the hill and this involved releasing your back foot from the board and walking like you had a clubfoot - in a walk, then drag technique. Once we were a third of the way up the nursery slope, we sat down and strapped ourselves in and then Dan instructed us how to get back up. This was not a good look, as the bum had to be waggled in the air to manoeuvre into the right direction. Once in position, you could slowly push yourself up and glide down the slope. I waited until the other two had gone and then I slowly pushed myself up. I expected an immediate fall but I stood up and with my hands out, like a surfer, I sailed down. Yippeee!

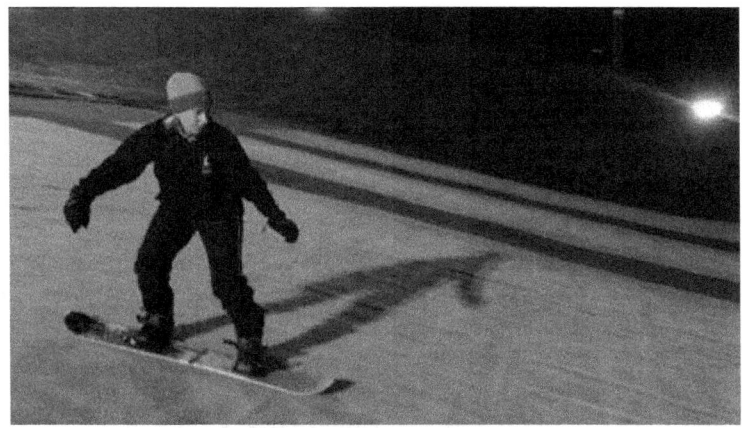

Looking like a pro

I couldn't believe how well that went and how balanced I felt. I hot-footed, club-footed up the slope and under Dan's behest, went straight to the fabled top of the mountain/small nursery slope. I strapped in, arse in the air, and then slowly up and off I went again. Straight down, no issues. It felt exhilarating and like a small kid on a slide, I just couldn't get back up quick enough. Dan tried to make us include a small jump, halfway down but I decided that this would undo my good work, so I half-heartedly attempted it but for somebody with balance-itis, that introduction would have to wait.

I absolutely loved my time on the board and was sad when the hour was up. I think the apprehension before the lesson, mixed with the exhilaration during the lesson, made for quite a chemical reaction and I felt absolutely pumped all the way home. Paul was pretty astounded to hear how effusive I was about the whole thing. Maybe there'll be a ski holiday in the future after all, but he will be on the skis and I'll be on the board.

TyreFit – Number 79

Next up is the potentially pun-tastic TyreFit, created by James Latus of Kernow Martial Arts. I make no apology for the list of puns I will try and scatter throughout. If you're looking for a high-brow critique of this new type of cardio and strength class, you will be left deflated. Boom tis!

I turned up at the class feeling pumped (boom tis) – OK, that might be annoying, so I'll stop for now. On entering the class, it looked more like a Kwik Fit garage, with various tyres strewn across the floor. The idea of the class is to work around the different stations in a circuit training type way, completing 4 lots of 2 different exercises.

I was partnered up with Bailey, a young, lean, fighting machine, who also knew what was required for each station. After James had run through what was expected on each station, the music started and the timer counted down. The first 30 seconds involved swinging a standard car tyre from one arm to the other. The next set was lifting a tyre above your head, then down and up again. The first 30 seconds were fine, but this was repeated four times and it was starting to burn.

Using tyres is quite an inspired use of equipment; it is easy to grip and it provides a challenging weight to swing about. The only downside I could see as the class went on, my hands started to look like those of a seasoned mechanic!

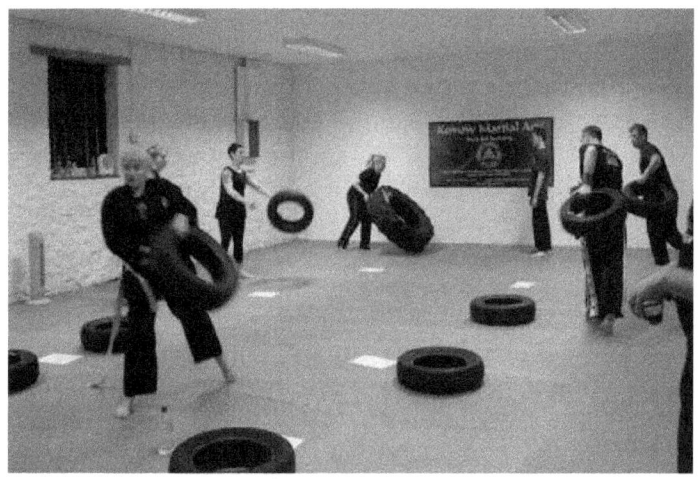

The Gym looks like a KwikFit Garage

There were five further stations, each with two exercises on each. My favourite was picking up the tractor wheel and lobbing it to your partner, in a Jeff Capes style challenge. Who knew that there was so much to do with a tyre? We progressed onto pushing them, skipping in and out of them, jumping on them, doing sit-ups holding them and using them as weights. Tyres are a versatile bit of kit. I am considering buying one as a gift for one of my children for their birthday. Imagine that; the look of anticipation on their face as they behold the sight of a large, beautifully wrapped, present, with the promise on the gift tag stating "it will give you super-human strength." How delighted they will be!

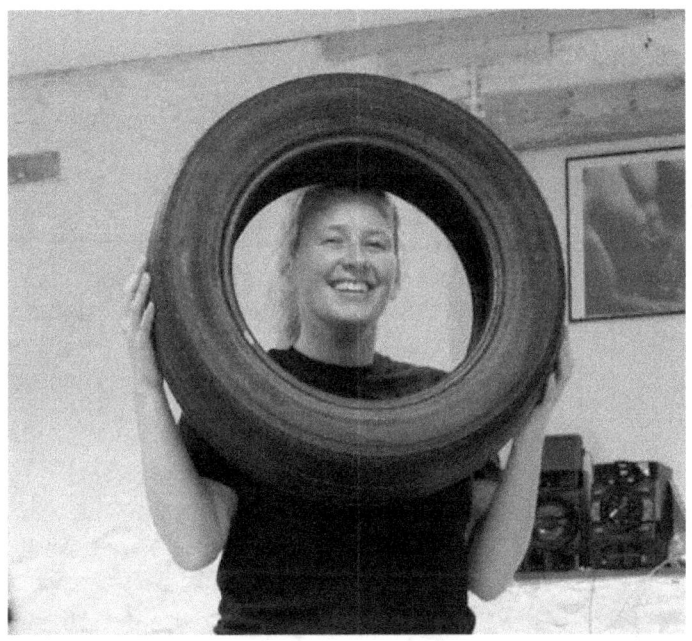

Look what Mummy has bought you for your birthday!

The class was relatively challenging for me but the hour went by really quickly. I enjoyed mixing the cardio with the strength exercises and I managed not to let go of any tyres whilst swinging them above my head, which was a bonus. I think that class would work wonders on my personal spare tyre, so it is definitely a class I would recommend. The one thing which I have been surprised with throughout the course of the challenge is the change in my feeling toward strength based exercises. Before, I would only want to do cardio, as I had accepted that I had very little upper body strength and I was happy to embrace the bingo wings but actually CrossFit, TRX, Kettlercise and TyreFit have shown that there is potential there and it is something I've enjoyed working on.

The class finished with a song which required us to squat whenever the lyrics "Up" or "Down" were mentioned, which turned out to have more mentions than The Grand Old Duke of

York and Tubthumping's "I Get Knocked Down" combined. So we ended on a burn and at that point, I re-tyre-d. Boom tis.

Dance – Number 80

Next on the list is dance and not just any old dance - this was a six-hour danceathon at Wembley in aid of Comic Relief. I have to say I didn't really think it through when signing up but it proved to be yet another cautionary tale highlighting the perils of going onto Twitter whilst tipsy. Tipsy twittering is bad! On consideration (after pressing the sign-up button), six hours is quite a long time; you could fly to the Caribbean, Mo Farrah could run 2 and a half marathons or you could drive from London to Scotland in that time. Basically, six hours is a long time to be dancing for and if I'm honest, I wasn't quite sure I would be capable.

I travelled up the day before and stayed with my lovely hosts, Sophie and Graeme. I decided the night before the big day, I should "carb up," so off we went for pizza and prosecco. Don't worry, I made sure that I didn't overdo it; I am an athlete after all! The order of play for the day was as follows:

- 12pm – 70's disco - Yep, I have moves in the locker for that
- 12.30pm – Swag - Not sure what that means but my 12 year old daughter says it A LOT!
- 1pm – 80s Anthems - Right up my street
- 1.30pm – Musical Theatre - Iffy on that one
- 2pm – 90s Rave - Move over people, I have landed
- 2.30pm – Michael Jackson Moves - Got a moonwalk in the bag already
- 3pm – Funk - Happy with that
- 3.30pm – Diva Dancing - All over this
- 4pm – Bashment - What the hell is this?
- 4.30pm – Pop - Standard moves
- 5pm – Ballroom & Latin Taught by Dancers on Strictly - Enjoyed my Fitsteps class so this should be OK
- 5.30pm – Sixties Soul - I got soul in a bowl, baby!

When I got to Wembley, I joined the queue behind a myriad of brightly coloured participants. I looked wistfully at my tutu and wished I had made more of an effort. The whole event was to be hosted by the optimally fringed Claudia Winkleman and the stage was adorned by other celebrities, who were prepared to get their dancing shoes on for the day.

The arena filled with over 2,000 people and Claudia reminded us about the wonderful cause we were supporting. I spent this time thinking how I was going to get a lock of Claudia's hair, which I promised each person who sponsored me. The excitement was building as I found my dancing area (which was immediately invaded by a bunch of red feather head-dressed dancers - who seemed to find my presence magnetic, no matter where I went, over the course of the day).

The music started and on came tune after tune after tune. I assumed that although I would be there for six hours, I would be able to cheat a bit and go and eat and take multiple wee stops but I hadn't banked on the fact that I couldn't literally tear myself away from the fantastic tunes. I did the first hour and a half non-stop and went for a quick toilet break, through the first half of the musical numbers set. When I came back, I carried on until the halfway mark, when I started to feel tired. At this point, I thought if I stop, I won't be able to start again, so I made my way to the front and I went for it!

The atmosphere was fantastic and everybody was genuinely having a great time. My favourite sections were Bashment, which turned out to be a Caribbean inspired, hip rotating dance style, Diva and Rave. Sophie and Graeme had managed to equip me with a whistle and glow sticks that morning, which allowed me to convey to the people standing within 20ft of me, by the power of noise and sight that I loved the rave days!

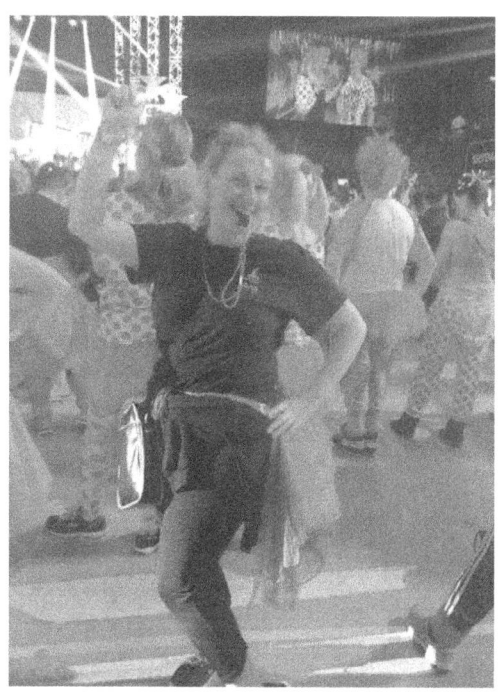

A hot and sweaty raver

The last hour was hard. I found I couldn't actually lift my arms above my shoulders, which was tricky for the final numbers. I gritted my teeth and felt euphoric when the glittery paper came down to signal the end. Claudia said we were all brilliant and I felt brilliant. The day was fantastic and I felt a real sense of achievement, not only for me personally but also because I was a little part of something which will hopefully make a big difference to people. I didn't become Claudia's best friend as planned but the 5-hour journey back to Cornwall didn't seem that bad after all that.

The Challenge So Far - Number 71 to 80

The end is definitely in sight but having already planned the next 10, my journey feels like it is resembling that of a mountain climber (which isn't one of my sports) and the closer I get to the summit, the steeper the mountain seems to get.

For instance, my next 10 include; Parkour (free running), surfing on an indoor wave machine (which seems fraught with danger) and also underwater hockey, also known as Octopush. Octopush is one of the sports which I use as a sound bite if anybody asks me why I am doing what I am doing. I usually chortle and say that I am documenting a breakdown, or I came up with the idea over a bottle of wine or that I was intrigued by certain sports I had never come across before, such as Octopush. The truth probably lies somewhere in the middle of all three.

As I come to the end, I am increasingly being asked about what I am going to do next. I'm not really sure how to respond, as I'm almost too busy fitting in each sport to give much thought to it. My instinctive reaction is to actually sit on a sofa and drink a lot of wine but maybe that would break the momentum. After my challenge, I will still be supporting my two youngest as they complete their own mini SofaDodger challenge through school, so no doubt, I will be travelling about helping them to sample different sports.

I am really excited about the opportunities with the mini challenge and definitely want to explore this further. Most of all, I am looking forward to having some time to reflect on what I have achieved. When people climb mountains, they get to the summit and they no doubt look around at the view and reflect on the journey they have just been through. I am looking forward to my own reflection, as I think about the people I have met, the stories I have heard and the experiences I have had. I have never climbed an actual mountain; maybe I will do that next?

Chapter 10 - Challenge 81 – 90

Personal Training – Number 81

Having tried a home exercise class and a plethora of fitness classes, the next progression would be a personal trainer. I've said previously said that a fitness instructor, I feel, brings out that little bit more effort from you and makes you work that little bit harder. I am slowly abandoning my tendency to cheat in fitness classes by stopping if the instructor glances away momentarily. I've weaned myself slowly off this urge to "cheat myself" but it's nice to know that it is always there in the locker if I need it. Clearly, though, with a personal trainer, you are given 100% attention and unless I paid a streaker, this attention will not be diverted and I will have nowhere to hide.

I met Mike from Priority One Fitness on a beautiful lunchtime in the park. We made our way to a pagoda at the top of the hill, which afforded the most breath-taking views. I asked Mike who would use a personal trainer and his answer was simply anybody who wants to achieve a goal, whether that is weight loss, fitness, a change of body shape or to break the habit of inertia and get them back into exercise. A good personal trainer will be able to understand your specific objectives and devise a plan tailored to your specific needs and should also include nutritional advice.

For me, I would probably want to work with a personal trainer to lose weight. People don't believe me when I say I haven't lost any weight through my challenge. The reason is simply that I probably snack too much, as a reward for all my hard work - that and we have a bread maker, which pumps out beautifully smelling, hot loaves, which glisten and sing to me once they are dressed with their buttery companion. I don't think I need a food scientist to tell me where the problem lies!

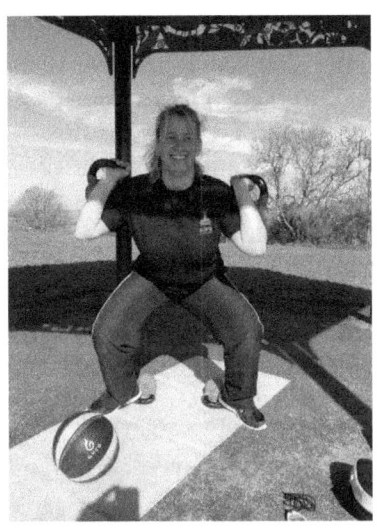

Why do I smile, when I feel the opposite?

After a full stretch, we did a lap around the park, as the birds chirped and various sized dogs bounded about. We made it back to the pagoda and to the smorgasbord of kit Mike had brought along. We started with the kettlebells. Mike's chirpy demeanour changed as my whining started to kick in. Every moan equated to an additional rep. Was that a cloud I saw in the sky? I watched a dog come over and cock his leg on one of the struts on the pagoda.

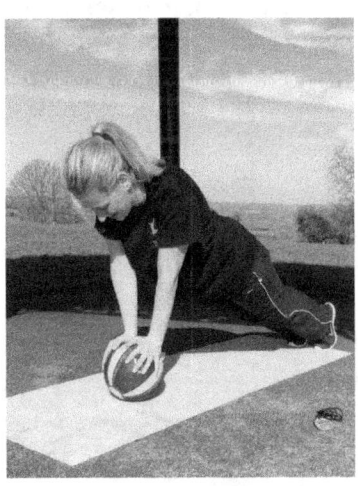

Planking with a ball

After a number of different exercises with the kettlebells, Mike browsed his kit bag options like a torturer inspecting his tools. He glanced over the TRX and medicine ball and went for the boxing gloves and pads. Woohoo! I love boxing now. I donned the gloves and Mike explained the sequence of punches. The sequences were hard but, Mike was constantly motivating me and counting down and getting that little bit more out of me. The boxing was hard and at the end of it, I was almost wheezing. Mike looked pleased.

Although personal training is a more expensive option, by cutting down on that extra bottle or two of wine a week or a takeaway, you would almost cover the cost. There is no doubt that 6 weeks with a personal trainer would help to achieve your goals, as your objective becomes their objective. So maybe, if I seriously want to shift some weight after this challenge is over, this could be just the kick start I need.

Parkour – Number 82

When I declared to my family at tea time that I was going to Exeter to try parkour, my children sniggered. The fact that Olly, seven, then proceeded to beg to come as well, made me worry that this might be more his thing than mine. Parkour, or free running, is essentially a way of getting from A to B by running, jumping and if you like, adding some tricks. You can see it in music videos, where cool, fit looking people run across buildings, jumping over stairwells and anything else which gets in their path. To watch it is pretty awesome, so although I was eager to see it in real life, I was pretty daunted by the prospect of trying it myself.

I met Dom from StreetMotion, who welcomed me to the club as I joined a teenage/adult class. Immediately I brought the average age up by a number of years...most of them must have thought I was there to pick up a child from the previous class. I was relieved to spot a fully-fledged adult, who told me that this was her second time of trying it. This put me at ease, as we got ready to warm-up.

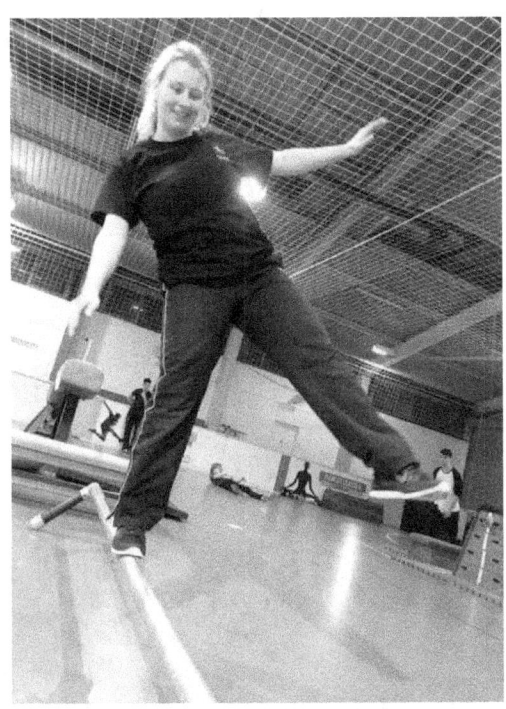

Balance and flexibility are not my greatest skills

I haven't really being writing much about my back but I'm suffering again from a lower back sprain, which means I'm a regular visitor to my chiropractor at the moment. The pain was particularly bad tonight, so I had to adapt the warm-up, as I was clearly not going to be able to walk on all fours. I added flexibility to my mental list of things I was lacking. I must admit, I did enjoy the warm-up game of "zombies," which was essentially a Halloween version of stuck in the mud.

Once warm, the coaches introduced us to and demonstrated each of the three stations which were laid out. It looked like they were walking on air as they gracefully skipped across the various obstacles. Momentum was definitely the key to this. I scrambled to the back of the queue and watched the people in front make their attempts.

I could no longer put it off and it was my turn. I accelerated up to the springboard and stuck out my foot to attempt to get to the top of the horse but as I put my foot out, my brain said, "you won't make that" and I pulled up, like a horse before a jump. I tried several times and did the same thing. I was then allowed to climb on to the horse and when this stubborn mule refused to jump onto the next horse (there was quite a gap), I was allowed to climb down from the horse and then climb up on the next one. This continued until I finished the course. My effort was pretty dismal, but I couldn't help being completely rational about what I could and couldn't do. I didn't look at the people in the queue, for the shame.

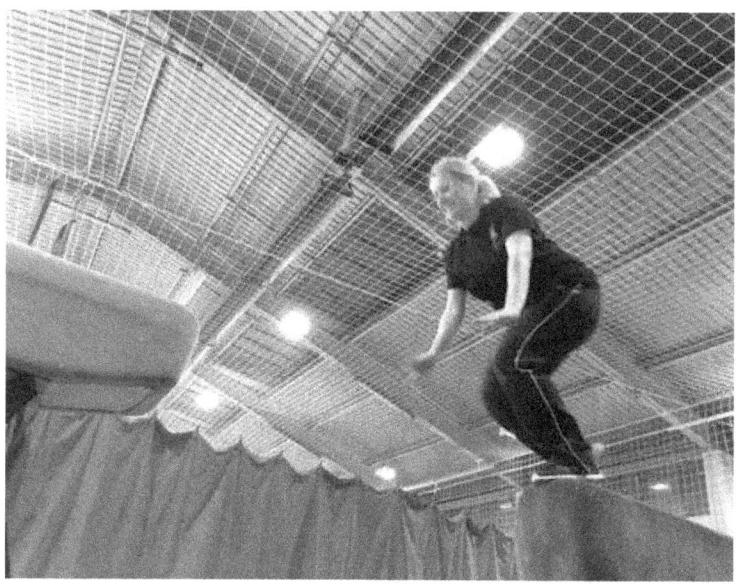

A jump too far

My back had rendered my movements to that of an old granny and my brain was disabling my ability to trust what my body could achieve. All of the coaches were very sweet and diagnosed me with "having the fear." As I was crippled with my fear, I watched my classmates, who weren't suffering from the same condition. They were having an absolute ball and each time they attempted their station, they would add complexities to their journeys and it was really mesmerising to watch their flips and runs.

I collected myself for the final station, which for me looked by far the hardest. This required me to jump off a rail and scramble up a horse, which was the same height as me, then walk across a steel beam (again the same height as me) to the next horse. Then jump from there to a horse, which was 3 ft. lower down. I tried my hardest but it wasn't pretty to behold: my arse flailing about, clinging on for dear life, until I got to "the jump." The same feelings from Coasteering came flooding back to me; essentially of

220

fear and impending doom. I made half a dozen aborted attempts to jump, as my hands were sweating and my heart started beating out of my chest. I am sorry to say that I couldn't do it; the fear washed over me and sent me crashing, beached on the shore.

I was annoyed with myself for not pushing that little bit further but I had to accept my limitations that time. Some of the class came over to console me and tell me about their first attempts and how they conquered their own fears, which was nice. Although I was much older, I know that if I wanted to go back and conquer my fears I could. It was a very welcoming class and what they do is pretty jaw dropping. I even got some kudos when I pulled out my new phone to takes some pictures. If I had known that it would take a new phone to give me some street cred, I would have pulled this trump card out at the start, instead of trying to impress with my lack of free-running skills!

Buggyfit – Number 83

Next up was Buggyfit and as I no longer own a buggy, or indeed a baby, I roped in my friend, Katie and her 5 month old daughter, Isabel. Buggyfit is a post-natal workout, which allows buggy wielding mums (but I am told that dads are welcome) to meet up and exercise, whilst not having to worry about putting your little one into a crèche or childcare. The thought of being amongst a group of ladies where I might have the strongest pelvic floor was a giddy thought. So with my baby procured and her mother in tow – just in case she needed a snack break - off we went.

Nel, the instructor, was extremely welcoming and we were introduced to the group and their offspring, who were all tucked up in little blankets and an array of winter suits...I was starting to feel a little broody. We marched outside into the park and Nel advised us on the best posture for pushing our buggy and off we marched single file up to the hill. I forgot how taxing it was to push a buggy. Katie smirked at me as I puffed my way to the top.

At the start of the class, I had myself down as a bit of a pro, what with being an experienced mother of 3 children. However, I haven't been in baby mode for about 6 years now and it showed, particularly at the top of the hill, when we stopped to do some lunges and I forgot to secure the brake on the pram. Luckily we were on a kind of level, but Katie did seem to be more watchful from then on.

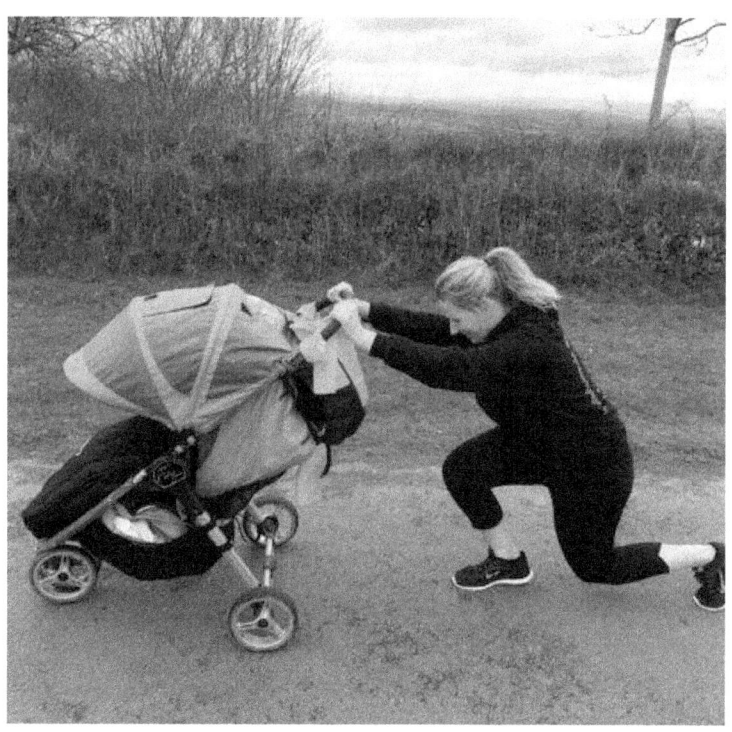

Buggy Lunges, or as I renamed them, Blunges

I am not sure what I expected from the class but if I'm honest, I didn't expect it to be so physically challenging. We were all getting a proper workout and definitely feeling the dreaded burn. I would have loved to do this when my eldest was first born. It's not just about getting back into shape but meeting up with other mothers and getting a change of scenery. When I was a new mum, I didn't really know anybody else with a baby, so this would have been a fantastic opportunity to socialise as well as exercise.

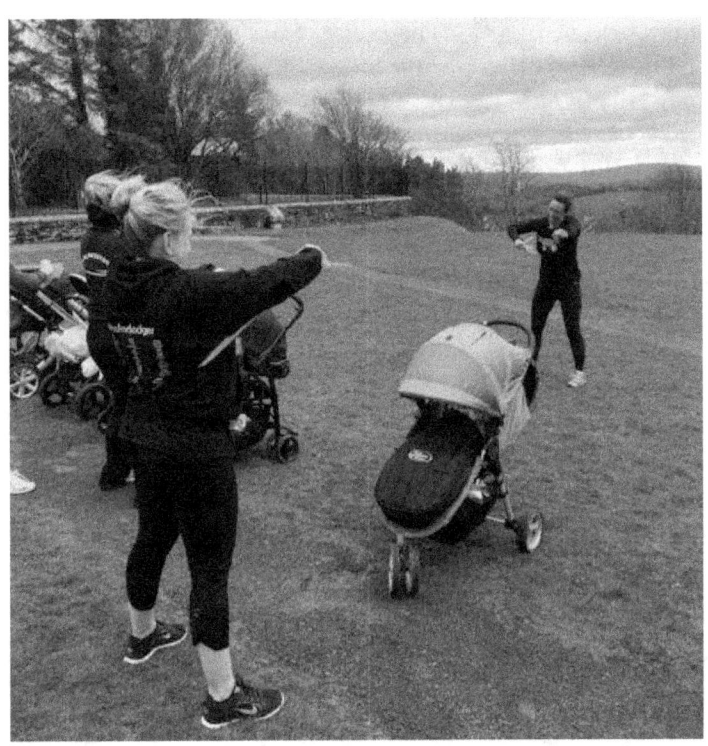

Upper body workout, with the brake fully applied to my buggy

The workout focused on all parts of the body, with the aid of a pink elastic band thing, which proved to be a very effective resistance tool. Although the workout was challenging, it was OK to go at your own pace and if you didn't feel up to certain reps, you could lessen the intensity. Between each set of reps, we would walk with the buggy at our own pace, then stop and do more reps. I know I am a bad person for saying this but it was kind of enjoyable watching Katie moan through some of the exercises. We have known each other since we were 10 and when she wasn't a county swimmer, she was a long distance runner and has also run the London Marathon. For the first time in over 25 years, I might actually be fitter than Katie. This is excellent news and a headline worth savouring and repeating to everybody who knows us.

Towards the end, some of the babies were getting restless, so they were being comforted at various pit stops. I was happy that my baby was sound asleep. That was until a barky dog came bounding up to the buggy and started yapping and I started to feel a familiar sense of panic. The owner apologetically came over and giggled "he doesn't like prams." I gritted my teeth behind my smile and mentally replied: "If that dog wakes my baby, I will kill someone!". Note: I was quite the irrational first-time mum, when it came to the possibility of something or someone stirring my sleeping child.

I didn't have to have a public breakdown about the dog, as Isabel slept soundly throughout. She continued sleeping until we stopped for lunch, where she proceeded to empty her nappy on me at the table, smile at me and then after her lunch, vomit all over me. I felt broody no longer as I handed Isabel back to Mummy and made a swift exit home.

PoolBiking – Number 84

Challenge number 84 will go down as my most arduous challenge so far. Me and four of my girlfriends abandoned our families and work for 4 days, and jetted off for a cheap break to Tenerife. I'm already behind with this challenge and if I am going to hit my May 1st deadline, I can't afford any more injuries or cancellations, so I have to be on the ball and holiday or no holiday, I had to do something.

In the hotel reception, I perused the leaflets and the options ranged from jet skiing to off-road quad biking. None of these appealed but I plumped for parascending – you know when the boat lifts the parachute out of the water and you are suspended in mid-air, contemplating your recent choices and rethinking why this seemed such a good idea. I convinced my friend, Harriet to join me and act as cannon fodder to see if a) she would enjoy it b) if she hurt herself and c) if she made a fool of herself in front a beachfront full of tourists. We booked in for the last day of the holiday.

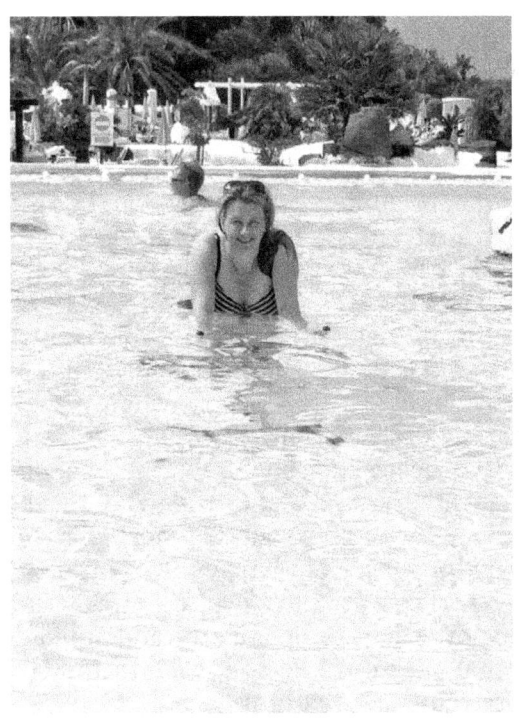

An Aqua Spin Class

Meanwhile, my friend, Sarah had spotted a fitness class – Poolbiking. The pool in question was approximately 2ft from my sun lounger, so at the allotted time, I rolled myself into the water and onto a specifically designed bike. Given that I had already drunk my body weight in Cava so far on the holiday, I felt a real sense of achievement to even manage that much. Whilst we got ourselves in place, I spoke to a retired gentleman, who told me he and his wife had already been on a 6k run that morning. He seemed keen to impart to me that if you go on holiday and eat all day, drink all night and don't move off a sun lounger, you will inevitably put on weight. I started to feel self-conscious and rubbed one of my newly emerging chins. With this new insight, I decided to put in the extra effort before I rolled back onto my lounger with my book.

Our lovely, multi-lingual, instructor guided us through the class. Initially, I was unconvinced that this would be of any benefit but when we got going, then rotated between fast cycling and standing up, and then reaching backwards and forwards, I did feel myself get puffed out and warm. Essentially, it was an underwater spin class but 100 times more enjoyable than an actual spin class.

Toward the end of the class, our instructor employed some yoga techniques and encouraged us to hook our feet around the bars and then lay back with our heads in the water, with our eyes closed. I spent about 2 minutes bobbing about, feeling the sun on my face and the water soothing my sore back. Waves of contentment and happiness washed over me. I felt so grateful at that point to be where I was. We slowly arose from the water and all happily chatted to each other in various dialects.

I returned to my friends, who hadn't made the challenging 2ft journey to the pool and instead intermittently peeked over their books to watch my progress. I waddled back to my lounger to join them but for that fleeting second, I felt really superior and went into full hunter-gatherer mode and trudged off to the bar. Instead of cocktails though, I bought a round of mocktails.

The parascending never did happen, as a mini-tornado seemed to sweep the resort for the next two days, which meant that the only extreme sport I had to do was try and sunbathe in 50 mph winds. I felt that including Poolbiking into my challenge was a push, but Extreme Sunbathing would never have passed unnoticed.

Athletics – Number 85

OK, no need to panic but I am getting really behind on the challenge and my back hurts...it really hurts! My lovely chiropractor, Liz continues to massage me, stick needles in me, pummel me, crack me and tape me up, in the hope that I will be able to give as much as I can to everything which is left. As I had a meeting in Bournemouth this week, I decided to search for a club en route to join for a session. That was easier said than done given as I have completed so many, there aren't too many left to choose from. On my to-do list, however, is athletics. I managed to get in touch with Dorchester Athletics Club, who happened to be training in Yeovil that evening.

I was warned that although it was billed as Senior Training, all of the participants would be teenagers and that I had the choice of training with either the endurance, sprints, throwing or jumping coaches. Hanging out with a group of teenagers no longer causes me any undue thought. Strange looks and questioning glances are

226

part and parcel of this challenge and after Parkour; I know that I have a secret weapon...my IPhone 6 something. Oh yes, they all love that.

After a two hour journey, I found my way to the track and I was enthusiastically greeted by the coaches, who quizzed me on the challenge. Apart from one lad, the rest of the teenagers were all girls. I am not sure what a group of pubescent girls are called but for writing up purposes and my own amusement, I decided to call them a gaggle, mainly because they giggle...a lot. So, the gaggle of giggling girls made their way onto the track. I decided I would probably need a real warm-up, so decided to jog the 400m floodlit track. I thought about going around another lap, which seemed a good idea until I got to 300m. I then joined in with the gaggle, which was in full flow, discussing who was with whom and, "didn't you hear about" and "you'll never guess what."

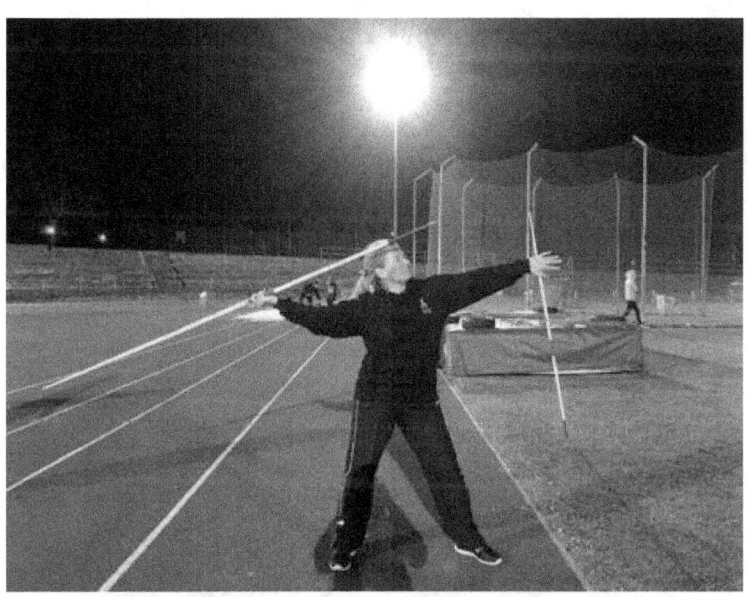

Getting the technique for the javelin

At this point, I looked at my options; endurance - I guessed would mean more running, sprints – I would like to hold on to some remnant of dignity, so throwing and jumping it was. Guy was the coach for throwing and he set about showing me the technique for javelin, which I tried from a standing start and then progressed to a bit of a shuffle, before I unleashed. I was paired with one of the girls, who turned out to be the South West Under 15s Girls champion and boy, could she throw. I was keen to measure my attempts but I sensed they only had long tape measures. I would say I threw a solid 5 metres.

OK, so I am no Fatima Whitbread but maybe my forte would be the long jump. I made my way over to Peter. He seemed to be trying to motivate a particularly wilful gaggle of girls, whilst holding a rake. I've watched enough Olympics to know that the technique is all about height, so from a standing start, I launched myself into the air and managed to plop slightly ahead of where I started.

The girls started to get interested in my T-shirt and set about reading all the sports I had tried. "What's AquaFit?"....I explained... "What's Petanque?"...I explained... "What's Bowls?" Really? Peter continued raking. Never mind, I had the girls on side and they would form part of my master plan. As stated in my gymnastics challenge, I will make no apologies for trying to emulate an Olympic experience. So, after a few more tries, it was time to take a run up. I decided to pretend that I was in an Olympic stadium and this was for the gold medal. I encouraged the girls to clap and off their own back, they clapped and chanted my name. I stood at the line and did that roll back on my back foot before bounding up to the board, like a demented elephant. I hit the board (in my mind the white flag went up) and then plop. Again, Peter wouldn't measure it but I think I cleared a good metre and a half. I looked around to see if the crowd was roaring, but they had got distracted and forgotten the cheering bit.

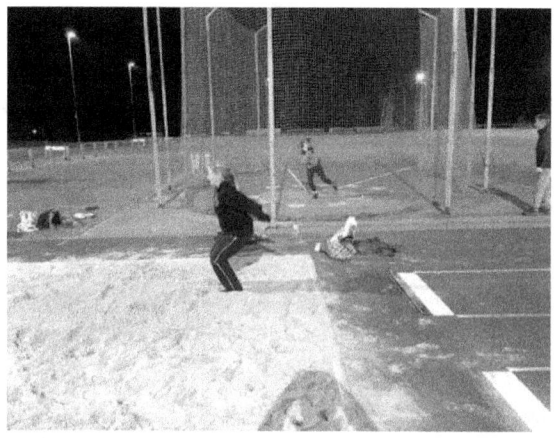

And the crowd went.....quiet

Before the end of this challenge, I might just purchase a mobile podium to put in the boot, which I can roll out at will. Maybe I could get the National Anthem on the IPhone and go the full hog. I had a great time with the club, who made me feel really welcome and you never know, some of those kids won't have to buy a mobile Olympics kit and could actually make the real thing!

Surfing – Number 86

Paul must have come to the decision that the only way to spend time with me, given his recent neglect and my self-interest over the past few months, would be to actually join me for a challenge. This time, it is surfing but not in the sea (which has proven too often to be my salty nemesis) but on a wave machine. The idea piqued my curiosity, so we went along to the Flow Rider at the Retallack Resort.

There we met Tom, our instructor for the session, and crammed ourselves into our wetsuits before making our way out to the machine itself. We were joined by a little girl, who was 10 but had already been on three times before. This was not a scene out of a surfing magazine. The Cornish mizzle had descended upon us and I was freezing, having opted for the summer wetsuit.

Tom invited us onto the machine and allowed us to bounce about, which all seemed very simple. We then went to the side, at which point he actually turned the thing on. Immediately, jets of water travelling at 45 mph thrust up to the top. I think I turned white, in abject terror. We were encouraged onto the top bar and to fall into the menacing water below. Was this a joke? I ushered the girl in front of me to show that it was possible and it wasn't some kind of setup. Children are strange and have no idea of self-preservation; she jumped straight into the oncoming torrent and somehow, with her legs and arms in the air, took on the shape of a parachutist. She survived and moved to the side.

Maybe that was luck and I was keen to push Paul to the front to verify. Paul has an annoying knack of picking things up, so it was no surprise that he managed it effortlessly. It was my turn. I stood on the top and just couldn't find a way of suspending my disbelief. I looked beseechingly at Tom. He encouraged me to kneel down. I talked myself out of it but then looked at the parents of the little girl and I met their eyes and they seemed to whisper, "get on with it for Christ's sake – we've paid for this!" I closed my eyes...I launched myself screaming into the current. It was a crazy sensation but I was actually managing to stay in position, which weirdly felt like I was flying.

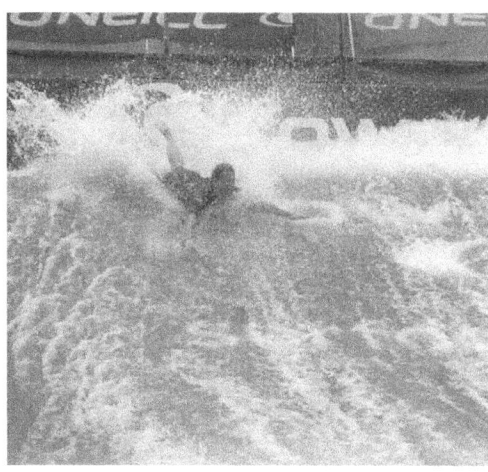

The picture doesn't convey the screaming which accompanied this manoeuvre

I washed up to the side and Tom gave us a body board each. Again, when it was my turn, I knelt down for the launch. Having the board was much better and I gripped onto it with my life. Tom encouraged us each time to progress to the next level. Paul and the little girl were attempting to roll about and go on their knees on the boards, whilst I was building up to not kneeling at the start and not drowning. I was happily going about my business and actually starting to enjoy myself, when Tom, sensing an increase in confidence, convinced me to push the board in front of me and catch it when it came back.

This had disaster written all over it but OK, I thought what the hell. I tried it and after a lot of screaming, managed to catch the board and get back on it. That is a tick in the box right there, so why, oh why did I feel cocky enough to do it again? I shoved the board in front of me and for some reason it took exception and blew up, crashed into me, wiping me out and sending me crashing to the top. My ego felt bruised and my poor back was certainly unhappy. Tom evidently was taken in by my sulking, as I was allowed to retreat to the hot tub, which was positioned at the foot of the machine.

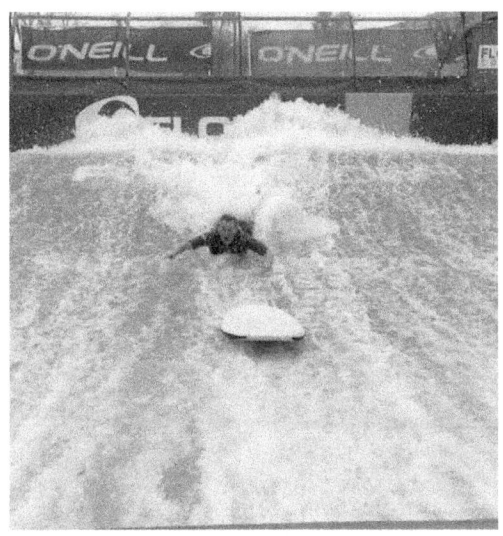

How not to bodyboard: Step 1, let go of the board

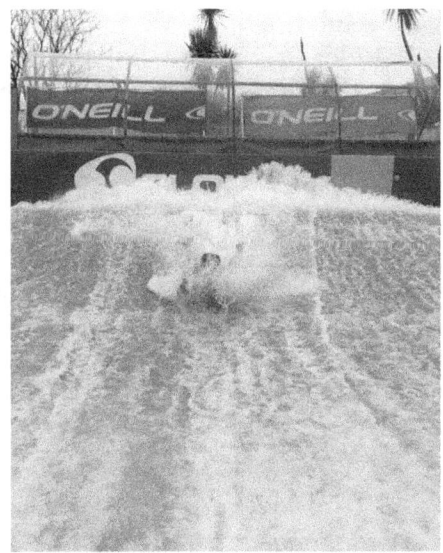

Step 2: Let the board smack you in the face

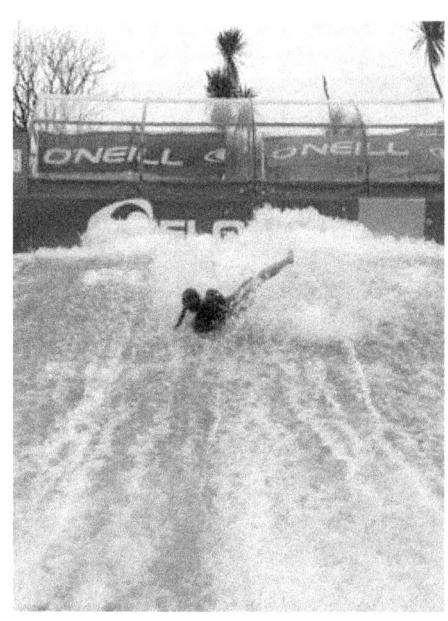

Step 3: Drown

I can't tell you how amazing it felt to get into the hot tub. It was everything the Flow Rider wasn't; still, hot and calming. I lay back and watched Paul and the little girl challenging themselves to go further. Tom implored me to try standing up but I was highly resistant. Doesn't he see I am born to be a hot tub dweller?

Paul came out and he was absolutely buzzing, talking about getting the guys down to give it a go. Then he clocked the bar, which sealed the deal on this activity. He listed all the friends and family who had to try it. I lay back listening, with my legs floating around and my face catching the falling rain. Yes, I could see myself doing this again but without the surfing. Hot-tubbercise is my new, most favourite, activity!

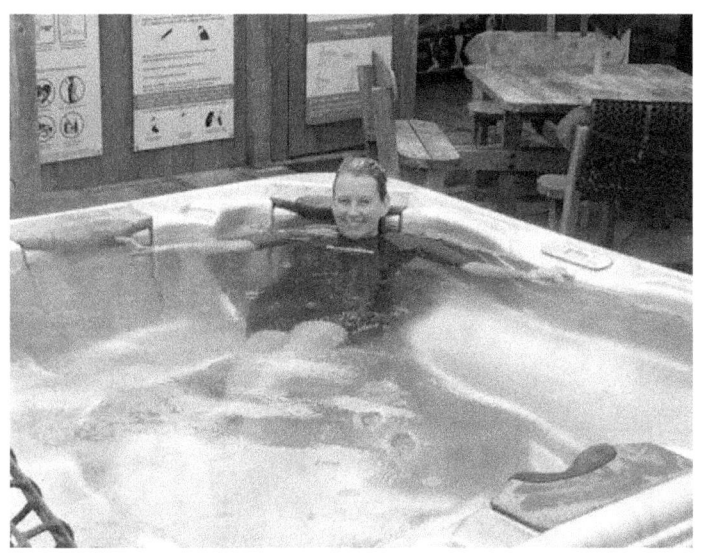

Hot Tubbing like a pro...

Capoeira – Number 87

Capoeira is my next challenge and I couldn't resist having a look on YouTube, to see what it was all about. I had already slathered a bucket of Biofreeze (I need to be sponsored by these guys) on my back and after watching two minutes of footage, I marched straight into the house and sprayed some deep heat onto the Biofreeze, for extra protection – which for your information, is not a good idea!

I made my way down to Falmouth and met with Josh and the rest of the class. Josh explained that Capoeira is a Brazilian form of martial arts, with its roots from Africa. Unlike other martial arts that I have tried, there were no bouts or belts to be had but instead, it included a bit of dance, gymnastics, music and acrobatics. I was keen to give it a go, but first to the warm-up.

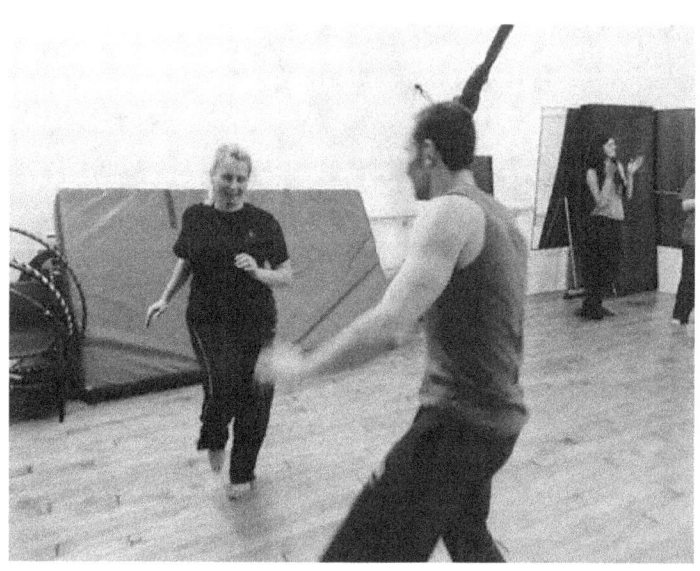

Learning the moves

As Capoeira involved a fair amount of kicking and bending, this is what we focused on. As this is number 87, I like to think I have experienced every sort of warm-up possible but I certainly hadn't warmed up in such a rhythmical way before and I was so glad there was a pro in front of me, who I could just about follow. Josh walked about praising us and encouraging us and to ensure we were getting down low enough, he would swing his bow and arrow type instrument over us, just to be sure. Nothing motivates me more than a mock decapitation! So I made sure I was low!

Capoeira isn't just about exercising or learning a routine, it encompasses a whole cultural experience and as well as working our muscles, we also got to work our brain, as we repeated a count of 10 in Portuguese throughout. I loved that but my brain seemed to take resources from my limbs, as these simultaneous tasks made me either miss a count or lose my rhythm, which is a worry, given that I pride myself on being a multitasker.

Next up was practising of the cartwheels, as this is quite an important part of it. This wasn't a full on run up, gymnastic cartwheel, which I nailed in gymnastics but more of a cartwheel from a standing start. We paired up, shook hands and facing each other, we rotated down the room. I can only imagine what I looked like but it really didn't matter, I was enjoying the atmosphere and the challenge.

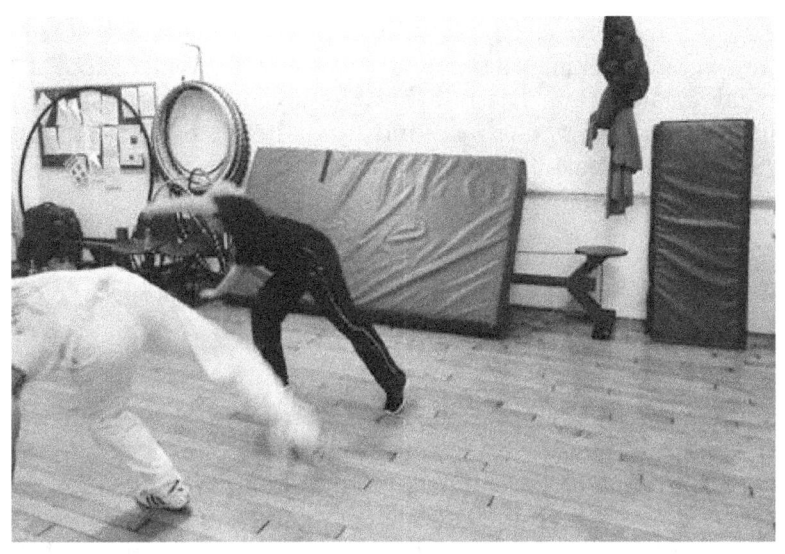

Cartwheels in motion...

Josh called us in and spoke more of the origins of Capoeira. He introduced an instrument and after explaining its significance, he began to play, as we provided a 3 clap beat. Josh sang and encouraged us to chant a word, at certain points. This was great. I love history and learning about different cultures, so I was in my element. My brain was just about coping with the chant and the clapping. As long as we weren't going to move about at the same time, I won't be shown up by my lack of rhythm. Obviously, the next step was to do it altogether, as we freestyled in the middle of the circle, whilst the clapping continued and a bongo drum came out.

This was a chance to put everything I had learned so far to the test. My partner, Peter was a pro and my assigned babysitter for this. We clapped and sang until it was our turn to take to the circle. Unlike a dance off, when you are pitted against each other to produce the best moves, this was a very fluid sequence, which allowed you to freely express yourself. If I kicked, Peter ducked and maybe cartwheeled out of the way and if Peter kicked, I yelped, panicked and jumped out of the way. Under the spotlight, I seemed to forget all I had just learnt and started to overthink it.

We each took turns to "play" in the circle and my brain really started to reject the amount of work I was putting it under, so my clapping rhythms went to pot but then in the circle I would remember some of the moves. Doing three things at once, was overload but I have to say, I really enjoyed Capoeira. Obviously, it wasn't really an ideal activity for my back but with each of the martial arts I have tried, I have enjoyed learning about the heritage but not so much the hitting or hurting – maybe I have found my ideal martial art? I just need to exercise my brain to take on more than one instruction at a time!

Gaelic Football – Number 88

"Come over and have one Margarita" read the last minute email that went round on the Friday evening. Surely one wouldn't hurt? I knew I had to be responsible as I had to be in Plymouth for 10am the following morning for my Gaelic football challenge but it was a bank holiday and a little Tenerife reminiscing wouldn't hurt. One turned into two...two turned into three...you get the idea. Jessica Ennis-Hill has a support entourage including psychologists, nutritionists and coaches. I have a rabble of tequila wielding drunkards in my camp. What hope do I have?

I made my way to Plymouth considering my friendship choices and chewing frantically on gum, which I hoped would conceal the fumes. I met up with the lads of Plymouth Parnells Gaelic Football Club and we made our way onto the muddy rugby field behind the leisure centre. I wasn't sure what Gaelic football was about but I was reassured the night before by Aussie Mat that it was like Aussie Rules. As I didn't know much about Aussie Rules, this wasn't helpful information. The team enlightened me and told me that you had to score points; if you hit the ball over the bar, you scored one point. If you scored under the bar, past the goalkeeper, you scored a goal, which is worth three points.

Unlike rugby, you can't carry it for more than four steps before you have to hand pass the ball, bounce it or solo it - soloing the ball is toe tapping the ball back to yourself. You can also pass the ball forward or backwards and there is no offside, so goal hanging seemed to be a viable option.

We started off with some drills, which involved hand passing, then booting of the ball and finally soloing. I struggled with the soloing but I enjoyed booting the ball about, as I sprayed it in different directions and as usual with team sports, I really enjoyed the banter. I find most teams start on their best behaviour around me and once everyone relaxes, the banter starts in earnest. The only problem I was finding was my back was really starting to niggle and I knew as soon as I cooled down from any running I would start to seize up. This happened after an hour of training and we moved onto match play. I stood out for the first drill but that five minutes of standing around in the cold made me seize up and as I didn't want to hinder their practise, I took on the role of cheerleader/ball retriever - although even picking up the ball was painful and I did start to wonder if ignoring the advice to rest was actually doing myself proper damage. I will consult with Liz the chiropractor in the week, who will give me my ritual weekly rollicking, before I am sent away again.

The match play was fast and furious, with fitness being a huge requirement, as the play was relentless. It is an enjoyable spectator sport and I would definitely go and watch a full game. With nearly all male only sports I have taken part in, I have noticed that they are fuelled by competition, which is in turn driven by testosterone. At one point, there were proper handbags going on in the game, which did make me smile a little and wish I had some popcorn to hand. Obviously, being a hockey player, I do see the competitive side of women too (maybe we have titosterone?) but blokes having a row with each other seems to be an inevitable by-product of team sports.

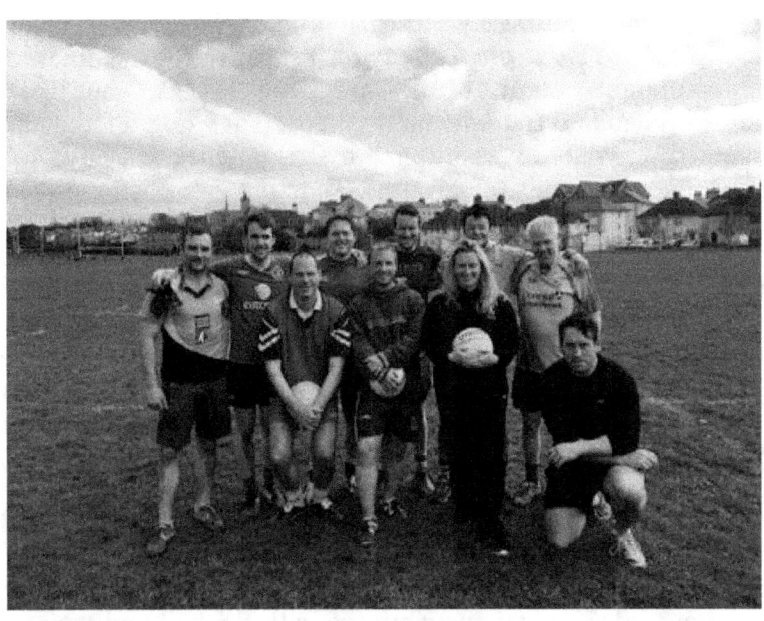

Me and the Lads

The drills ended and I could put my imaginary pompoms down. The guys were exhausted but told me that they were soon going to be soloing the Plymouth Half Marathon, which I can't even imagine. Fair play to them. I bid them farewell as I trudged off in search of carbs and more water. From Spain to Ireland in 12 hours...not bad!

Water Polo – Number 89

I made a conscious decision to leave Water Polo towards the end, as I figured that after all of my sports, I would look much better in a swimming costume towards the final few weeks of the challenge. Unfortunately, due to my long standing commitments to wine, carbs and the Easter Bunny, this didn't pan out as hoped but, at least, I have my snazzy tankini to cover some of the lumps and bumps.

I met up with the St Austell Water Polo Club at the Polkyth Centre in St Austell for an adult session. Leanne was given guardianship of me and as we were going to the changing room, she asked what costume I was wearing. *"How lovely,"* I thought, *to be entering into some girly chit chat.* I mentioned my tankini and was just about to point out the ruffles and tassles, when Leanne shook her head and told me bluntly: "No, that won't do, that could get ripped off you!" I was stunned by the potential assaults I may face in the water and was given not one but two costumes to put on, just in case one was ripped.

Whilst the rest of the team practised their drills, Leanne took me to the diving pit area to go through the basics and try some techniques. First thing to master was the "egg beater" method of treading water, which effectively meant your legs had to rotate like a beater, which uses less energy than the usual kicking. This wasn't an easy technique to grasp, but Leanne assured me it becomes second nature after a few sessions. Apparently, in an actual game, there is no shallow end and you have to tread water and swim continuously for four lots of seven minutes, which sounded exhausting.

I moved onto trying not to drown whilst throwing the ball, trying not to drown whilst swimming with the ball and trying not to drown whilst catching the ball. Leanne seemed pleased and we moved back to the group and joined in with some catching. I swam at great speed toward the safe bosom of the shallow end. After a

238

few drills (which all went swimmingly) I was parted from my mentor and invited to shoot at a keeper, which I was more than happy with, until it was my turn to go in goal. I managed a 100% consistency by not being able to save any of the 10 shots.

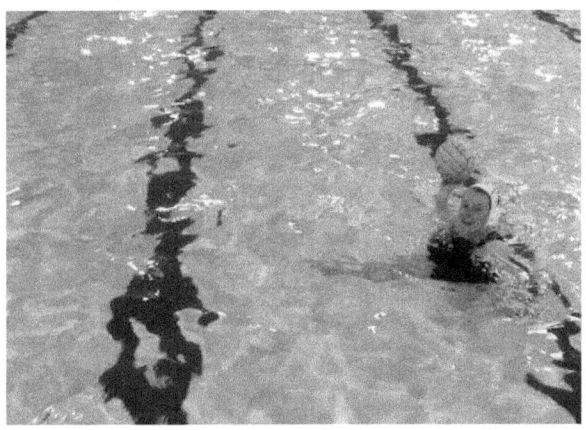

Shooting the ball

In the shallow end, I felt safe but then it was our turn to go to the deep end and work on attacking in the "pit." It is hard to describe what I beheld; suffice to say it looked more like attempted manslaughter than man-to-man marking, as the attacker swung limbs around whilst getting dunked by the defender. I copied by pretending to mock drown and apparently I did well.

Next was the game and again with team sports, especially with ball sports, I have an understanding of positioning and making space. However, this knowledge seems fairly dependent on having legs on the ground, as I found while trying in vain to keep up with the swim sprints and change of direction. It was fairly frantic and when the ball was in the open and everybody was swimming towards it, it was reminiscent of a frenzied shark attack. The pool turned white with frothing and splashing.

I subbed myself off and regrouped. It was time to employ my own strategy and play to my strengths i.e. using my legs. I subbed back on and this time I marshalled play in the shallow end, whether that meant I was an attacker or defender, I abandoned all the requests from my team to mark a man and instead employed my own zonal marking. Effectively, I patrolled no man's land and tried to hide the fact that I kept putting my feet on the floor.

Water Polo was really tiring but the session was great. The club were very friendly and my back enjoyed being in the water. To be

239

honest, if you wanted to get fit, you don't need to flounce about in an aqua class, go straight for this! I gave Leanne her swimsuits back, which were thankfully unscathed and I waved them off as they set off for a post-training pint. It seems that the more nervous about a certain challenge I am, the more I actually end up enjoying it. My next challenge in the pool is Octopush, or underwater hockey. I consulted with the guys at Water Polo and they were deeply concerned for me, which means in my logic, it will be my best challenge ever! I might have to ditch the tankini again, though!

Tennis – Number 90

Ahhh tennis...one of my favourite sports and this time in a venue I am familiar with and people I know. This is a luxury challenge for me. I have spent a lot of time over the past 11 months falling out with the sanctimonious Sat-Nav lady, practising my 3 point turns in various towns and villages and peering at signs in the dark. To nip down the road to my local leisure centre is an absolute joy.

I met Jackie and Steve the coaches and the rest of the beginners' tennis class, with my own racquet in tow. Apart from cardio tennis, which didn't actually require you to hit the ball in the court, I haven't picked up a racquet in anger for nearly a year now and I have missed it. When I say played "tennis in anger," I mean I used to be the sub in the over 60s double matches, opposite the church in the village. That setting should be one of quiet enjoyment of a not-too-competitive game but if there is one sport which gets me angry, it is tennis. I usually spend the whole match trying not to swear, shout and curse at myself and instead I silently, violently, grip my racquet and make mini swishing noises with it, whilst gritting my teeth and murmuring under my breath. I love the game, but I get frustrated by my own ineptness.

Previously, in an earlier chapter, you may remember that I have a wicked backhand, which I seem to be naturally gifted with. When this thing works, this stroke can really unleash. To compensate for this blessing from Mother Nature, I am also saddled with the world's worst forehand and a non-existent serve. It is like having twins, where one is gifted, pretty and charismatic and the other is the complete opposite. It isn't fair and it isn't balanced. This makes me OK at doubles, as I patrol the backhand side and only have to serve one in every four games but it makes me rubbish at singles.

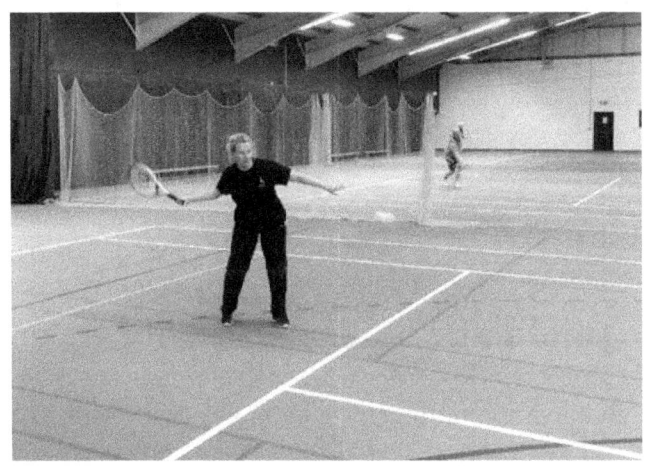

This return will end up either in the roof or in the net

Consistency is also a big problem and I also tend to scream or stifle screaming a lot. I wasn't sure what side of my game was going to turn up to this practise and by the look of the returns I was spraying all around the court in the warm-up, the rust had set in. After the warm-up, we were split into teams as we had our own mini Davies Cup competition. I was paired with Andy first up. I apologised profusely in advance and seemed to make it my mission to put him off as much as I could, on what I can only call Operation Hindrance. If I wasn't messing about finding my optimum position at the net, I was looking to go towards his ball, which would make him miss. We narrowly lost 3-2 but I was starting to get more comfortable and less annoying to my partner.

Next up was Sarah, who had already been mockingly given code violations for her on-court potty mouth. Of the five games we played together, between us we must have gone through the whole dictionary of expletives. It felt good to properly let it out and the more I did, the more my backhand started firing. I am a fairly selfish team player at tennis and although it is nice to win, I really need to come off court feeling like I actually properly belted the ball and connected with some shots. We lost 3-2 but the bigger headline was that my backhand was back.

I went into the final match in full confidence but I stopped swearing with my new partner and the backhand went AWOL. We got thrashed 4-0 but the games were played in good spirit. Jackie

241

told me that I should come back and get the forehand fixed, as I was evidently quite an unbalanced player. I would really like to be coached to improve this massive weakness in my game.

One thing's for sure; I will definitely go back to tennis after the challenge has ended, as it has reminded me how much I enjoy the sport from a social aspect, as well as the game play. Who knows, with a bit of coaching and an improvement in my technique, I might stop swearing so much and racquet swishing...but I effing doubt it!

The Challenge So Far - Number 81 to 90

Oh, my god, I am finally down to my last 10 sports! I cannot believe that I am so close to the finish. 80-90 has been bitter sweet as I've really struggled with my back. I first sprained my lower back in the 20s, but managed to take a couple of weeks off to rest it and thankfully got back into the flow. Then I hurt it again at the end of the 70s, which has really hampered me both physically and in my enjoyment of what I'm doing.

The problem is that my back needs to rest and not be doing all of these different movements which I am forcing it to do. The other week for instance, I was chucking around a javelin one minute, doing cartwheels the next and then wiping out on a boogie board. This really isn't normal behaviour, my back and my chiropractor are both loudly complaining. At one point recently, I seriously thought about extending the challenge and resting but the headline of "100 sports in 13 months" isn't quite as catchy. Mentally, I really need to get through and finish. I plan to spend the month after the challenge just resting, with a bit of swimming and to be honest, I need to spend a bit of quality time with my family and thank them for their own sacrifices while I have been here there and everywhere! I worked out the other day that I will have travelled nearly 10,000 miles over the course of the year to get to all of the venues I have been to.

I have filed away the thought of putting the challenge on ice. I have used that ice for my back and am going to employ mind over matter for the remaining 10. The last 10 have been booked up already and I will finish the challenge on the 30th April 2015 at Kernow Wakepark with Wakeboarding. I have invited some journalists down to the finale. My dignity has been ditched long ago, so the thought of wakeboarding with a bad back, whilst having the spotlight solely on me in front of a group of strangers, will be a very fitting crescendo to my adventure. Other plans for that day will be to drink lots of Prosecco and to stop dodging the sofa.

These last 10 will need to be done in 20 days, so I'm going to find fitting it all challenging if nothing else but I'm still excited to meet new people and discover their sports. My list of things to continue with after my challenge (and rest) continues to grow and I'm look forward to these new adventures, which I should be able to share more with the family.

I'm also looking forward to going up to the National Blog Awards in London next week. I've been shortlisted in the lifestyle category. I've checked out the people in my category and I have no chance of winning, unless bribes are accepted, or if all 9 of my fellow nominees decided to give up blogging as a past time. Never mind, it's a chance to put on a new frock and get to meet some proper bloggers, who are at the top of their game. I, in turn, will try and disguise the fact that I am a complete charlatan!

So, here's to the finishing line!

Chapter 11 - Challenge 91 – 100

New Age Kurling – Number 91

I don't think it will sink in exactly how many sports I have tried and what I've personally achieved until much later on, but one of my regrets is not being able to make it up to Scotland to try curling. I really fancied trying it but alas, time has beaten me. I was therefore delighted to receive an invitation from Terry at the Cornwall Special Olympics to try New Age Kurling. I readily accepted the invitation, as I'd already had the privilege to come down and play Boccia with them. The group meet every month and enables people with learning difficulties and their families a chance to come down and have a go or compete at a range of sports.

As soon as I got through the door, I met with Rose, who I had spoken to before. Rose was thinking about attempting every horse-based activity going - apparently there are over 50 - she was putting me to shame! I bumped into lots of other people, who I had met previously and were eager to get an update on my progress.

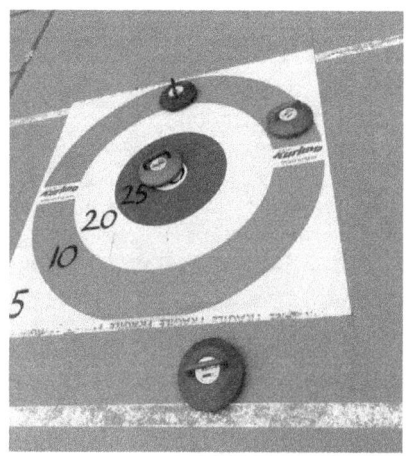

Scoring with New Age Kurling

Archery, badminton, football, boccia and new age kurling were all laid out in the hall but nobody seemed to be around the kurling area, so I circled it a few times but was invited to play boccia. I was mid-game when a tribe of cub scouts came marching in and dominated the equipment. I finished the boccia and tried to muscle in but they were not having any of it. Did they not appreciate that I have my own sports badge to aim for?

From a distance, I could see this type of kurling looked a lot of fun and was certainly keeping these kids entertained. Just like the senior sibling sport, you had to push the pucks towards a target but as the hall was bereft of ice, the pucks had little wheels on them and could be pushed. Finally, after what seemed like an eternity, the kids ran eagerly off to pick up some bows and arrows and I had it to myself. All I needed was an opponent. Obviously, I looked pathetic enough for a girl to come over and play with me. We played the first game but neither of us could get enough purchase, so we agreed that I would move the target closer to us. After more practise, we both made it on to the scoring zone.

We started to attract more players and I managed to play a couple of other people, including David who had Downs. He was an absolute gentleman and congratulated me on my wins and high-fived me if I made an impressive shot. I really do enjoy my time with the Special Olympics crowd. All the activities are played in the right spirit and I am a huge fan of people being able to have the opportunity to try a range of sports, no matter what their ability.

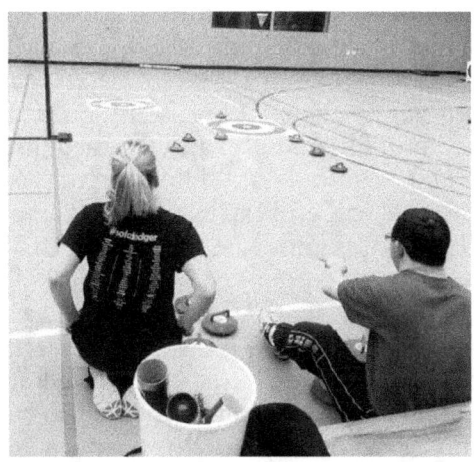

Eyeing up the target

It is close to my heart as well, as my brother-in-law has his own learning difficulties and I would love for him to come down here and show how competitive he is at sports. There is such a world of opportunity, if he wanted to embrace it.

I was sad to say my goodbyes so soon. Driving back, I made a vow to fulfil my wish to go to Scotland try curling, as this version really whetted my appetite. With less than 10 sports to go, I guess I will have a lot more time on my hands to consider that as a realistic possibility.

Sailing – Number 92

As previously mentioned, the person who benefits most from my sports challenge is Liz, my chiropractor. Most weeks, I have limped in, bemoaned my failing body, received a lecture and then have been massaged and taped up and sent on my way. In my recent patch-up session, Liz mentioned that her fiancé liked to sail and had a boat. *Jackpot!* I thought. I still needed to cross sailing off the list and given the time of year; none of the clubs I had approached were training yet, so this was my golden ticket.

I declared that, as an extension to her customer service, I required a sailing lesson. I expected to be rebuffed but it went well and after speaking to Simon, we agreed a date and time to meet. This was the business, alright; a medical practitioner who was already aware how sore my back was. If I played my cards right, I could be sailed about, whilst having a beer with my feet up. I might even get a free back massage.

We made our way to the boat and were joined by Liz's friends from her rowing club. I met Simon and thanked him for letting me go on the boat, as I positioned myself in the discussion as more a passenger. For the sake of embracing the experience, I would have to do the odd thing but mainly just for the pictures - I could make the rest up.

Liz took on board a trolley full of booze in preparation for an imminent voyage to the Scillies as I made my way onto Simon's pride and joy, the "Lady P." I was really eager to look around downstairs, as I admired how homely it was. I think I might like a boat. I took in my surroundings, on this beautiful, if not blowy day and yes, I definitely think I could take up sailing.

All of my dreaming did encompass the fact that we were still firmly moored in the harbour, so I was keen to get going and seal the deal on my new life plan. I sat down and started chattering, whilst Simon beavered about. Ropes were untied and things were pressed and off we went into the open water. I was invited to "help" by untying this and that and putting away things. I am not sure the memo went around about my master plan of how the day was to pan out. Liz told me to come up and unfurl the sail (I think there was a technical term). This sailing malarkey was starting to be hard work. I started moaning about my back and put myself on the subs bench.

The sail went up and the engine went off and there we were actually sailing. The trouble was, it was a bit windy, so we were bobbing about quite a bit. I was happy to listen to their sailing stories and what their typical weekend entails on the boat. Simon then elected me to take the helm, just as the beers came out. My instruction was to pick a point on the horizon and aim towards it. This is easier said than done, as I went into full learner driver panic mode. I wrenched it forwards then backwards and felt the boat almost tip when I caught the wind. I didn't like it. I didn't like it all.

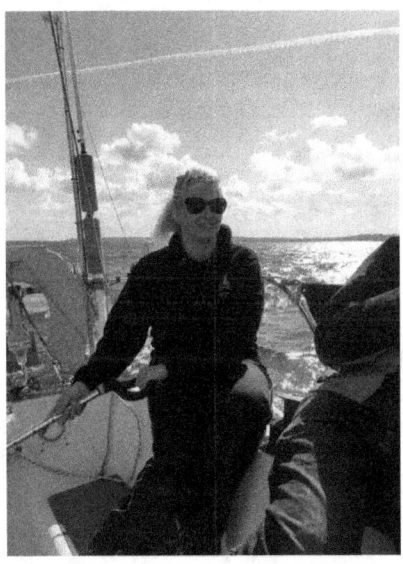

A very nervous driver

Simon regained controlled, as I whimpered in the corner with my bottle of beer. I thought it would be easy but there's a lot to think about. Liz enlightened us with her new found knowledge with her recently gained sailing qualification. I looked wistfully at a speedboat motoring by. Whether it was the bottle of beer, the sun coming out from beyond the clouds or the fact that we had turned around and had a smoother ride back but I went back to enjoying myself. I proved myself inept at the helm, so was only given menial tasks. I was even given a crash course in knots, which I made a right hash of.

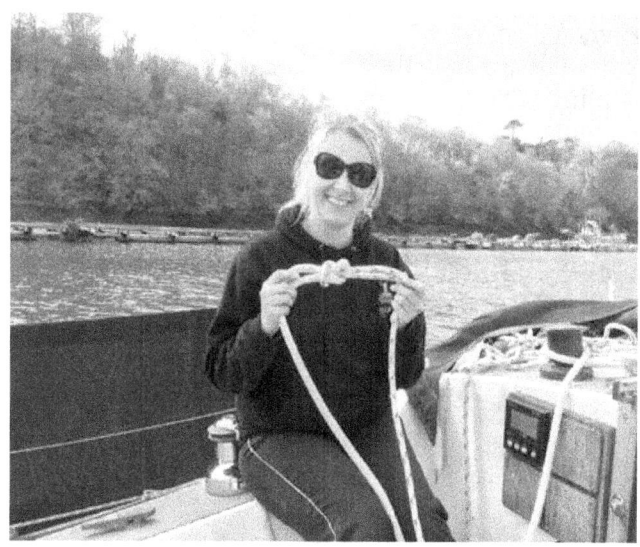

Crash course in knots

As we got back to the dock, I decided that the idea of having a boat is awesome (oar-some – I know). As a family, we could sail out and find remote beaches and then have a BBQ and swim in the sea, (probably with dolphins) but the reality is that sailing takes concentration and physical exertion, so instead I figured I might just have to keep getting my back fixed and occasionally muscle in on Lady P as part of a customer loyalty scheme.

Ultimate Frisbee – Number 93

I'm a huge fan of team sports and especially keen to be on land again after Water Polo. With all of the clubs I have visited so far, it is generally a stock formula as to how the visit will go; I make introductions, I am assigned a babysitter, I practise the techniques, I am coached in the rules and the objectives of the game, once my mentor feels that I have achieved a basic level of competence, I am released back to the group where I have a go at some drills and at the very end, we usually end with a small game and I get an invite to the pub after. These are tried and tested steps and form part of an internationally recognised method of being introduced to a new sport.

What hasn't happened before is that I turn up on Mini-League night, get given a pink shirt and a typed-out rule sheet to read on the side line before I am subbed on. Obviously, I am embellishing the truth slightly, but I did get a baptism of fire!

I will rewind slightly; it is true that I made my introductions and yes, I did get my babysitters (Jam and Afro Pete) to teach me how to throw and catch. I felt fairly confident with the backhand throw; obviously growing up in Cornwall, I have had my fair share of experience chucking a Frisbee around on a beach. However, the big headline was that when you catch a Frisbee, you don't pick it out of the air with one hand; you have to crocodile snap catch it, with one hand on top and the other on the bottom. Of course, that makes sense. The forehand was not a technique I had ever tried and whilst everybody was warming up, I watched this throw and it looked fairly simple and certainly fairly stylish – if I wheeled that move out on the beach, I would look like a proper pro. Pete told me to whip my wrist, in the same manner you would whip a tea towel to inflict pain...I thought back to my childhood. My forehand Frisbee is as bad as my forehand tennis though and like tennis, it would seem that I would be heavily reliant on my backhand to get anywhere in a game.

I had a good ten minute practise before I was given my team pink shirt, handed the 10 commandments of the game and put on the side-line, ready to sub on. I shouted after them, what "sport is it like?" I've amassed quite a bit of sporting knowledge over my challenge, so aligning it with other sports might help me get it. "American Football and Netball" came the answer. OK, that made sense to me. I quickly scanned the rules and watched the play. As soon as one team scored, I was beckoned on. I donned the part of the headless chicken and thankfully, my team scored in spite of my presence. I subbed off. This time, I really watched what was going on and actually it was a fairly simple concept; attackers threw the Frisbee in any direction and once caught, they couldn't move but had 10 seconds to release it. The idea was to get it to the scoring zone. If you dropped it, the possession was lost. The revolutionary part of the sport was that it was self-governing; a concept utterly unfamiliar to me.

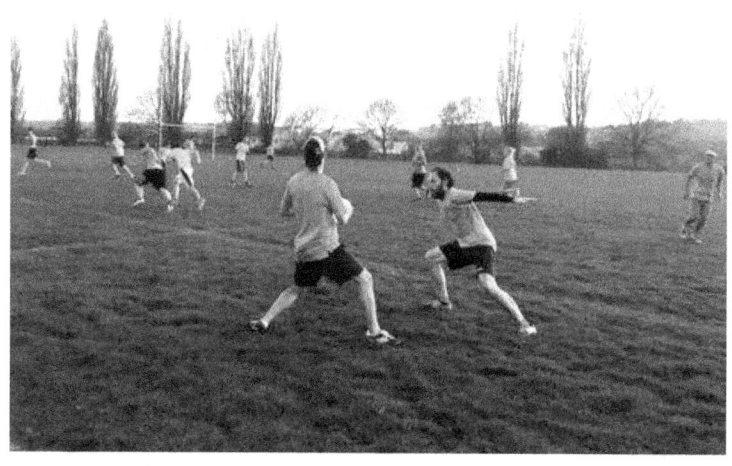

It's a fast moving game

I subbed back on and listened more to my team, as to what I was to do and made myself available for a pass. My teammate threw me the Frisbee and I actually caught it. The ten second rule didn't faze me, as I have perfected the old Hot Potato technique, so I chucked it back like the damned thing was on fire! That was the high point of my Frisbeeing foray. We drew the first game but when I saw the brown team trudge over, they looked like absolute giants, so I felt my cheerleading skills were a much better deployment of my skills. I also had the scoring board to deal with, so I was kept more than busy, as my poor pinks got thrashed. I felt justified in my decisions side-lining myself.

I loved my time with the Devon Ultimate guys and girls. The whole self-governing, honesty part of the game was very refreshing and ensured that the matches were played in a competitive but enjoyable spirit. Everybody was really welcoming and loads of people came up to ask me about my challenge. The fact that it was a beautiful evening, in a freshly mown park, by a river and just a hop, skip and a jump away from a beer garden all added up to making Ultimate Frisbee one of my favourite team sports so far.

Underwater Hockey – Number 94

There are two sports which have been giving me butterflies: American Football and the yet to be completed Octopush, or Underwater Hockey. Nobody seems to have the foggiest about what Octopush is and where there is doubt, tales of fiction are created, including the necessity for scuba gear or free diving. One of the Water Polo guys told me that he knew somebody who played and could hold his breath for 12 minutes! On reflection, the guy's friend was either a Merman or he was taking the mick out of me. Either way, I didn't think my own hockey skills would be of much benefit in this particular situation.

I don't know what was making me so nervous, but I was thoroughly daunted by the prospect. I drove the 50 minutes to the Life Centre in Plymouth and the radio stations must have sensed my trepidation because I kid you not, the songs which played included Bonnie Tyler's "I need a Hero", M People's "Search for the Hero" and finally Queen's "We Are The Champions." I just needed the theme tune to Rocky and I would be suitably buoyed. I applied the lyrics to my own situation and remembered that this was an opportunity to experience somebody else's passion and it's a privilege to be invited along.

I met the Kingsbridge Krays Octopush Club poolside. We were going to be in the diving pit, which Tom Daley uses. I peered up in the rafters to see the diveboard he jumps from and shuddered at the thought of that being on my list of sports. Anthony was my contact and after introductions, he went off to fetch me some flippers and snorkel gear. I wasn't sure how I would get on with the mask. I am really claustrophobic and I couldn't even have the gas and air mask on my face in labour, so I was feeling really apprehensive but I put my game face on and put the thing on my head. I didn't really have time to cradle my phobia, as I was too busy taking in the ridiculous vision that I must have made, waddling about like an aqua clown in my flippers.

Swimming with my flippers was a very odd sensation. Swimming backwards seemed to be easier than forward for some reason but Anthony told me that backward swimming wasn't that useful in the sport. I did a few lengths of the pit and then on went the snorkel and mask. I remember snorkelling as a kid and I loved it, so on it went and surprisingly it felt kind of OK. After some wading about, taking in the sub-aqua world of the dive pit, it was time to try and dive to the bottom. The pool floor was 3m down and seemed an awfully long way down. Anthony gave me some techniques, which didn't go very well, but after a change of tack, I managed to swim downwards but the pressure hurt my ears. There was a lot to think about: holding your breath, popping ears and trying not to swallow. I continued to try and I must have got to 2.85m but I couldn't reach the bottom.

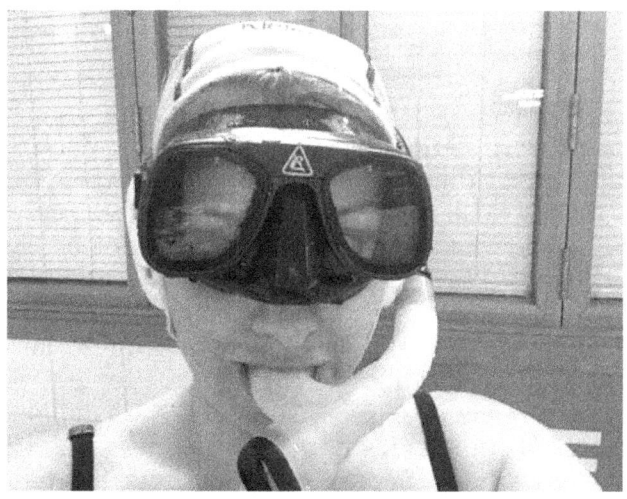

Then on goes the mask

Anthony left me to practise, as they went into a match in preparation for a big tournament. With my snorkel gear, I was able to watch the action, which was fascinating. The play happened at the bottom of the pool, where both teams fought for possession of the puck and to score a goal. Obviously, players would have to come up for air and would have to come out of a tackle or make a pass and then come to the surface, before submerging again.

It was a completely different world and a sport like nothing I had never seen before. As a team sport it is incomparable, as you can't call for the ball or shout a formation. Everything is done with a kind of knowingness of positions and play, which I guess comes with experience. Some of the team were GB players, so I was watching the best.

As I couldn't get down to the bottom without my ears feeling like they were going to explode, I watched with my head underwater. I tried to emulate their flipper action and decided my time was best spent not only mutely cheerleading but also trying to practise becoming a mermaid. This would go well, until I would swim along, get excited about something and then swallow a snorkel full of water...you never really saw Darryl Hannah gripping onto a rock, gasping for air and spluttering out sea water, so I have a long way to go before I become a fully-fledged mermaid.

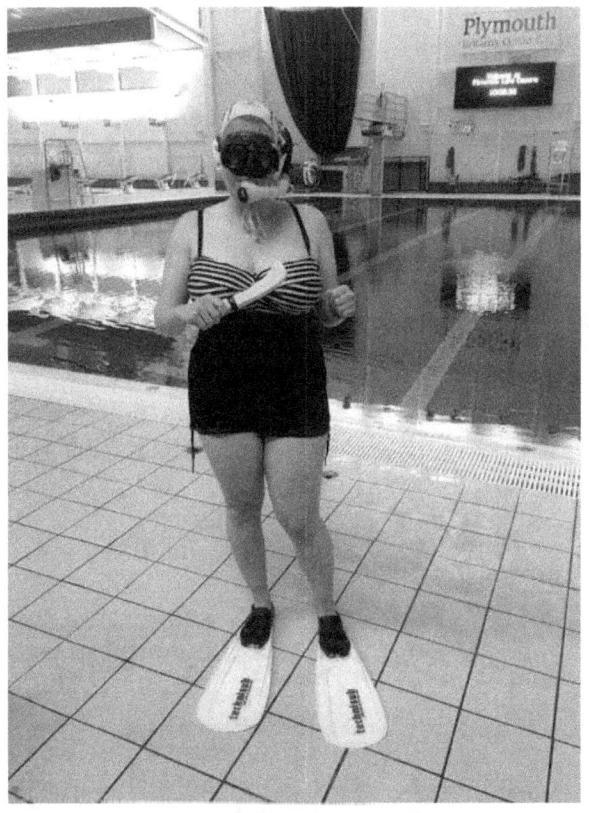

I am a very good surface Octopusher!

Shooting – Number 95

Next on the list, as I get to the end of my challenge, is shooting. Originally, I naively thought I could rock up at my local shooting club and start firing some weapons. Apparently shooting isn't like a basketball session, where you can turn up and start shooting stuff. When I enquired, I was told that I would have to complete a 3 month police and history check. For the purposes of my challenge, that seemed a lot of effort to go to, so I set about finding a clay pigeon shoot I could try.

I found Lower Lake Shooting Ground and arranged a lesson with Bill. When I arrived, it was a glorious day. We went into the club house where Bill took me through the main steps of shooting. This included the stance, the way you hold the gun and also the gun and cartridge itself. I wasn't sure how I would get on with this sport. I do have decent hand-eye co-ordination, which is one of the positives I've discovered along the way and I vaguely remember shooting an air rifle as a teenager but I wasn't sure whether I would actually like to fire a gun now. As previously noted, I am much more of a wuss than I was before becoming a mum.

Bill took us down to his special firing area in the woods. First things first: we had to work out which was my master eye. I remembered that this was something which had to be ascertained back at Archery. At the time, I was diagnosed as being "Cack Eyed" but I couldn't quite remember what that meant. Bill went through the procedure of coming up with his own diagnosis, as I pointed at things with alternate eyes shut. Yes, it was concluded that the second opinion verified the first and although I am a right hander, my master eye is my left. All that being said, Bill insisted I shut my left eye and rely on my right eye. I decided that if I didn't hit anything, I would be wheeling this out as my excuse.

I was given my ear muffs and shoulder protector and Bill showed me where the "bird" would come from. After some final instructions and adjusting of my stance, I shut my better eye and nervously glared up to the tree area, where it would be fired from. I followed it and fired. I had no idea what happened but the adrenaline started coursing through my body as my hands began to shake. I still couldn't hear properly from my underwater hockey challenge, where the water hadn't quite vacated my ear canal, so I took my ear protectors off and waited for Bill's commiserations but none were forthcoming; apparently I hit the thing! I did a set of 5 shots and for each one, I was prepared to prove that the first was a fluke but I hit all 5.

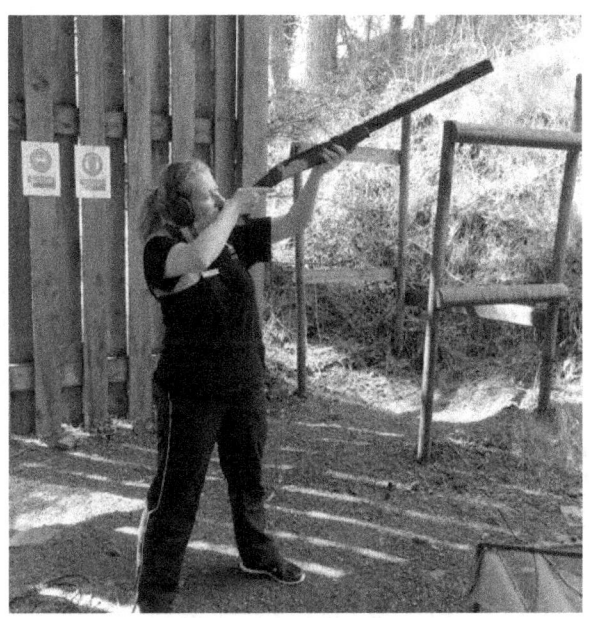

Bullseye!

I didn't quite understand what was happening. Maybe Bill had a remote control explosive hidden in the clay, which went off, just to make me feel better? Bill was congratulating me but my heart was beating out of my chest and my hands continued to shake. We moved on to firing the clay pigeon, which was moving away. I only managed to hit half of those, but Bill felt I was good enough to progress to the next level.

We moved across to the range, where the "birds" were fired from right to left and then left to right. This added complexity as you had to fire into the space where the target was travelling to and you couldn't get your sights on it. Again, I hit all of the right to left birds. I couldn't quite believe what was happening. I had gone out of the fluke area of the graph and was heading into the skilful range. How bizarre? I was brought down to earth slightly when the target moved left to right. I found this much trickier and only managed to hit a couple of those.

We ended on a high, as I shot the last two birds. I was absolutely thrilled and surprised by my performance. This is the beauty of my challenge; by having the opportunity of trying so many sports, I can really nail down what I am good at. It turns out that I am naturally gifted at golf and now shooting…2 out of 95 aren't bad!

Gig Rowing – Number 96

I am not going to lie; sometimes in this challenge enthusiasm has to be manufactured to even get out of the door and in this instance, to get out of bed. If I could bottle that feeling after I've done a sport or worked out and spray it on me before I go out, I wouldn't feel so resentful of the bed dwellers in my household on this Sunday morning. After a quiet breakfast alone, a stern talking to myself and a look out of the window at the beautiful, sunny morning, my resentment slowly started to turn to smugness. I was getting to enjoy more of the day than any other family member.

I set off to meet the Padstow Gig Rowing Cub at Padstow harbour. I have been to Padstow hundreds of times but today, I was day dreaming on auto-pilot and found myself driving to our favourite beach. Panic! I got into the car park with 5 minutes to spare, to find out that I hadn't brought my purse and there was no change in the car...Proper Panic! The phone started to ring as my friend Liz, who was part of the club, tried to locate me. I whizzed the car around to where they were and ran after them, as they started to put the boats into the water. "Hi everybody, I'm Sammmmmmm!" That was a literary interpretation of me sliding on algae covered stones and falling flat on my arse in front of everybody. What a complete prat.

Thankfully my bum is so big, it managed to take the full force of the impact, without so much as an "ouch" but my pride and dignity, which were in short supply already, were bruised. Everybody was lovely and confirmed that it was very slippery. I hauled me and my red face into my assigned boat and I was put at the back to observe technique, before I was let loose with oars.

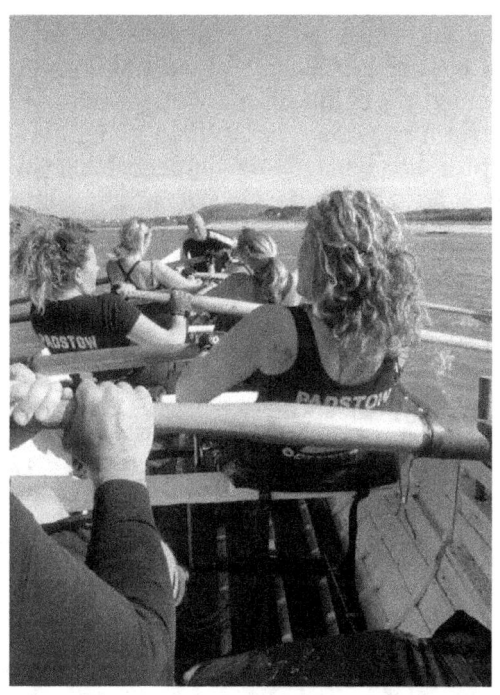

Row, row, row the boat

As my boat rowed out of the harbour, I started to feel myself relax, as I took in the beautiful surroundings. The Camel Estuary is very familiar to me and either side of us were two of my favourite beaches. As my team rowed out, I felt like Lady Muck being carted around, whilst I relaxed and took in the surroundings. Steve, who was in front of me, showed me how to hold the oar and pull it back towards your body. As we got further out, we started to get bounced about by the waves and as the boat dug in and increased the speed, I could tell my time was nigh.

After a rest, I swapped with Steve and took the oar. My focus was timing. Unlike my previous rowing experience in the river, I had a team to worry about. It was essential that I didn't start hitting other people's oars, as this would affect the synchronised strokes. As soon as I started to get a rhythm, I was given helpful instructions by Steve, which made me engage my brain, rendering my limbs abandoned of focus and thus, I would either tap somebody's oar or completely get me out of time. Steve stopped giving me tips after a while.

I was swapped back again, as the boat practised their starts and sprints as we turned back. As Pete the cox called instructions, I could feel the boat really motor. The girls gritted their teeth and gave their all. I watched intensely. My initial problem seemed to be that I was re-enacting being on a rowing machine and instead of pulling the oar into the body, you pulled it slightly to the side and then really pull it back. I swapped back with this new understanding and this time, I did much better. My timing improved and it felt much more rhythmical.

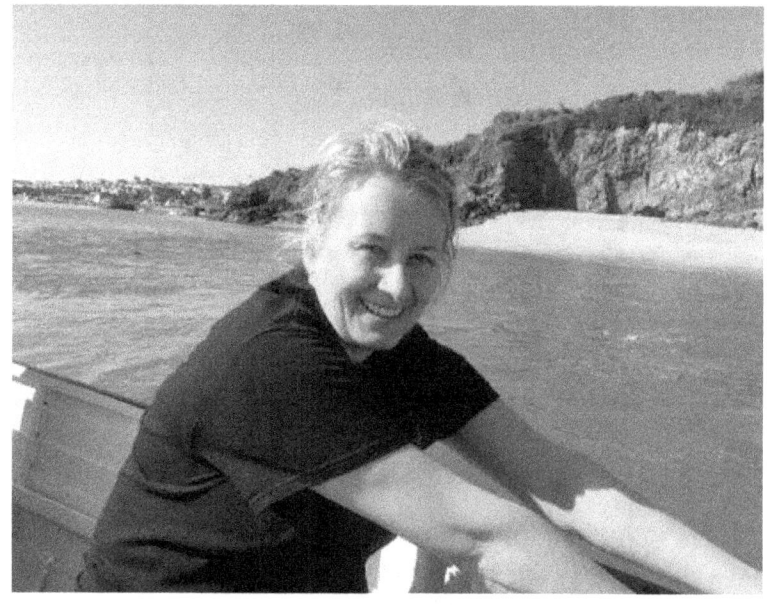

Feeling Oar-some!

We got back to land and I felt genuinely privileged to have had that experience. I used to see their boats from the beach and always wanted to give it a try and guess what: it isn't difficult to try it out. If this challenge has taught me anything, it's that if you've always harboured a desire to try something, go ahead and do it! Everybody is always very friendly and everybody has to start somewhere. After helping put the boats away, I waved goodbye to everybody but unlike my entrance, I made a very slow and mindful exit. It is one thing to make a fool of yourself in front of a dozen club members but something completely different with a town full of tourists.

Floorball – Number 97

Floorball is my next sport and I am excited to try this one, as it looks a little like indoor hockey. Mysteriously, me trying to be a mermaid in Octopush last week appears to have miraculously eased my back pain and it feels kind of normal, which is fantastic news, as it was really having an impact on my enjoyment. The only problem with this challenge is that it involved a five hour round trip drive to Bristol and back in an evening. It will be my last major journey for the challenge, so I figured I would use the time to take stock and reflect on my journey, whilst being on a journey. Actually, I just ended up singing along, at the top of my voice, to a medley of tunes on the radio.

I made it in good time to the leisure centre and met the guys from the Bristol Floorball club. Floorball is apparently very popular in Scandinavia and the Czech Republic and is one of the fastest growing sports in the world. Back along, when I was writing about my Ultimate Frisbee adventure, I mentioned the rules of trying a sport; introductions, techniques, drills, gameplay, invitation to the pub after. I was shocked in Frisbee to have skipped the drills part and gone straight into their mini-league. Floorball topped this altogether by skipping technique as well, as I was given a stick and a bib and assigned a team to play in!

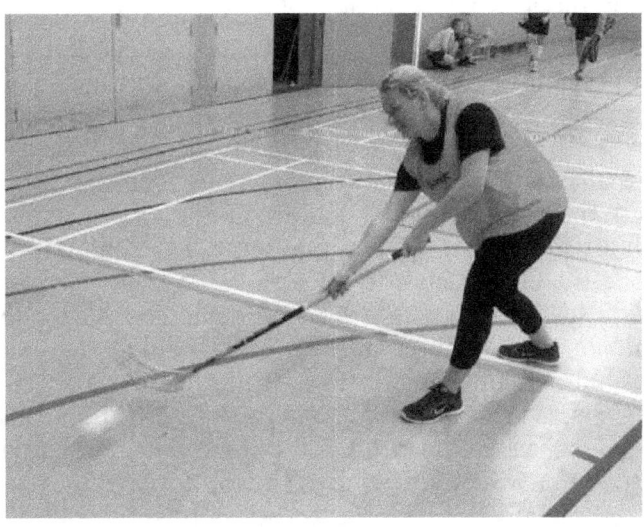

Getting used to the stick

I had to learn on the job. My first issue was being able to use both sides of the stick. That seemed alien to my hockey playing self, as I fumbled to turn my stick over to receive a ball. The whole game seemed to reflect that of ice hockey, but without the ice and all the gear they wear. The goals were the same size and you could play behind the goal. Playing the ball off the wall was also a useful gameplay technique. It was certainly fast and furious and some of these guys were extremely nimble, as they twisted and turned past me.

In hockey, if you are in a bit of a cul-de-sac, one very valid and used play is to put the ball on your opponent's foot for an immediate foul. I tried this early on and quickly found out that this rule doesn't apply in Floorball, as the ball can legitimately come off the foot. Rats! I have been perfecting that for 25 years. I searched my back catalogue of other weapons I could deploy but none came to mind, so I figured that I might actually have to go back to basics and run, receive and pass.

I was finding that receiving the ball on the stick was a 50/50 situation. Either I managed to collect it and pass it on or I completely missed it altogether. I understood the positioning and making space part of it and even felt confident enough to call for it a couple of times. At one point, I called and received the ball and even managed to score a goal, which had to get over a sports bag which was acting as a makeshift goalkeeper. Before the goal, the opposition didn't really try and tackle me that much but after that, I felt I was treated more equally. It was nice to feel that I garnered some respect but a shame for my goal tally, as the shots became harder to come by. In fact thinking about it, in all of my team sports, when it came to playing a game at the end of the sessions, I haven't really scored a goal, a try or a basket in any other of my forays into them, so this was a definite first!

The hour flew by and I really enjoyed Floorball. It's a shame that this is the closest club to me and it is 150 miles away. Given the miles I had to cover to get home, I made a reasonably swift exit. The journey home was long and I didn't get back until midnight but actually, I definitely felt that it was worth it. I really enjoyed the sport. No wonder it was gaining such popularity. I fell asleep as soon as my head hit the pillow, but my last conscious thought was that sweet little goal in the top corner.

Cycling – Number 98

I hate bikes! There you go; I said it. I hate everything about bikes but I especially hate the seats. My bum, with its inbuilt cushion, should be able to deal with it but no, the last time I went on a bike was 10 years ago and it killed after. The time before that was when I was 8 or 9 and I had a nasty fall on the way to school. We moved fairly shortly after that but I didn't get back on the horse/bike and thus I am deeply suspicious of these wheeled monsters.

It's a real shame, given that where I live are some of the best cycle routes in the whole of the UK, including Lanhydrock, The Camel Trail and Cardinham Woods. My previous forays onto the bike in my challenge have been in a spin class and poolbiking in Tenerife. These had all gone well and I hadn't fallen off those bikes but they were attached to a floor and not capable of moving, so I had to step it up a notch.

My friend Sugar, of Badminton fame, agreed to take me around one of the off-road trails at Lanhydrock. I see my friends on Facebook going there all the time with the kids. I see the lovely pictures and the smiles on their faces...sometimes there are picnics; sometimes there are stories of how little Tommy managed to ride without stabilisers. I usually skip over them, as I know the truth about bikes but I am curious, so after cramming my neighbour's teenage child's bike and hat into my car, off I went.

I had five minutes to unload the bike before Sugar arrived, so I donned the helmet and tentatively started to roll around the near empty car park, which actually felt kind of acceptable. Sugar met me and after a quick catch up and an inspection of my bike, we made our way to the trail. I explained to Sugar that I specifically wanted to go on the family trail, which is what they all talk about on Facebook. She agreed that this would be a good start, as children with stabilisers can achieve that. Give me the stabiliser route any day of the week. This route was the green route, so I'm not sure why we lined up at the blue route. Maybe the blue route was actually green in disguise? Maybe the blue was easier?

After adjusting the 21 gears on my bike (which is frankly too many for any vehicle), I fixed my helmet and off we went. I launched myself downhill, whilst screaming expletives all the way. My white knuckles clenched the brake, which only seemed to work on one side. I prepared to die and held on for dear life. Somehow, I managed to navigate my way to the bottom and the flat part. I could hear Sugar giggling ahead, saying something about the start being the hardest bit. I felt deceived but also relieved that we had the place to ourselves – I'm sure the sight of a screaming, swearing, swerving, nutcase would make any little Tommy in the vicinity, cry.

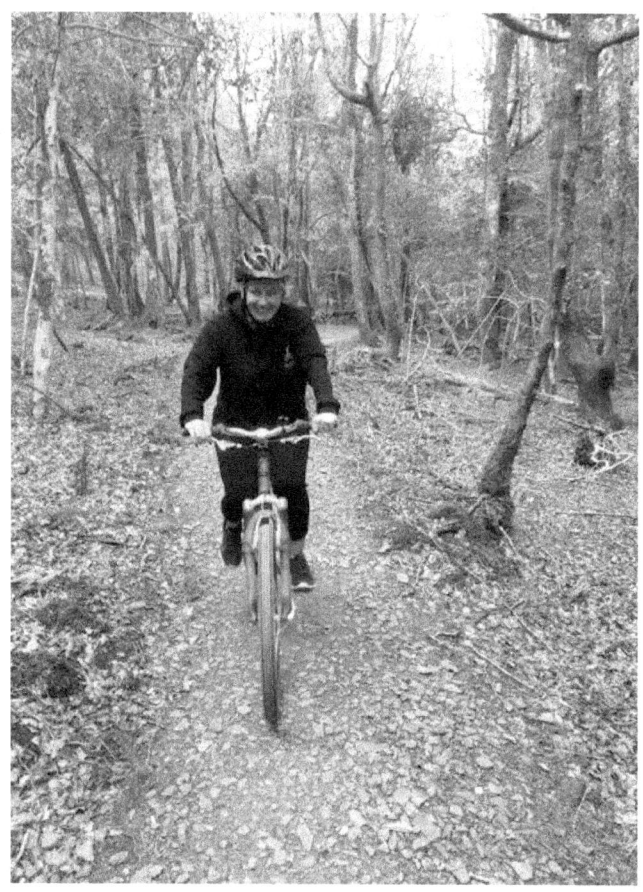

Managed to find some flat ground

I managed to compose myself around the flatter parts. Right behind bikes on my list of things I hate is hills, namely up hills, and there were a few of those going around. We finished the blue run, with me managing to stay on but that didn't seem to be enough for Sugar, as I was led to the "skills" area. I felt I had shown sufficient skill to actually stay on the bike, but apparently this was not enough. The course consisted of humps, jumps and bumps. I cycled up to the first hump I encountered, only to find myself not quite at the top and slowly going backwards. I managed to scream and put my feet down. Apparently more momentum was required.

Sugar told me to not look at the thing you want to avoid i.e. a large stone, a pothole...apparently, if you give it the luxury of attention, you will be magnetically drawn to it and hit it/fall into it. It was soon time to test this theory as I had to traverse a narrow bridge; either side of it was a slight drop. My eyes were drawn to this huge crater I perceived in my mind and I wobbled (whilst screaming) across the bridge. This was the last of my skills test, which I failed miserably. My bum was sore, my adrenaline was pumping and I felt battered by the experience. Maybe if I stick to empty car parks, I would start to enjoy cycling again but other than that, I am afraid to say that I still bloody hate bikes (apologies to all bike enthusiasts!). I did however like the cup of tea and cake afterwards. Every cloud and all that...

Bootcamp – Number 99

If there's one fitness class, which even by its very name makes people supportively wince, it is Bootcamp. It smacks of military-style discipline and fitness. I was provided with extra "Good lucks!" as I made my way down to the Bootcamp, ran by Martin Rowe of Limitless MPR at Pentewan Sands. Yes, this bootcamp session, would have the added dimension of sand.

Although I had my usual self-preserving amount of caution, I was ecstatic at the thought of not having to do another plank or burpee in this challenge after tonight. After everybody was accounted for, we made our way down to the beach. I said it before with the personal training but when the outside is as glorious as this, why would I consider a gym after this experience? There was even a rainbow (apparently these aren't guaranteed or part of the payment).

First thing's first and the warm-up, which was a run up and back. I know from handball that running on sand, is exhausting, especially the fluffy dry sand, which is pretty to look at but a *beep* to run on! I was properly puffing and blowing when we got back and after a stretch, Martin had us racing in twos, around a circuit. He advised us to find a similar paced partner. I asked if there was a chubby, slow person and there were no takers, so I ended up with a lovely lady, who turned out to be as fast as a cheetah on steroids! The guys were predictably competitive but it was done in a great spirit.

Martin then introduced us to a kind of assault course, where you had a different type of exercise to do at each station. First up were 10 burpees, then 15 press-ups, then 15 pull-ups, then 15 squats and 15 planks type things. This was to be repeated 3 times. By the second set, my press-ups looked like I was essentially dry humping the beach and I don't even know what kind of interpretation of a plank I was doing. Oh, and I may have decided that 14 was the new 15! I know, I know – I'm just cheating myself!

That was hard but although, it is named Bootcamp, there was no drill sergeant shouting orders. Good instructors give encouragement and praise but build you up within your ability, so although I pushed myself, I knew my limits and the limits of my newly rejuvenated back and Martin was great about adapting anything I was struggling with.

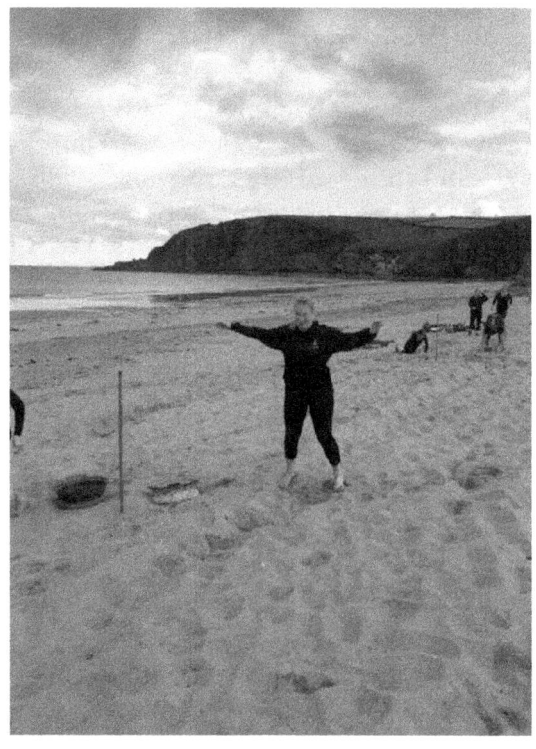

Instead of lifting, it was adapted to star jumps

After a bit of a breather, I became very suspicious of the equipment being laid out next. There were massive metal cotton reel-looking things and straps attached to them. I didn't like the look of this and made sure I was at the end of this particular queue. We had to put the straps over our shoulders and drag them as far as we could. Then move onto the next one, which had two metal things and then finally a large tyre. After the other two, the tyre felt like I was carrying a handbag. The first two, were near on impossible for me to drag, as I pulled with all my might but only manage to cover the distance of an ice cream cone.

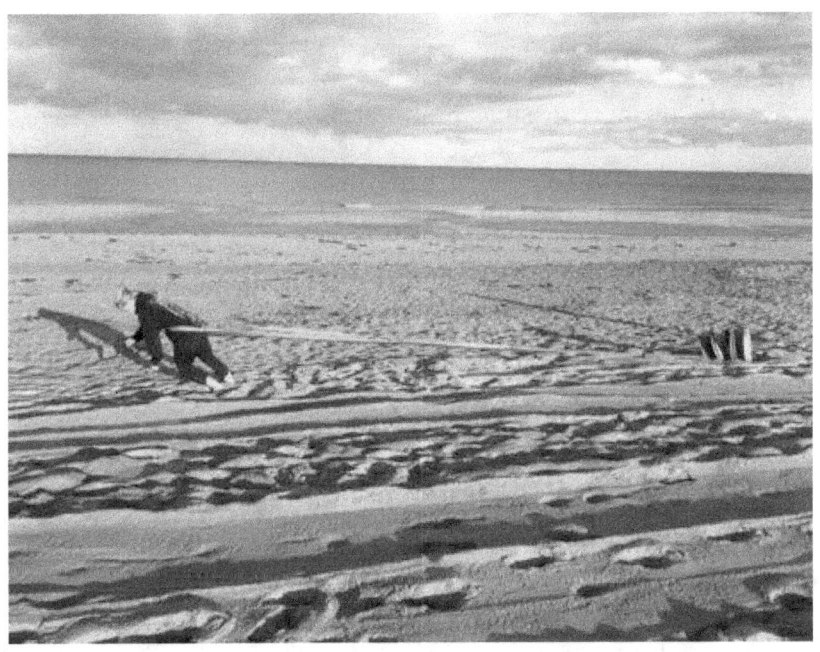

Managing to pull them a full 6-7cm

After some core work, which I adapted, on account of my back, we warmed down and finished. I even managed a little leap for joy, as I told everybody that I only had one challenge left to do. I explained that it was wakeboarding and even the bootcampers consoled me and wished me good luck. It seems like the unknown gets people into a panic. If I had listened to all the detractors before, I wouldn't have even made it down to this session tonight and although it was challenging, the setting was beautiful, I had a proper workout and I might not have passed out with flying colours but I did manage to survive and feel good after – oh and did I mention that rainbow and the fact that I have ONE MORE LEFT to go?

Wakeboarding – Number 100

So one year to the day after embarking on my 100 sports and fitness class challenge, I was finally at the end. I decided to end on wakeboarding, as I felt it symbolised everything I have gone through i.e. trying something completely new, something which sounded a bit scary and offering a high chance of making a fool of myself.

To add further possible humiliation to this last challenge, I decided to invite some reporters to the event and then topped it off by having Paul, Isobel and Oliver come and watch as well. I was imaging the scene of being dragged along, face first, screaming for my life, then looking up to see the shame on my family's faces as they watched, whilst all this was recorded and transmitted to an evening TV audience! I was playing for high stakes, people. By the time we made it down to Kernow Wake Park in Penryn, I was a nervous wreck.

I couldn't have chosen a more scenic backdrop than this old quarry, though. The sun was shining and the water was glistening. We were made very welcome, as I nervously paced and babbled my way through the introductions. Two reporters made it down to the event; one from a news service and one from ITV news. My pacing and babbling increased as I got changed into my wetsuit and everything was set up outside.

Katy was my instructor, who was very calm and chilled out and almost soothed me into thinking it would all be OK. I had also phoned her up a few days before, whining about how scared I was. She had reassured me that she controlled the speed and all would be well. Once I was ready, she calmly conveyed the safety elements and I started to breathe and feel more confident.

I was attached to the wakeboard, which is not dissimilar to getting on to a snowboard. Then I was lowered into the water, whilst I clung to the jetty. Katy gently got me to let go and trust that I would float on the surface. I closed my eyes, let go and sure enough, I floated. Next, I had to cling onto the handle, which was attached to the cable, which went across the diameter of the lake. I had to keep my arms straight and when I started lifting off, I had to make my legs go underneath my bum as I was pulled up.

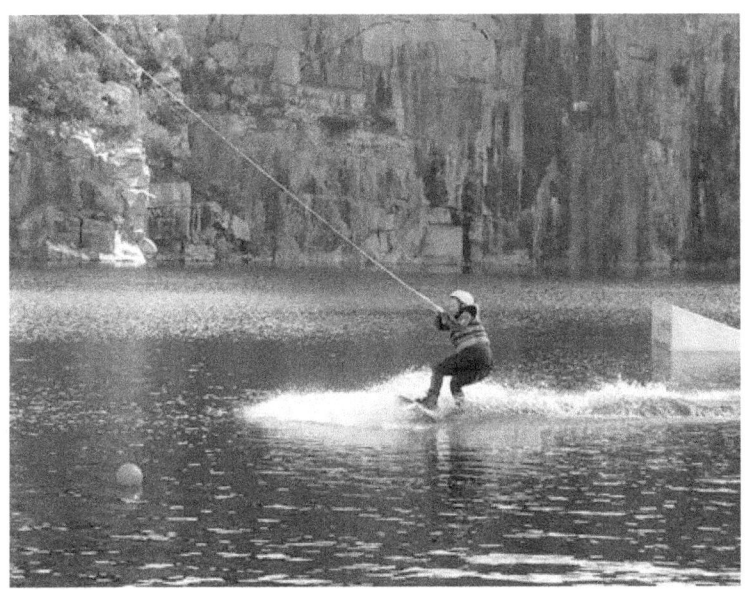

I'm up and actually wakeboarding!

I am not very good at taking multiple instructions at the best of times but it is amazing how having a camera thrust in your face makes you concentrate. The first attempt saw me crashing out into the water. Katy told me what I had done wrong and off I went again. This time, I tentatively got up and turned my body and managed to stay up. I got to the other end of the lake and then I came back again. There was much action from James the Photographer in the boat and I was delighted to be able to come back in, facing the camera, standing tall, feeling confident and smiling. I could hear my family cheering. This felt fantastic!

I managed to get up and back a few times. It was only the last go which saw me lose concentration and face plant in the water a couple of times. I knew that I was tired, so wasn't going to push it. I came out feeling exhilarated and jubilant. The thought of having achieved this feat made me well up and get very emotional. I popped some champagne, posed for pictures and indulged in all of the accolades.

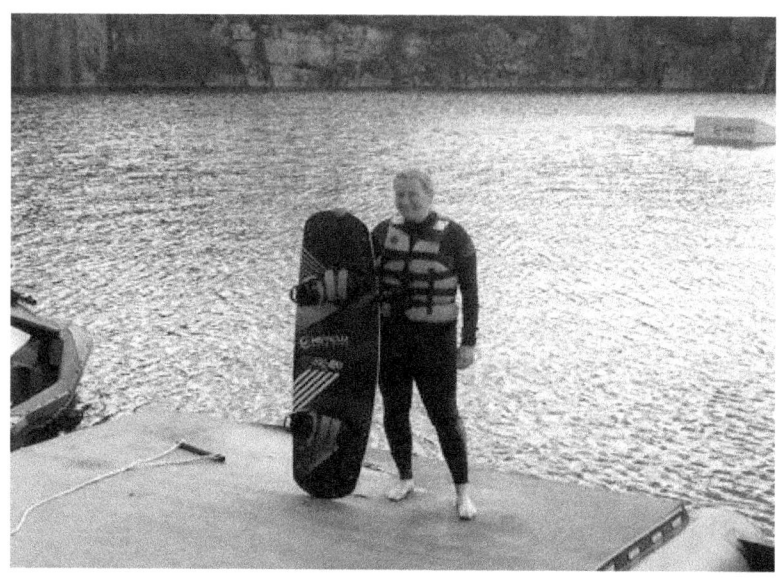

Posing for snaps

On the journey back, the kids said that they were a little disappointed that I hadn't done any jumps whilst on the board and when I switched on the news that evening, the footage was not of my triumphant cruising in on the board, like bloody Boadicea. No, they had me and my fat arse waggling about in an ill-fitting wetsuit, getting dragged about in the water, from one of the rare times I fell.

No matter though; the footage summed up the challenge really. Just me giving it a go, not giving a damn about what I look like, having really helpful instructors or coaches around and a smile on my face. Whatever you are into, that is what sport and fitness does for you: it makes you smile.

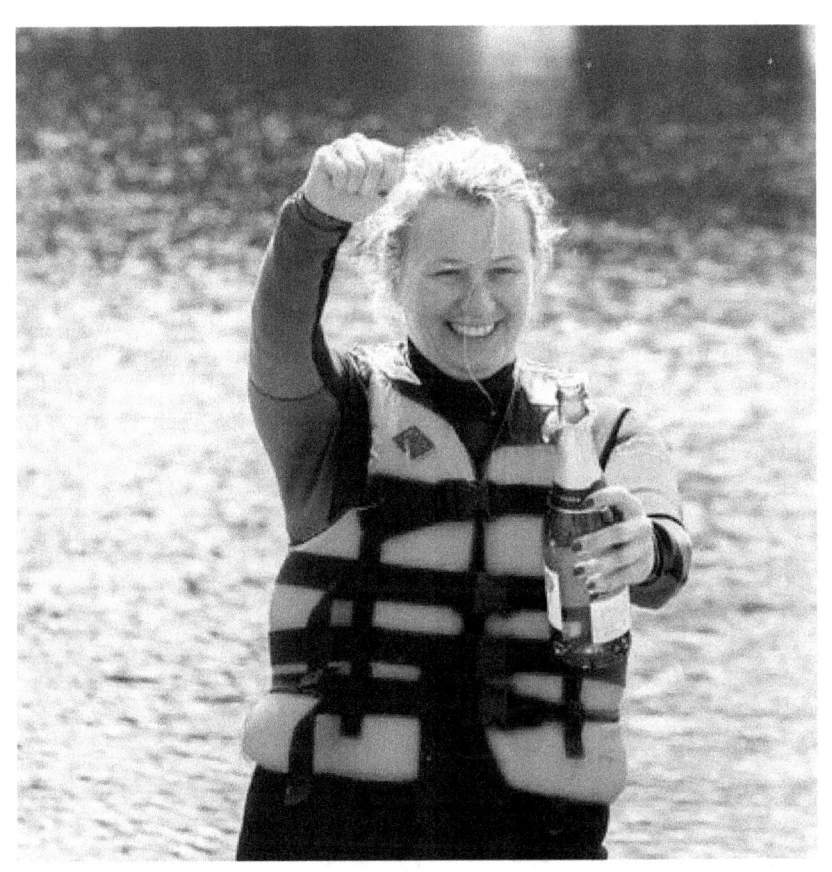

I've done it!

Chapter 12 - My Five Minutes Of Fame

It's been just over a week since I finished the challenge and I've been inundated with lovely messages from friends, family and the clubs and instructors who helped me throughout. I've also had messages from complete strangers who have come across my story via the media, which has all been a bit overwhelming.

Gym-phobic mother completes 'sofa-dodging' challenge... taking part in 100 sports in just one year (including hockey, wakeboarding, yoga and pole dancing)

- Sam Taylor, a self-employed mother-of-three, finished her challenge today
- She travelled more than 10,000 miles in search of new activities
- Ms Taylor sprained her back twice and says she is 'relieved' it's over
- She took between two and five classes per week

By TOM BEVAN FOR MAILONLINE

PUBLISHED: 15:38, 30 April 2015 | UPDATED: 17:15, 30 April 2015

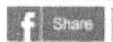 **337** shares 5 View comments

A mother-of-three has gone from a couch potato to an all-action hero after competing in 100 different sports in one year

Sam Taylor, 36, from Bodmin, Cornwall, previously described herself as an unfit 'gym-phobic' but wanted to challenge herself to get off the sofa and live a more active life

Her epic feat, which she finished today with a wakeboarding session, took her more than 10,000 miles around the country and involved sports including Gaelic football, pole dancing, croquet, hockey and yoga

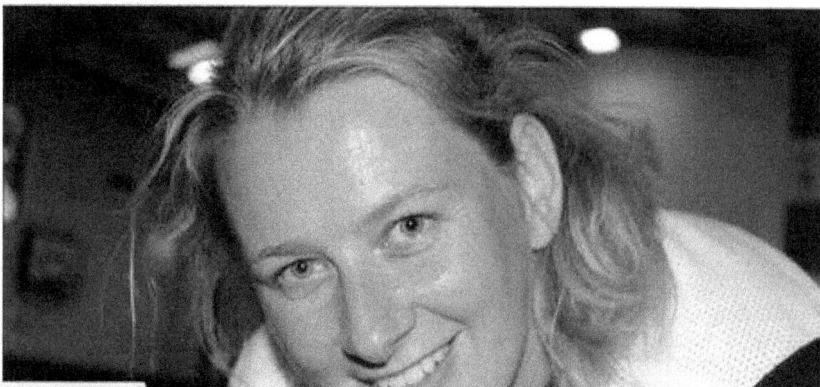

They changed the headline from Unfit Mother to Gymphobic Mother!

The story made it into the regional press and TV, care of ITV Westcountry News. I had a couple of interviews on Radio Cornwall and Heart FM and the story even made the Daily Mail website. In the comments, I even like to think that I had my first "troll," who questioned whether as an "unfit mother of 3," I should be allowed to do such things! I think they were confused by the story. Either way, it made for a very exciting week. My friends threw me a party, complete with a hundred balloons, a bouquet of flowers and a bottle of champagne. I was very touched.

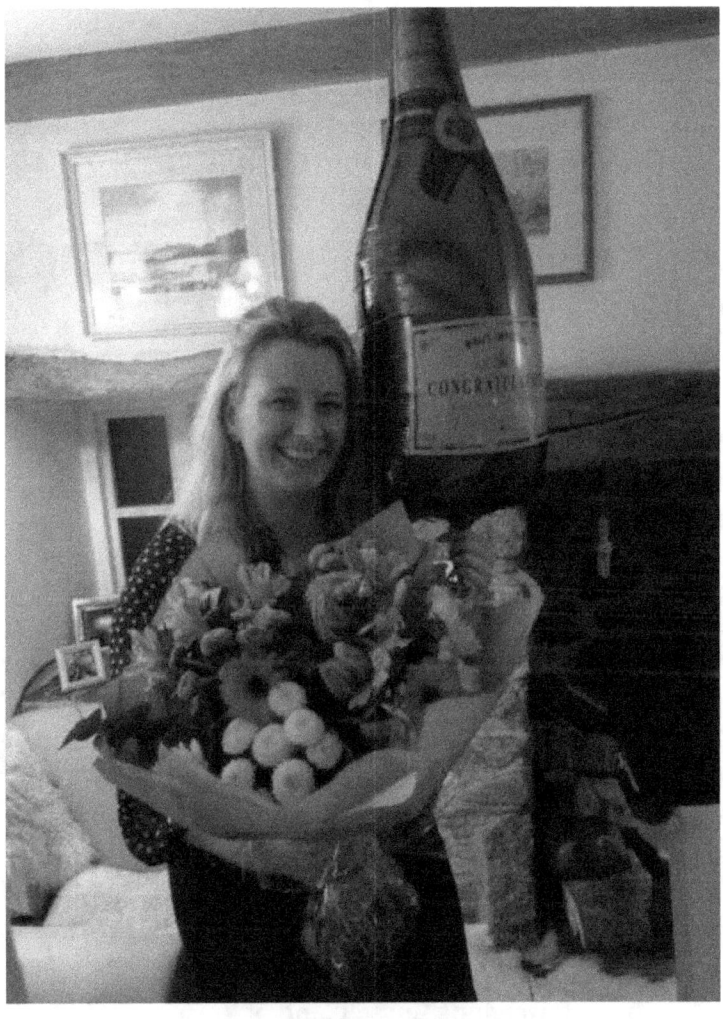

At my "I Survived!" Party

Olly asked me the other day, "are you famous?". I replied that I wasn't but just fleetingly, it was quite exciting and within my hamlet, yes, I probably am a celebrity (behind the horse, who won a rosette in a national competition the other year). Other than a bit of recognition, there have been no other notable indicators of celebrity; there are no paps at the door, nobody has sold a story on me and no Premiership footballer has been in touch for a date. So yes, my 5 minutes of fame have been and gone.

However, what hasn't gone away is the repetitive question posed by nearly everybody I meet. The question, which I should have a well-rehearsed answer for, is "What next?" This question follows me around and when I am not being asked directly by somebody, my subconsciousness takes over and I wake up thinking, *What next?* I have a flippant answer of "sitting on the sofa and trying 100 different wines" but that is only proving to be a stop-gap, before I have to answer properly.

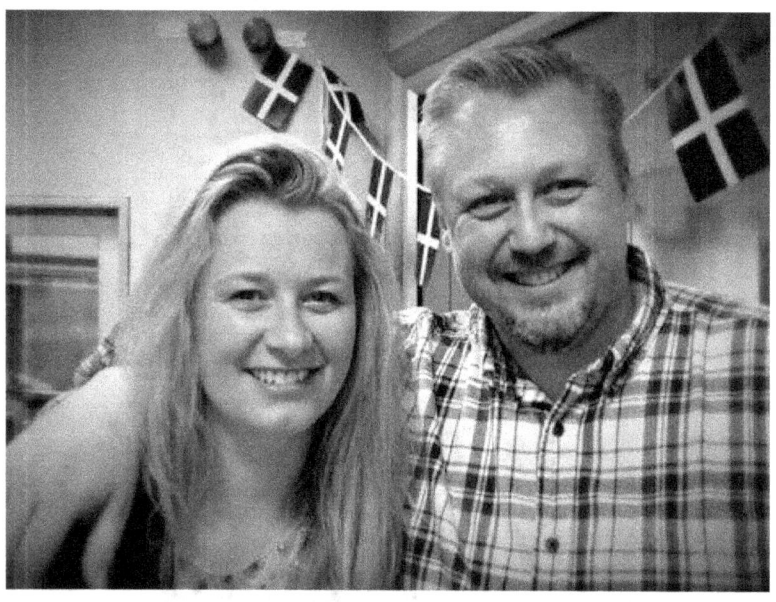

After my interview with David White at BBC Radio Cornwall

I do know that I can't stay on the sofa for too long, as I've gone to the bother of weighing myself and it turns out I am not a professional athlete and I didn't need to carb up for snooker and bowls. I'm quite excited about reminiscing back over everything I've tried and actually going to a class or joining a club and sticking around and making friends, rather than rocking up, doing something once, taking some pictures and then going off again.

Also, I've been approached by five different schools to talk in their assemblies about all that I have tried and all that is out there. My message will definitely be "if I can do it, you can do it" and I really want to spread the word that people do not judge you. If you've taken the brave decision to try something new for whatever reason, whether it is to make friends, lose weight or get fit, in my experience, people only encourage you, they don't judge you. You just need a sprinkle of bravery and a smattering of enthusiasm and I can promise you smiles at the end of it. I'm hoping primary school kids and teenagers take to this message and don't just sit there judging me, but that could prove to be the biggest challenge I've faced yet!

Chapter 13 – My Favourites

Martial Arts

Two of the questions I'm constantly asked by people are "what did you enjoy the most?" and "what will you carry on with?" It's truly difficult to answer those questions as I enjoyed each and every one of the activities I tried but because I did such a varied lot, it is hard to compare them. For instance, it is difficult to compare trampolining with climbing. The only similarity between the two is that I nearly wet myself doing both! Therefore, I've decided to categorise them into the following: team sports, martial arts, individual sports, fitness classes, dance fitness classes, racquet sports, adrenaline sports and water sports. I will then review my experience to come up with my own top 3 favourites in each. It will be my version of the Oscars but unlike the Oscars, it will have little meaning, no red carpet and no Oscar!

So first up, I decided to review Martial Arts and combat sports. Having tried karate, boxing, Capoeira, judo, Kickboxing, KravMaga, Tai Chi, Tang Soo Do, Wrestling and Aikido, I have decided that I am a partial martial artist. The problem I specifically found with these was the differing techniques which were required. One week, I had to punch with my fist, then the next I wasn't allowed to punch but to cup my hand and strike somebody's ear. The chopping, punching, slapping, then reverse chopping, kicking and slapping turned me into a fighter with no discernible skill. The one thing I learnt from all of them though was that the first defence in all situations is to run!

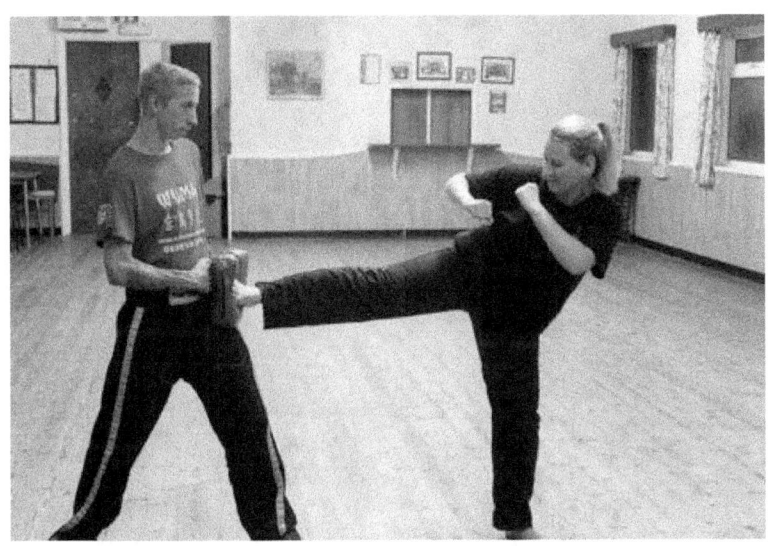

I'm a Nervous Ninja

Although martial arts is not something I will probably carry on with, on account of being a wuss, I really enjoyed being around such a disciplined and respectful environment. This is especially good for kids as they learn respect for their instructor, the heritage of their discipline and it makes them aspire to gain their next belt and continually improve. This was a lovely thing to witness throughout my travels but there was one martial art which stood out for me and that was Aikido. I thought that the movements looked graceful (apart from when I was doing them) and I enjoyed how defence was turned effortlessly into offence. Sensei Jack, my instructor, looked like Keanu Reeves from the Matrix, as he swished about swiftly disarming and nullifying his assailant.

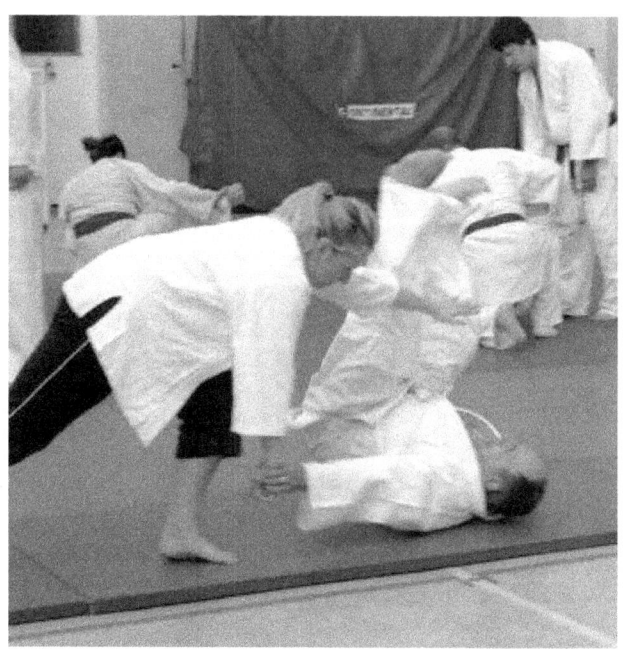

Aikido, My Favourite Martial Art

Next is Capoeira, although this stood apart from the rest, as it included gymnastics and dance, which is probably why I enjoyed it. Also, as there wasn't any contact, I didn't get hurt, which was a big endorsement in my book. So my first two martial arts are fairly "pretty", unlike my next favourite Krav Maga. This couldn't be further away from the first two. Krav Maga, in comparison, is a "get down and dirty" type of affair, derived from the military and adapted to real life situations. I think that self-defence is an important skill to learn, especially as a woman, so it appealed to me.

Extreme Sports

Next up in my review of my favourite sports and classes, I am reminiscing on adrenaline sports or extreme sports if you prefer. Being a self-declared wuss, my definition of an adrenaline sport would be much different to others. For instance, in my experience,

I would class cycling or dodgeball as an adrenaline sport but for the purposes of my review, I've included climbing, Coasteering, ice skating, karting, parkour, rollerskating, Segway, snowboarding, skiing, and wakeboarding.

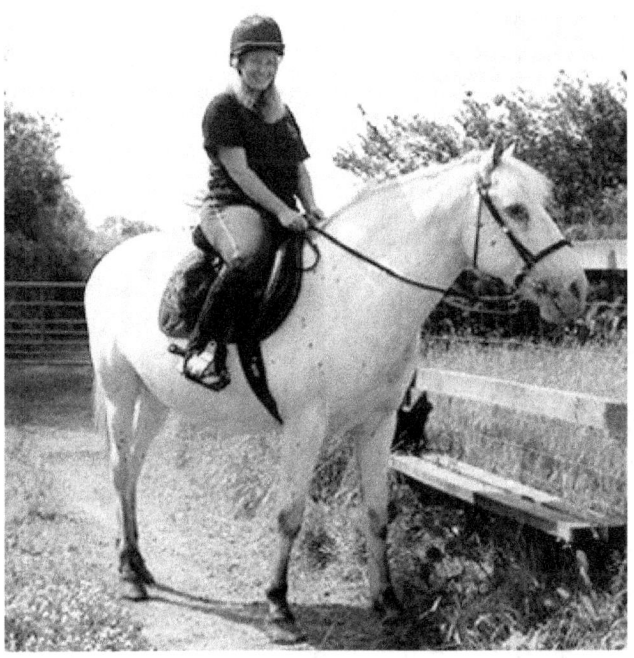

I consider this an extreme sport!

Previously, I thought that anybody participating in an extreme sport was devoid of fear and in my book, frankly unhinged but actually the people I met varied so much, it's hard to define an "adrenaline junky." The more you practise an activity, the more skilled you become and the greater the gap between what people view as extreme. If you are a Coasteering instructor and you jumped off cliffs every day as a living, you would become skilled in that, trust your experience and be able to jump from higher and higher cliffs.

With everything I did, I really tried my best but anything with heights proved to be a real fear. From jumping off a (small) cliff ledge, to climbing a wall, to getting on a horse or standing on a gymnastics beam, these all represented mini challenges in themselves. The only thing I remembered which I couldn't/wouldn't do was on my Coasteering challenge. We stood on the side of a rock pool, which was only as big as a large hula hoop but apparently it was extremely deep, so the instructors dived in and the rest of my fellow coasteerers jumped or bombed into the pool. I stood over the pool and all I had to do was suspend my belief and take a step into the unknown but that unknown was too much for my brain to risk. After many aborted efforts, I conceded defeat and chalked up my first concession to my fears.

However, when I did manage to conquer my fears, the feeling it gave me was absolutely mind blowing and I can see how you could become addicted to that. Considering all that I have done, I would probably say that my favourite was actually snowboarding. I assumed that because of my lack of balance and how rubbish I was at stand up paddle, that this would be an absolute train wreck but for that one hour, I felt that I owned that nursery slope! So not only did I enjoy the activity, it made me re-evaluate my preconceptions.

Followed closely in second, was my very last challenge of wakeboarding. By this point, I was happy with a board and although the press were there and showed my "worst bits" both in terms of my ability and my body parts, the truth of it was I actually did quite well and stood up for most of it. Coupled with the beautiful setting at Kernow Wake Park and the fact that I was going to drink some champagne not an hour after it had finished, I'll always think fondly of wakeboarding.

Last but not least, a height based challenge is in my top 3 – climbing. On paper, it should have been my worse experience but given the encouragement and the instruction I was given, I really broke through a few mental barriers and made it up to the top of the wall. If I think back, that gave me the greatest sense of achievement and exhilaration when I got down to the bottom.

My tips for fellow wuss's is that there is no such thing as "Can't" (apart from when faced with a rock pool) and also that you have to trust your instructor implicitly. If you follow those rules and ensure that you have frequent toilet stops leading up to your activity, you can get through it and actually, you may even enjoy it.

Individual Sports

My next category is the individual sports I tried. I know that some of them can be played as a team but for the purposes of my categorisation, I have included; angling, archery, athletics, bowls, croquet, cycling, fencing, golf, gymnastics, horse riding, orienteering, petanque, running, shooting, snooker and trampolining.

As somebody who has played team sports most of my life, I'm deeply suspicious of individual sports. The onus is completely on you to perform and there is nobody to hide behind or "blame" if you're having an off day. It's like a footballer having to take a penalty for a whole match. No, I am happy to share the limelight and the highs and the lows. Throughout this challenge, I have found that under my own steam and with my own pressure applied, I tend to scream like a pterodactyl – imagine the pressure shot I played in croquet, where the adrenaline got the better of me and I made a noise of a prehistoric bird....very unprofessional.

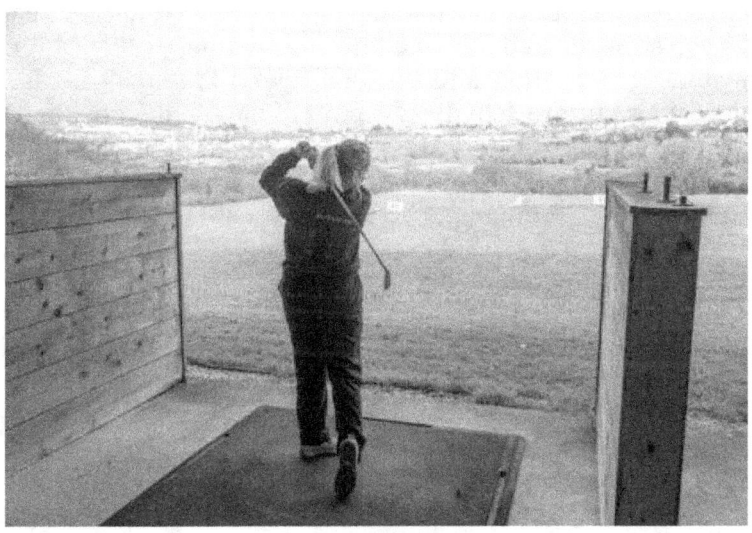

Swing battabing!

As much I started off with my misgivings, I actually enjoyed every single one of the individual sports I tried, so it is hard to pick my top 3. However, there were two which I turned out to be quite good at and those are golf and shooting, so they have to make it on to the podium. I really enjoyed my time playing golf. I enjoyed the release of smacking a ball and have vowed to take myself off the driving range and actually play a full round. I am sure I will spend more time in the sand and water than a toddler at a beach, but it definitely piqued my interest and I might actually think about taking it up (if the round goes well!).

Shooting was my second favourite individual sport. Again, mainly because I was quite good at it – I don't think I could put myself throughout the continual torture of taking up a sport, say fencing and actually being quite rubbish at it. I would get too frustrated with myself, so I'll start with an advantage and go with a bit of natural ability. I didn't think I would get on with shooting, as I am "cack eyed" i.e. my left eye is my master eye, but I am right handed. The first shots which I fired gave me a huge adrenaline rush, as my brain attempted to process all the senses which had just been assailed.

Picking the last sport to make my shortlist was really, tough, as I genuinely enjoyed them all. I have crossed petanque, croquet and bowls off the list, simply because after the pterodactyl screech, I tend to drop an expletive and these sports don't really fit with a deranged, foul mouthed, frustrated and sulky player. They require patience, strategy and playing the long game, whereas I need immediate gratification and personal glory. Trampolining is also off the list as a future activity, given that I have a 36F bust and that after three children, I have the pelvic floor strength of a 70-year-old woman.

Looking at the remaining pelvic floor friendly activities, there is one which sticks out and that is orienteering. Although I was fairly rubbish at it and my daughter and her friend Lily literally had the ability to find all the posts, until I dragged them "off-road" into brambles and bushes, I do plan to do this with the family, as it is essentially a competitive walk (although it is mostly run to get the best times). I think this will be a really fun thing to do together and be an easier sell than a standard walk with the family.

So there we have it, my top 3 individual sports are golf, shooting and orienteering. I just need a country estate so I can do all three in my own back garden!

Team Sports

Choosing 3 favourite team sports out of the mahoosive number I tried is a mahoosive challenge in itself! In total, I tried 20 (land based team sports) and they were:

- American Football
- Baseball
- Basketball
- Cheerleading
- Cricket
- Dodgeball
- Floorball
- Football
- Gaelic Football
- Handball, Hockey
- Korfball
- Lacrosse
- Netball
- Rounders
- Rugby
- Ultimate Frisbee
- Volleyball
- Walk Football
- Wheelchair Rugby.

When asked about my favourites, I usually dig around this fertile ground for anecdotes, as there are rich pickings. Turning out to play American Football with a dozen daunting looking dudes, was a memorable experience, as was trying to keep up with the guys in wheelchair rugby as they raced around me. In terms of extremes, I went through every weather system imaginable; from playing lacrosse in the torrential rain and then driving 300 miles home to playing handball on a beautiful, golden sandy beach on a hot, sunny day. No matter the weather, what couldn't be dampened in any club which I visited was the banter. Obviously, there was time for being serious, when drills were being practised and the games were being played but before and after, the jokes flew!

This is why I love team sports and to pick just three out of the 20 is not easy at all. My third favourite would probably be floorball, a sport which is familiar to me as a hockey player.

Floorball is essentially indoor hockey, or as I described it; ice hockey without the ice. It is not widely played in the UK – my closest club was a five hour round-trip drive away but it is gaining popularity and growing fast.

My second favourite team sport is another minority sport, which isn't widely known and that is korfball. Korfball is a mixed sport and is reminiscent of netball. I really enjoy netball but Korfball gives it a different dimension as it includes guys. The play was fast and furious but actually quite easy to pick up. We only had a small introduction and some drills before me and all the other newbies were subbed on to play a practise match. It was a very friendly club, so therefore it grabs my silver medal. With my silver and bronze sports, they are kind of like long distance romances, as there are no clubs in Cornwall. Actually, they are probably more like holiday romances; you got hot and sweaty for a bit, you remember them fondly but chances are you aren't going to meet up again. I will, of course, stalk them on social media and keep up to date with what they are up to, but the liaison was sweet and brief.

However, my gold medal goes to a more locally played and more popular sport, which is...drumroll...cricket! To take the romance analogy on, cricket and I are childhood sweethearts. From the age of 11, I was an avid cricket watcher and in the early 90s, that represented true commitment, given the middle order batting collapses you had to painfully and regularly witness. To be interested and knowledgeable about a sport from the safety of an armchair is very different from actually picking up a bat and ball and actually playing, so I was a little nervous that my illusions might be shattered. However, I really enjoyed playing. I was rubbish at catching and bowling the ball but I enjoyed batting and throwing, so overall it went well and I am so glad that I managed to eventually play the game I love to watch. It was slightly tinged with regret that I didn't take it up when I was younger and had the opportunity but there you go, I decided to be a mediocre hockey player instead of a mediocre cricket player!

I hope you can see from my list that there is a veritable smorgasbord of team sports which you can try and just to let you into a bit of a secret...no matter what your age or ability, every amateur club will welcome you with open arms, as they all need players, supporters, officials, volunteers and committee members to survive and prosper. So don't be like and me and leave it 25 years to play something. If you fancy giving something a go, just go ahead and try it!

Water Sports

I have always fancied being a mermaid. I started dreaming about this ambitious vocation at around 3 and a half. It was then firmly cemented as my ideal career after watching Darryl Hannah in Splash. After that film, I spent a lot of time perfecting various warbles around the house and I insisted on buying a hair crimper with my birthday money.

Apart from my wavy hair, I never really progressed in the other skills required, such as breathing underwater, being a strong swimmer, developing a tail and generally evolving into an amphibian. As I grew older, I abandoned my idea as impractical but I have always had an affinity for water; in times of stress, I find staring at a puddle quite relaxing. So, I was really looking forward to becoming at one with water and water-based activities.

I tried, with various levels of success, Canoeing, Gig Rowing, Sailing, Rowing, Stand Up Paddle, Surfing, Surf Life-Saving, Water Polo, Wild Swimming and Underwater Hockey, otherwise known as Octopush. In surmising my abilities in this category, I would say it varied. It turns out that I have set criteria for being at one with the water and that is, I don't like falling into it i.e. losing my balance on a board and wiping out and I don't like it if it is too cold.

Taking these factors into account, I, therefore, proclaim that my third favourite water based sport was Water Polo. The gameplay is easy to pick up and it is a fantastic way to get fit. My second place spot would definitely go to Gig Rowing. I had the most beautiful experience of rowing out on a gorgeous, sunny morning on my favourite part of the Cornish coast. Although I didn't fall in the water, I did fall down before I got into the boat, but I have decided to not mark it down because I am unbalanced.

However, there is a standout favourite and that would be Underwater Hockey. Before I took part, I had really serious back pain and it was severely hindering my ability to carry on with my challenge, as well as being able to do my washing and other menial tasks. I tentatively got myself into all the gear at the pool and although I couldn't properly take part, as it takes some practise diving down 3m to the bottom of the pool, I did hover on the surface, with my snorkel and flippers and watch what was going on underneath. I swam up and down and tried a bit of diving, whilst trying to emulate the action of a mermaid, and when I got out, my back was completely and utterly and miraculously cured! No more pain, no more wincing, I was fixed. For that,

Underwater Hockey has to be my most favourite and most memorable water sport. My mermaid, fairy godmother must have remembered me and waved her magic tail!

Dance Inspired Fitness Classes

Before I started my challenge, I was completely phobic about fitness classes. I had attended approximately 3 or 4 in my life and each time, I never went back. I found that anything which involved rhythm thoroughly off-putting. I felt like a spotlight would mysteriously beam straight on to me, so that my lack of co-ordination would be magnified and that people would judge me or snigger behind my back.

If I am grateful for one thing out of my challenge, is that my misgivings have been completely blown out of the water and I now love shaking my big booty in a class. I have even taken to freestyling at points because I have learnt the secret...nobody cares what you look like! When you embrace this truth, it really does set you free and Sista, (or Bruva) you can set about shaking what your Mamma gave you!

For my dance-themed fitness classes, I tried Clubbercise, Fitsteps, Zumba, BarreConcept and I danced for 6 hours at the Comic Relief Danceathon in Wembley. I have to say that a dance fitness class is now going to be part of my life. When I look back at each of them, all I did was smile throughout and the atmosphere was fantastic.

I would have to say that my favourite was Clubbercise, just because I am a 90s chick at heart and can't get enough of a bit of rave music. I loved the fact that the class was so different, given that it was set in a darkened room; so again, you didn't have to feel self-conscious at all. There were people of all ages and sizes in the class which I attended, all busy waving their glow sticks and having a good time.

Second favourite in this category would be Zumba. Zumba has been around for ages and for the reasons previously stated, I veered away from it, fearing the dance steps required. When I went to the class, I was a little fuzzy headed from the night before but boy, did this wake me up. I absolutely loved it. Given that there are no Clubbercise classes down my way at the moment, I will be finding my local Zumba class to get my groove on.

Close behind Zumba was FitSteps, which is the Strictly Come Dancing themed class. Again, I went in with a suitcase full of preconceptions about not being able to pick up the steps and looking a fool. I think it was in this class that I learnt the secret – remember; nobody cares what you look like. You want to sit down, mid track and take a breather? Sit down – nobody cares! You want to fling your hands around a little bit? Go for your life – nobody cares! Note: This does not apply if you suddenly want to set off the fire alarm or decide to fart loudly in time to the music.

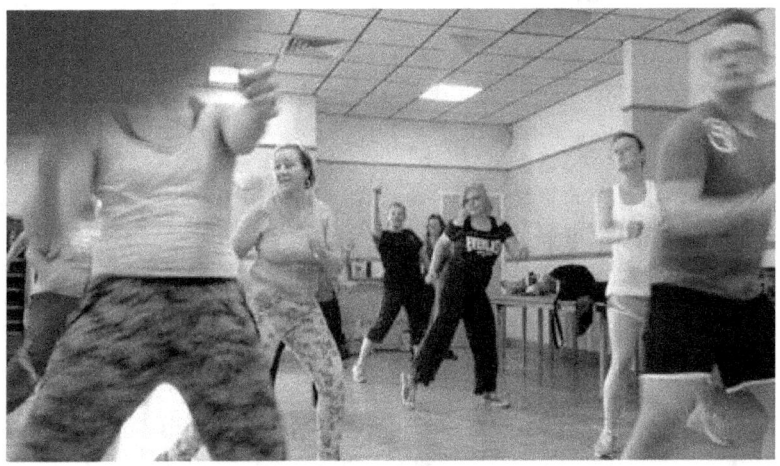

Yeah, I'm out of time!

You get what I mean though. These classes are about getting up, getting out and having fun. If you are like me and need to be tricked into getting fit by mistaking exercise for enjoyment, then get yourself into one of these classes and give it at least four tries, smile and remember the secret!

Fitness Classes

So, this is my last review of my 100 sports and fitness class challenge and I end on fitness classes. When I first started the challenge, I thought I would just be adding aerobics and step on to my list of possible fitness classes but it turns out that we don't live in the 1990s anymore and this century has thrown up a plethora of different fitness classes to try. In all, I tried: Aqua Aerobics, Body combat, Bootcamp, Buggyfit, Bums, Tums and Thighs, Cardio Tennis, Circuit Training, Cross Fit, Insanity, Nordic Walking, Online Exercise, Personal Training, Pilates, Piloxing, Pole Fitness, Poolbiking, Powerhooping, Spinning, TRX, TyreFit, Yoga, Kettlercise and KickBoxing Aerobics. I had a go at all of those classes and there are still dozens which I didn't get around to!

How do I go about choosing my three favourites out of this lot? Well, taking out yoga and Nordic walking (which were two of my favourites) but aren't really classed as a fitness classes as such, I have to look at the pros and cons of my experience to find my perfect fitness class. If I was to make up a lonely hearts advert for my long term class, it would say: "Fuller figured, 30 something, mother of 3, with questionable pelvic floor muscle strength, past commitment issues and a loathing of floor to ceiling mirrors, seeks local class with GSOH, challenging but fun and calorie busting. Burpees and plankers need not apply."

The one class which fulfilled the criteria was Kettlercise. At no point did I think that this would be my knight in shining armour class, given that I have always laughed off having bingo wings and no upper body strength but although I found the class challenging, I finished it feeling that not only had I had a proper workout but that I really enjoyed it. We just clicked. I had to kiss a lot of frogs but in the end, I found the class which got me hot and sweaty.

My second favourite class was Cardio Tennis. I really like the idea of a sport making a fitness class version, on the basis that I really enjoyed a various number of sports but I wouldn't want to play them competitively on a weekend. I just want to enjoy an hour a week playing and getting fit at the same time. I am a big fan of tennis, so this was right up my street, not that it particularly mattered, as it wasn't about getting the ball back over the net, it was about running to get the ball.

There are a number of other fitness classes which I enjoyed but in terms of having a GSOH, I would say that my 3rd favourite would be Powerhooping. It took a little while to master the old hoop but I know that in two to three classes, I would be twisting with the best of them. The class was very different and because it was so unexpected, it is one that sticks out in my mind.

When I finished the challenge, I decided to give myself the month off to recuperate and take stock. Once the month had finished and my local off-license had seen a massive upsurge in business, I decided that my next course of action was to write up my favourite experiences in each category. As I typed this, I was still thinking of what to do next before I actually commit to a new regime and I find myself back where I was before I started; finding it difficult to get off the sofa!

Admittedly, I have started walking the kids to school twice a week, which is a four mile round trip but they break up for holidays soon and then what? I tell myself that I am so busy, which I am but I know that I have to find the time to exercise. 26% of women in the UK are classed as inactive and I know that I have to fight my desk-bound lifestyle to ensure that I don't end up as one of those statistics. So even knowing what I know: that working out makes me smile, that those endorphin things are really cool, that people are friendly and non-judgemental and that I have found my perfect activities, I still have to change my mind-set, ditch my excuses and actually get on with making a long-term commitment, not to the fitness regime but to me and to my health.

Chapter 14 - What Next?

OK, so it has been three months now since the end of my challenge. At the end, I did say I was going to take a month off before starting my timetable of activity, which I was going to take up post-challenge. It has now been three months and I have essentially spent the time eating, drinking and being extremely inactive, citing "tomorrow" as the day to start my new life.

All of this procrastination and gluttony has meant that if I carry on in this manner for another three months, I could feasibly audition for Jabba the Hutt's understudy in the upcoming Star Wars Movie. Excuses like "my body needs a rest" and "it's the summer holidays" all came to a grinding halt at the weekend, when I went to a friend's party and all I felt comfortable wearing was my "fat dress" and the pictures I saw after was devastating, so it starts tomorrow, not "tomorrow"!

Apart from turning myself into the size of a small building, I had the pleasure of awarding my Mini SofaDodgers at the local primary school with their certificates for achieving a certain number of sports in two terms. For 10 different sports, you received a bronze award, 15 a gold, 20 was platinum and for 25 different sports, they received the accolade of being the Ultimate SofaDodger. The poor mites who achieved this were probably expecting a cape or something but they too got a certificate, just with a different colour on it.

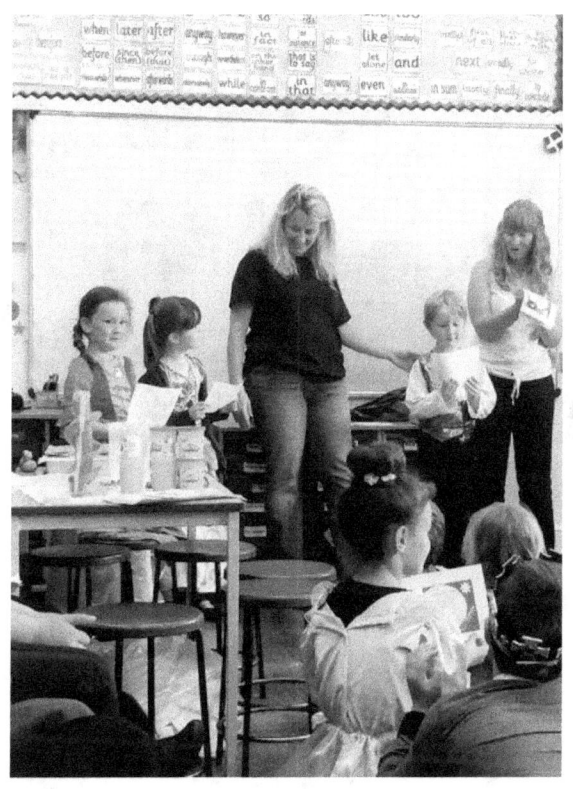

Mini SofaDodgers Accepting Their Certificates

In two terms, the Ultimate SofaDodgers tried everything from rock climbing to table tennis to ultimate Frisbee and they seemed to enjoy keeping a track of what they had done in their own booklets. The school will be carrying on the theme of trying new sports next term, as they have more yet to try – this is fantastic and definitely what it is all about. Trying something new and finding out what you enjoy. These kids are really lucky to have such a supportive school which enabled them to try such a variety, especially as this is set against a backdrop of PE budget cuts in state schools.

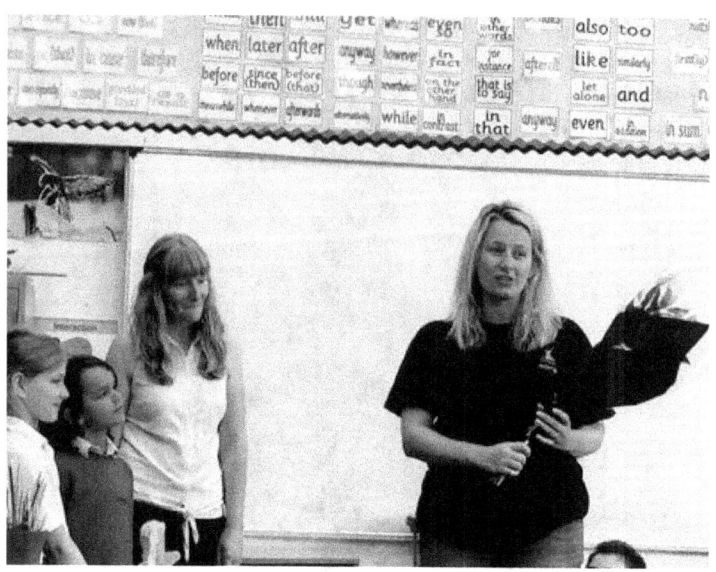

Here I am telling the kids not to be afraid to try new activities

However, what I think was great with this challenge is that you were not judged on your performance, but rewarded for trying something and I think that is very important. Kids who show a talent at a particular sport, can then take it up further and then be judged on ability i.e. getting selected for a team, badges for swimming or gymnastics.

What is required, I feel, is that kids are given the opportunity to sample as many different pursuits as possible. As I found in my own challenge, it is easy to talk yourself out of something by saying "you can't" do something, or feel that trying something will make you look silly. By trying something early, children will hopefully not take on a certain preconception of an activity into their teenage years and beyond.

Now that I am done, I am inspired to talk to more children and more schools about the fun and all the positives you can get from sport and being active. Like Coach Smallworth, who I met at the Cornish Sharks, said, "everybody has a gift." I believe that and I believe that everybody has their perfect sport or activity – some will have more than one but it is the part of school, government, national governing bodies and parents to help them find their favourites. Sport and fitness is good for your health, good for your mind and good for your soul. I went to a recent conference and the Health Minister said: "Show me somebody active and I will show you somebody who isn't lonely". This reflects my experience and what I have witnessed throughout my challenge. I have met all kinds of people, from all walks of life, all ages, all sizes and shapes and all with differing abilities. Some of the people I met will compete in Rio 2016; some people will feel the achievement of leaving their house for an hour a week to go to a fitness class. Both the Olympic contender and the average Jo or Jane started their own journeys in exactly the same way; they got off the sofa.

Chapter 15 – The People Who Inspired Me

I was fortunate to have met and been inspired by so many people across my challenge. What I soon realised shortly into my adventures are that these people were the real story; they teach people how to get the most out of themselves, they volunteer their time to run our sports clubs. They bring on the grass roots, they develop our potential; these people are the silent heroes behind sport and fitness in our communities.

I not only wanted to write about my own adventures but I went back to the people that helped me with my journey and asked them what made them take up their own activity and what it means to them. I would love to share, in their words, their stories:

I began Nordic Walking over 4 years ago. I'd had enough of being overweight and not having the energy to enjoy my life. Diets alone didn't work for me and I hated gyms and classes as being overweight I was very self-conscious. I found a Nordic Walking group and before long I decided that I really enjoyed it...it wasn't a race, there was no competition and no one was looking at me thinking how awful I looked because we were all too busy out enjoying ourselves. Not only was it good for my confidence and health, but I found that I was getting some "me" time too, being a mum I needed a break now and again and didn't realise it. I decided to buy a set of really nice poles; I wanted to make sure I kept on Nordic Walking so I thought if I buy these poles I will HAVE to use them. I started to calorie count as well and the weight began to fall off. I walked twice a week for roughly an hour each time. In about 8 months I had lost a total of 4 stone.

Now, I get to share my passion for Nordic Walking with my walkers who range in age from 35 to over 70, both male and female and of all shapes and sizes. I notice on my Beginners Workshops that Nordic Walking seems to give people confidence and all those insecurities and worries about exercising vanish as we walk along chatting and enjoying the beautiful Cornish countryside. On a weekly basis my walkers Nordic Walk, in their own words for the camaraderie, fitness, escape, exercise, support and to feel revitalised, invigorated, exhilarated and healthy. Every time we Nordic Walk I hear "I didn't feel like coming out today" then by the middle of the walk "I'm glad I came out today" and by the end someone has said "I feel better for that." It's great to know Nordic Walking is making people feel better and get healthier!

Kelly, Owner at Walk Kernow

Short mat bowls is a sport enjoyed by participants from school age to those over 90 years old. Being played indoors, it avoids the vagaries of the weather and can be played night or day. Most clubs have equipment to enable those wishing to give it a try a chance to participate without initial outlay. One golden rule for every club is that in order to play one must be wearing totally smooth bottomed footwear. This is essential to protect the mat. Most beginners start by wearing thick socks before buying their own bowling shoes.

Our club was started some 10 years ago with a membership of 14. Over the years numbers have grown to our current membership of 26. We have practice sessions, referred to by aficionados as 'Roll Ups', twice a week in the afternoon. Currently of our 26 members, 16 pay their affiliation fee and are eligible to enter County competitions. The remaining 10 members just enjoy the comradery and regularly turn up for Roll Up sessions and participate in the social events organised by the club. The average age of our members is in the mid-70's and ability varies between those playing at county level, beginners, and those with physical disabilities that means they struggle to keep their woods on the mat. No matter, all participate in our Roll Up sessions and the encouragement offered to those that struggle is always enthusiastically given and received.

Richard, who suffers with severe arthritis, finds he is unable to bend and has to rely on a walking stick to support his weight when he leans forward to release his wood. He still manages to bowl a number of very accurate woods each session. Although not a member of this club, my friend Henry, who last year had to have a colostomy and now has to live with a bag, is back bowling and has recently been selected to represent the county in a match against an England select team. A factor in his recovery was his determination to resume his bowling and the encouragement from his many friends in the bowling community to do so as quickly as he felt able. I have played with and against players in wheelchairs, carrying oxygen cylinders, registered blind and amputees. Proving that many physical disabilities can be overcome when it comes to playing short mat bowls.

My first experience of a competitive match was an eye opener. I was 62 at the time and playing lead in a two wood fours event. The lady lead for the opposition was obviously of advanced years. At the conclusion of the match, in which I had struggled and she had out bowled me by a wide margin, she approached me and enquired as to my experience and time bowling. I responded I had been bowling for 6 months and this was my first competitive match. She replied, "I am 92 and have been short mat bowling for 45 years, keep practising." I later found out she continued competitive bowling for another 3 years.

The message is simple: whatever your age, if you feel you would benefit from gentle exercise, improved social life and a new challenge then contact your local short mat bowling club who will welcome you with open arms.

George Loveridge, Blisland Short Mat Bowls Club

I started enjoying cricket at a young age as my dad used to play. I became a regular scorer for his team 'Pickwick' in St Issey as I approached my teens but I never played myself. School and teenage years took over and I didn't really get involved until my children started training at Wadebridge CC from the age of about 8. Before long we were going to matches and I became heavily involved with the club and subsequently dragged onto the committee. Given the opportunities that the club had given my children, it was a way of thanking them and I actually enjoyed making a difference. I became part of the 'cricket family'.

Now my eldest is almost 17, her cricket has progressed to a national level and we are regular travellers across the country. There can't be many cricket grounds or service stations for that matter that we haven't been to! Wadebridge CC is also still a big part of our lives and we have made some very close friends. Cricket is still very male dominated and although mindsets are changing and it is fair to say that women's cricket has had a moment this year, it is important that this continues. There is a big problem with gender and salary inequality despite countless women achieving excellence and achievements men can only dream of.

Recognising this, in 2014, I set up a women's section at Wadebridge CC. We quickly became established and joined the counties women league where in our first season we came 3rd. This year we were a close second and hunger that first place next year! We had winning success in the winter indoor league and had the opportunity to compete in regional finals. Our team is made up of girls and women from the age of 12 however we encourage girls of all ages to join in on training nights....our youngest is only 7! Building relationships and creating opportunities for the girls is very important to me and I would encourage everyone to join in and become one of the 'cricket family'.

Lowenna Roberts, Wadebridge Cricket Club

I am sat here typing whilst one of my trainers (also a qualified nurse and fitpro) is delivering a Neurological fitness class to a group of human beings. The humans in here consist of a young woman with dementia and Huntington's Disease, and an elderly chap with Parkinson's, a husband and wife, both with Parkinson's and both with a stroke and an amazing woman with Multiple Sclerosis. There are 14 souls in this class, all with stories and in spite of their disease or disability; they have spirit, cheekiness and vigour for life.

Sam asked me how being an instructor has changed my life and has it changed the life of my clients.

I remember being sat in a conference for long-term conditions back in 2009, sobbing when a client stood up to speak and claimed I saved his life. I am para-phrasing but his words were: "Without Helen I probably wouldn't be here today. She gave me confidence and the will to live". This really struck a chord with me and made me sob, not because I was sad but the reality that being kind and giving a little bit of yourself can truly make someone's day.

It's not all about the aesthetics and being body beautiful. It takes all colours to make up a rainbow. Fitness and wellbeing isn't rocket science, however, studying the human body and brain is a vast science and that is essential. The delivery of classes and personal training often looks easy. We are constantly checking, tweaking and progressing movement patterns, yet the client thinks they are simply swaying.

As for me, I have found my calling in life. I can't imagine being in any other industry. Inspiring the next generation of instructors and observing incredible evolutions in clients is enough. Over the years, I have watched less confident clients attend my classes that have crossed over to the dark side and become instructors in my beloved profession. I have seen transformations and huge mind-set changes. I have observed utter joy in my classes and watched people develop and grow. I have seen girls grow into great women, with great careers, curves to love and not to mention some radical body makeovers.

As a mum, wife, carer, friend, goddess, business owner- with curves and clearly no shame; I apparently am a realistic role model. I have created a persona to my customers that my work is easy and I can juggle it all. The Fitness profession can be really tough especially as music has ruined my life. If the beat has 8 counts in it, I can do anything with it. Everyone song I hear has a home in a step class, Zumba class, Age Defying Fitness, Body Balance. I never intend to stop learning. I am fascinated by anatomy and want to encourage anyone to move AND keep moving. We need to evolve our movement patterns as we age and keep things appropriate to our aging processes for great hormone balance.

For me health and wellness is more important than just exercise, followed by decent laughter, good sleep and daily meditation. Oh, and the perfectly good glass of wine with best friends.

Have I changed lives? I hope so. I intend to be provocative and create thought inspiring subjects. I want my clients to leave me feeling fabulous and motivated. I want them to get lost for one hour, debt free, not a wife or a mother but just being in the moment, utterly satisfied and happy. I want them to go home and re-enact their experiences or better still, just be happy.

Life is tough these days; we are so driven and influenced by social media and crap icons. I want to be a better version of who I am every day, which enables me to help and make other people be a better version of themselves; then I can die content.

Helen Tite, Core Health Consultancy

My first experience of petanque – the French game sometimes called boules – was in Brittany on the very wet afternoon in July 1998 when France won the World Cup. I was at a birthday celebration for two Breton friends. At some point in the festivities,

I found myself in a borrowed waterproof, with three boules in hand, plus a large glass of wine and a huge cigar, playing petanque with other guests on a narrow and very rough strip of gravel alongside an adjacent country road. Any small success by the new player was cheered wildly; setbacks earned commiserations and a refill. That was my first experience of petanque as a social and convivial game, and I loved it!

This impression was reinforced when a few years later my partner, Susan and I found that the game was played at the pub near our home in Tregony, Cornwall, and were able to start taking part regularly. Again, it was very social, great fun and accompanied by lots of laughter, but we also became aware of the skills involved. It took several months before we won a game but with advice and help from other players, we began to get the hang of pointing – lobbing your boule to roll close to the small wooden 'jack' – and of shooting opponents' boules out of the way when they got close. Cornwall was for a time home to Paul Lancaster, a former member of the Great Britain petanque squad, and coaching from him, plus regular practice, made a big difference to our playing skills, our ability to 'read' a playing surface and a game, and our understanding of tactics.

We also joined Kernow Petanque, the Cornwall region of the English Petanque Association (EPA), and in addition to our weekly club nights in Tregony, moved to the Sports Club, we were able to take part in summer and winter leagues, county competitions and matches against other regions. We even won a few regional trophies. The annual inter-regional competition organised by the EPA, with more than 700 players coming together from all over the country, became a regular fixture on our calendar.

The Internet makes it easy to watch top-level competitions from France, often live. The best players have a level of precision in their play which makes some games quite awe-inspiring. At the same time, it's comforting to see that even top players can suffer the same mischances which afflict us! It has also been a pleasure to go to watch major competitions in France: there's nothing quite like sitting among a knowledgeable French crowd when big-name national players are competing and every successful point and shot is applauded. At the other end of the scale, we have also had a great deal of fun playing in local village competitions while on holiday, winning enough games to gain a friendly regard for 'les anglais' playing the locals at their own game.

Back in Tregony, there are still regular week-night sessions, plus occasional informal play at weekends. It's great to see new players coming along; trying what seems, at first, a ridiculously easy game but then starting to appreciate the skills involved and getting hooked. It really is a game which can be played by anyone from eight to 80 plus, but the abiding problem is bringing younger people into the sport and, once involved, encouraging them to stay in the face of so many potential counter attractions.

Quite what it is that makes petanque so enticing is hard to define. The mix of skill and sociability is certainly a factor, but so too is developing a rapport with teammates, understanding your own and others' strengths and weaknesses. The tactile 'feel' of the boules themselves is addictive. Each is a hollow steel sphere weighing roughly the same as one-and-a-half pots of jam: throwing them effectively to gain a point or to smash an opposition boule out of play is very satisfying! In principle petanque is also a game which ought to be played when the sun is shining, the air is warm and just being outside is a pleasure. Being Britain, of course, that's not always the case: not infrequently you find yourself playing with wet feet, a steady trickle of rainwater down the back of your neck and the jack beginning to float on a puddle. But that just underlines quite what a hold this game can take.

Graeme Kirkham, Tregony Petanque Club

I started attending a Yoga class when I was 26 and my second son was about 6 months old. My back ached and I was super stressed out. Various people I knew had been attempting to get me to try a yoga class for some years, I was extremely reluctant as I was far too rock and roll for that kind of hippy malarkey. It wasn't until things started to hurt that I started to listen to them. I also think now, looking back, that I knew they were right in more ways than I was prepared to admit. I wasn't a proper rock and roll legend as my outer façade was attempting to suggest, I was actually, probably, the biggest hippy around and deep down I knew that if I started to make the positive changes that Yoga offers I would like it and my rock and roll years would be over forever.

I went to a weekly class on a Tuesday evening for 6 years - well, I actually got kicked out of my Tuesday class when I was about 4 and a half months pregnant with my 3rd child – my teacher was not maternity trained and I was a bit gung-ho.

I was really getting into the practises and so was annoyed to be asked to find a pregnancy class but it was absolutely the right thing for her to do! I went straight back to my lovely class when my new baby was about 12 weeks old - it was sacred 'me' time. The only hour in the week when I wasn't up to my bleary eyeballs in mumness.

When we moved to Cornwall in 2006, I lost my familiar weekly group and started to look for new Yoga classes. I had tried various classes but always continued with my first teacher. I decided that one of the best ways to learn more was to start doing courses and pretty much the only way to get to learn about the philosophy and the theories was to start a teacher training course. Which I duly did for the next 4 years – part of the process of training to teach involved setting up classes- I hadn't really thought this through as I didn't really want a yoga teaching job, I just wanted to learn. I set up a class, and then ended up with another class and then another and in hardly any time at all I was teaching 8 classes a week.

When I graduated from my training course I opened a little studio in Truro, Cornwall and ran classes there as well as driving round teaching my usual classes some of which I'd then been doing for 4 years. The studio was cute and I loved it –the ceiling was bit low and there were a few issues with access and it was a little hidden so I started looking for a little place that was easier to find with higher ceilings! I found our current venue- it was about 4 times the size of what I was looking for but I thought it was great for the job so thought 'what the heck- let's give it a go'.

So - What is Yoga?

When people ask me this I usually say 'UMMMMM.'

I have an idea that they already think they know what they want me to say- something about exercise and breathing- that's a nice a simple explanation and to be honest it's the one I normally give.

It's always a little unsatisfying to leave it at that, though. I want to say more... how long have you got?

I attend a fair few business seminars, talks and events- I am familiar with the concept of 'strap lines', 'elevator pitches', pithy, clever, concise and combined with eye-catching branding this is the way to SELL something. I have given considerable thought to this and so far I have been unable to find a way to say something that sums Yoga up in way that make it sounds like you gotta do it!

What is it? It's a process of searching for something inside yourself, the thing that stays with you when all else is lost. It can only be found in quiet moments when the everyday clatter of stuff and thoughts is blown away by a surprising breeze through your head. It's not a quick process, it's not easy, it takes courage to start that journey and the only way to navigate is to keep coming back to stillness, and ask nothing. It's not fun, it's not glamorous, it's not pretty, and it's not a journey that takes you anywhere- despite what you might hear or see Yoga is not really a journey towards being able to stand on your head or balance on your hands. If that's a journey you're interested in taking I can take you on it – no problem. When you are balancing I will wonder is there space? Is there is peace? Is there contentment?

Yoga for me is not something I chose - I was compelled to it. It chose me. I have fallen out with it, I have thrown it away, it has broken me and it has put me back together.

It has given me my life, it has taken me places I would never have dreamed, it has brought the most wonderful people through my door every day!

If you were to ask any number of the students what Yoga means to them you are likely to get as many different answers as the number of people you ask- 'it helps with my back', 'it strengthens my knees', 'it helps to prevent headaches'. The only thing that many will agree on is that if you come and practice after an hour you leave somehow feeling better.

I quite often say 'It's not rocket science- you just have to do it'. It's not rocket science but it is a kind of magic.

Aimee Blackman, Cornwall Yoga Centre

My life with horses started when I was about 3. My Mum took me to the riding stables that she used to go to and that's how my love of horses developed. I have a lot to thank my mum for. Even though at the time I thought she was very hard on me. She used to gallop off and say follow me; I would scream all the way. But if she hadn't of pushed me I would probably still be on the lead rein now.

I have had the privilege to own a couple of wonderful horses in my lifetime. Therefore, I have some wonderful childhood memories...going to local gymkhanas and competing in games against friends, hacking for miles. Taking a picnic to Cardinham woods and being out all day. Trying to get my pony to swim in the river which I only managed once, but had tried many many times. I had so many adventures.

Now as an adult, I own the most kind and gentle horse who would try to do anything you ask of him. I sometimes say this horse saved me. Meaning he kept me going when all around me life was slightly crazy. I love being with this horse and sharing hairy, scary moments. I enjoy the adrenaline rush I get from galloping over the moors or jumping a jump and realising I can still do it. I guess I relive some of those childhood memories as an adult.

I have met some lovely people through our common interest in riding and some of those people I have been friends with for 25 years. We now are lucky enough to go on horsey holidays together. The adventures continue.

I guess every rider gets their thrill in different ways. But for me, it's being with good company of the human and animal kind.

Nina Rogers, Spot's Mum

Back in 1999, Truro Fencing Club was a typical local recreational club – a few youngsters and a few retirees who had made their way to Cornwall, getting together once a week to enjoy the sport of fencing. One or two members made the long journey up A30 and the M5 now and again to take part in regional or national events, but no significant results were coming the club's way, or were expected.

That was soon to change. As the club's Head Coach Richard Bonehill (a stuntman and fight choreographer) was selected for the 50+ GB veteran's team and worked to develop some of the younger members of the club, his assistant coach Jon Salfield began to compete at national level, and after a surprise result in a major event in 2004 qualified for the European Championships in 2004. The snowball gathered momentum and by 2008 the club was a major power in British fencing with a number of Commonwealth medals and many youngsters competing at international level in the GB youth team.

In 2009, now under the leadership of Head Coach Jon Salfield with Richard Bonehill as President, the club established their High Performance Programme, backed by private sponsorship, and began a full time training programme to prepare athletes for London 2012. Now 6 years on, Truro Fencing Club is the country's leading sabre club, boasting dozens of international fencers, numerous national and international medals, a dedicated fencing centre, full-time coaching and management staff and over 100 members.

Truro Fencing Club owes its success to years of hard work by many volunteers, but the incredible achievements of Bonehill (who became World Veteran's Champion in 2011) and Salfield, who became GB national coach for the London 2012 Olympics, is a testament what can be achieved by thinking the unthinkable and dogged determination to prove the doubters wrong.

Whilst the club has Olympic level fencers and a multitude of international fencers, and attracts athletes to train from around the world, it still values its recreational section highly, and runs regular beginners courses, school sessions and clubs for 5-7 year olds wielding plastic, rather than steel, weapons.

Bonehill sadly passed away in 2015, leaving an extraordinary legacy of a club truly for all. Salfield still leads the club, now regarded as one of the most successful Cornish sports clubs ever and Britain's most successful sabre club.

Louise, Truro Fencing Club

My name is Dianne and I have been working in the fitness industry for 20 years. However, before I found my true vocation in life I had several jobs from 'working as a waitress in a Wimpy Bar' to being a shop assistant in 'the wonder of Woolworths' and then ended up as a Civil Servant. I can't believe I worked for the Inland Revenue being in an office environment for 13 years! Unlucky for some and especially me. I was very unhappy, I dreaded going to work, the pressure, the targets, the abuse from customers and yes bullying from staff, I lost the plot and cried a lot. I was fortunate as I've always been employed but I hated my job.

Outside of work, I attended some community fitness classes. At the time I really enjoyed a Step class which was led by an instructor who looked very much like Halle Berry. She was amazing and also my inspiration to get out of the rut I had been stuck in for so long. I had that light bulb moment and thought that's what I want to do; I want to teach fitness classes and so my direction changed and my pathway on my fitness journey began. I booked myself on to my very first training course, Exercise to Music at Morley College, Westminster. I loved everything from the Anatomy & Physiology to the choreography. Although I hadn't really thought about the getting up and teaching the people bit. Scary **it zone! I passed with flying colours and that was in 1995, a life-changing milestone. I didn't quit my job straight away but the day I did hand in my notice felt soooo good.

Since then, I've run community classes and also owned my own successful Rosemary Conley Diet & Fitness Franchise in Essex. I have also completed many more training courses and kept up to date with all the latest developments in the forever evolving fitness world. I've taught a variety of fitness classes in clubs and leisure centres and have gained lots of knowledge and experience along the way. My favourites are Body Balance by Les Mills and Powerhoop, fitness with a twist using a larger weighted hoop. The best bit is meeting lots of lovely people and having lots of fun every single day. I enjoy what I do for a living. I am happy. It doesn't feel like going to work. I love moving, I love music, I love my job and I love people. Especially people who make me laugh.

Looking back, I used to do all this as a child. I was a gymnast, the girls' 1980 champion at the Sovereign Youth Club, happy days. I used to dance, it was always inside me waiting to be unleashed, and it just took me a while to find my path.

Approximately 5 years ago, I took the plunge and launched 'Funfit Exercise Classes' and I needed a motto. 'Bringing Fun into Fitness & Fitness to 'YOU' in the community. Yes, I know a bit cheesy. However, it binds everything together nicely. I love fitness, I love to teach group fitness classes and I love to have fun at the same time. I want to be able to share this with others and have an influence to be able to help others enjoy fitness and enjoy life, to 'Experience Fitness the Funfit Way' more cheese...

The other day I bumped into a class member who hadn't been for a while and she said it was lovely to see me, I'm always smiling and she couldn't wait to get back to my class. I do hope that I am able to inspire and motivate the people in my classes the way I was motivated and inspired all those years ago.

Dianne Trower, Funfit Exercise

When I first walked into the local sports hall aged 8 wearing one of my mum's old PE skirts, I was petrified what I might be letting myself in for. There must have been 50 to 60 children from 8 to 16 eagerly playing badminton with shuttlecocks flying in orderly lines.

Before long, I was getting stuck in on court one with all the other beginners. From the very beginning, I loved it, and head coach Eunice explained the importance of practising and if I practised very hard I could move up to court two one day.

Within a couple of years, I made the under 12s team and got to play matches against the other local clubs and I loved it. Over the next few years, I played more and more matches and tournaments, making the county squad at age 15. Unfortunately, county badminton clashed with county hockey too often so I didn't continue with this but for most of my teenage years badminton filled much of my time, (2 or 3 evenings, and all day Saturday and some Sundays).

I couldn't wait to go to Badminton training and matches, I had the same teammates from age 10 to 17 and in many ways we were the best of friends, but more than friends, because there was an unwritten rule that you would never let each other down. The harder I trained, the better we became and we became the under 15 ladies county champions, mixed county champions and singles county runners-up.

Badminton taught me a lot about teamwork and discipline, but it also taught me a lot about how valuable volunteers are in sport, particularly children's sport. Every single one of the coaches and officials were unpaid volunteers, and without them, I would not have had the many fun hours on the court and made those lifelong friends.

As well as the skills I learnt and the friends I made, badminton gave me something else, fitness. Between the ages of 8 and 17 I played anything between 2 to 12 hours a week. I got fit and stayed fit without trying, it was fun, all I want to do was chase the shuttlecock, it really does beat going to the gym any day!

Michele Poynter

I started rowing back in 2002 when a group of friends and I decided it would be a good idea to go and give gig rowing a bash in my old home town of Looe in Cornwall. Rowing was a sport I instantly loved and this consequently resulted in me spending on average 3 nights a week during the summer periods smashing the boats around at sea. As we were only a little club at the time, we never used to get on particularly well in the local regattas, but that didn't really matter as it was more the social side of the racing that I enjoyed.

As I grew into my later teenage years, I decided to move to Southampton to start university. This was where I got my first taste of river, slidey seat rowing (river boats are far narrower, fast and much lighter and are usually raced, as the name suggests, on rivers or sometimes lakes). This was the point in my life where rowing changed from a social sport to a physical daily challenge. From the ages of 19 to 22, barely a day would go by where I didn't do something rowing related, be it a rowing machine workout, weights or a row on the river.

It was whilst I was in university that I got into coaching. I started off with complete novices as at that time, I was still relatively novice myself, before getting involved with younger juniors and senior adults. These days I am now back in Cornwall where it all started and rather than going back to the old Gig rowing ways, I have decided to join one of two river rowing clubs in Cornwall.

Castle Dore Rowing club is based in Golant on the River Fowey. I regularly spend between 3-10 hours every weekend coaching and supervising junior rowers at the club. I coach these days because I feel I have a duty to keep the amount of juniors throughout our local club flowing. Most of the guys of my age at the club have usually moved away with work or, like myself, have gone on to university. I enjoy watching the juniors develop from complete novices, who really haven't got a clue what they are doing, into technically brilliant little rowers.

Rowing isn't really a hobby in my opinion; it becomes more of a lifestyle. 90% of the people I still keep in contact with from university were people I rowed with or coached at university, these are the people that would also be the people I turn to for favours and vice versa. No matter where they are in the world or what they do with their lives, there will also be a connection there and we will always keep in touch.

Robin Mills, Castle Dore Rowing Club

The first time I ever tried a martial art was when I was eight in Nottingham and I started Karate lessons. My real memories of this are unclear (now 21 years on) but I remember being used as cannon fodder for older and higher grade students, as I was a white belt and I was being swept to the floor by brown belts. This must have left a distinct impression on me as I left a few weeks later when I was nearly ready to take my first belt. So my start was not what I had hoped after running around as a youngster flinging kicks out just like the movies!

When I moved down to Cornwall at thirteen years old I was interested in starting Karate once again and I saw a poster for the local Camelford Club. It was run by a pleasant man in his 30's who had the energy like me but skills far beyond anything I had seen, I was inspired and couldn't wait for the session each week. Then the same Sensei (Roger Tarrant) introduced me to Aikido with a short demonstration of one technique and once again I was blown away. He said "I think you will be really interested in Aikido" (an art I had never heard of) "I'm opening a new club in Camelford soon. You should try it!" He was right, I attended the first session along with 30-40 other participants at the opening night and we were all blown away. Sensei would do a technique on a man bigger than him and they would hit the floor. I couldn't believe it! I thought this cannot work, there's some trick because it looks like magic. As I looked down the line of students I noticed it that it wasn't just me with my mouth wide open.

Where am I going with this? Well, this was my start in martial arts and it taught me you need the right club for you. And the instructor's attitude is paramount to your success. You may try one activity and not enjoy it as I did with my Karate (I could have been perturbed about trying Karate again but I took the chance it may be different and I am so glad I did as it opened up an entire new world to me!) or you could try and look for a different club and teacher as this could make all the difference in your enjoyment.

The key to anything you are looking for you must have a passion for it, a desire to try it, a need to do it! As long as the passion is there then forget if the fitness, ability or look you have is not good enough - just get started! At Karate, I remember very clearly not being able to pick everything up and Aikido was just the same. Although Aikido does not rely on any strength, I constantly found myself not achieving what everyone else could. As I was a young scrawny teenager in an adults' session and where my technique failed I had nothing else to help me get my opponent to the floor whereas the adults of the club (predominately men who were all taller and wider than me) used strength and put me down every time. There were several times I thought of quitting but my desire to learn with my teachers influence I kept going and I am where I am today thanks to that thought of let's keep going once more and once more etc!

Yes, I have moments of thinking I could stay at home, the weather is rubbish or too nice, I don't feel great, the kids are playing up, missing one session won't matter etc all the excuses in the book come up from time to time, but you push past them and you find yourself thanking your will power in making you go, because all those sessions add up.

The human race is made to feel in competition with each other but we are not. How can it be a race when we don't all start at the same point in life and we certainly do not all finish at the same line? Just enjoy your time. So my story is very ordinary and rather like so many others, I have not battled any great problems or overcome anything other than the norm but I have gone through all these major times in my life with the martial arts philosophy which I feel has put me in great steed for the rest of my life!

For me, it has given me everything! At every point in my life, the highs, lows, good times and bad situations my training has always been there and remains to be there. So much so that I am now making my passion in to my work, as I have started personal martial arts lessons and hope to continue this as a job.

What has martial arts meant to me? Over the years, the answer has constantly evolved from something to do to stay fit to gain skills of defending myself to now it simply being my passion! One which I would like to share with others so that can share the life-changing benefits with me. Over my ten years of teaching, I've seen the arts I teach give all sorts of things to my pupils – confidence, purpose, and passion are the biggest gains I can think of. I've helped students to overcome anxiety and nerves, including one student, who, after a few years of karate, began putting his hand up in school to answer questions. For himself, and his family, this was a major step. For others, it's a chance to focus in on one thing instead of worrying about the rest of their lives.

I have and still do teach 6-year-olds to people in their 60's and more; when I was a student one person started Karate at 70! There really is no barrier. If you are unconfident, unfit, inflexible, shy, have a lack of coordination martial arts taught in the right way of connecting the mind, body and spirit will improve all these areas and more!

With the traditional arts, there is little competition with others; the main competition is with oneself to improve! Personal achievement is one of the biggest rewards you can reap.

Therefore no matter what activity you take up make sure you are passionate about it and look at your own achievement and where you have come from rather than who is ahead of you and one day you will be the inspiration for others!

Sensei Jack, TBBA Aikido Cornwall

I started 'wild swimming' 10 years ago when I swam using a normal wetsuit. After a short time, I found I preferred swimming without a wetsuit as the spring water I swim in is beautifully soft and made my skin feel amazing! I have a diagnosis of mixed connective tissue disease with Raynauds. After a couple of years, the benefit to my health was quite remarkable; when I came out of the pond or the sea for half an hour or even a whole hour I didn't ache at all - this to me was remarkable and I started to see my regular outdoor swims throughout the year as part of my 'medication'.

Now, if I go without an outdoor swim for more than ten days my health deteriorates and I simply have to go for a swim. Curiously building my cold resistance has also meant I no longer feel the effects of my Raynauds on a day-to-day basis. I have no idea of the science behind this, however I explain the healing in this way; swimming outdoors, 'kick starts' my immune system to work for me rather than against me. The pond I swim in has a light green tinge, so it may be that there is copper in the water which has a medicinal effect? Who knows, what I do know is that I will keep doing this and it will help to keep me well. I love outdoor swimming!

Lin Chapman

I was first introduced to American Football in 1965. My father worked in the aerospace industry and as a family, we were moved over to America for his work. As a youngster with dyslexia, school was hard for me. Teachers labelled me as disruptive and made me sit in the corner with a Dunce's Hat, telling me that I wouldn't amount to much. I was asked if I played any sport and I said yes "football." I was delighted to be told that they played football as well and that I should turn up to training. The following week, I enthusiastically arrived with my shorts, boots and ball. The coach took one look at me and said: "What are you doing?" I was completely confused and it took a while for us to understand that the sport was lost in translation but that is my first introduction to football – American style. I fell in love with the sport and it helped me cope, with what was a tough upbringing.

When we returned to the UK in the 70s, there were no American Football clubs and it wasn't until the sport was televised on Channel 4 that it started to gain popularity. In 1983, I started the Heathrow Jets. I placed an advert in the paper looking for players and the first session attracted over 160 people – with just me as the coach! The club started to build and in our first game, I had 100 players and with a crowd of 12,000 spectators. I went on to coach the GB squad in 1991, where we won the first and currently only, Euro Championship.

For me, coaching is something I love. I have coached people from all kinds of backgrounds, with all sorts of problems but I firmly believe that everybody has a special gift; you just have to find it. Whatever your background, your size, your ability, your gender or the size of your ambition, I think it is important to be inclusive and I have always seen my team, as my family. It is a place where you can come and not feel victimised or singled out and if you need help, you get it. Everybody is equal and I make myself available to anybody if they have a problem.

I have been honoured to be named Cornwall's Participation Coach of the Year, South West Community Coach of the Year and placed in the Top 3 nationally, along with two Hall of Fame entries in the States.

In reality, I get back so much from my sporting family. In 1993/1994 season, I sustained an injury so bad that the Doctors didn't think I would ever walk again. I walked. In 2007, I was hospitalised 44 times; 11 of which were airlifted and four times I ended up in intensive care. Throughout my own personal problems, I have had the support of the club and the sport. I went through a particular trauma when my staffy dog turned and killed my collie dog. 15 players came to my door and spent four hours helping with the clean-up and helping me with my own devastation. I have given a lot to my sport but I have also got a huge amount back from it.

As well as the Cornish Sharks, I now spend time setting up taster sessions in schools and I also get the opportunity to coach other coaches; not only in my sport but from other sports too.

I have two mantras; you only have one life, so it is important to live it and there are only two things in life you can't change - the weather and referees!

Coach Smallworth, Cornish Sharks

I remember my first Martial Arts class vividly. It was so very alien, lots of noise, an unforgiving wooden gym floor at my primary school, sun streaming in through the high windows and commands shouted in a foreign language. It was not my choice to be here, and if it were up to me I would probably have never gone back.

My parents saw the local Karate class as a chance for me to regain confidence and learn valuable self-defence skills after a recent bullying attack which saw me pinned down by one assailant and punched repeatedly by another. Very vicious at such a young age (10).

Now, years later I see their point and thank them for doing what they did, then I did not see the value, I did not want to train, I did not want to go back, and I certainly did not want to don the 'Pyjamas' every week. However, things changed pretty quickly and this became a way of life for me.

After being forced to go back and knowing there was no way out I decided to give it everything, if I was going to have to do it then I may as well put heart and soul into it and be the best I could be, and in doing so quickly developed a healthy interest in the activity along with quite a talent, progressing through the ranks at a decent pace and becoming one of the 'regulars'.

It was a shock when the Instructor, still one of the most influential people to me in the Martial Arts had to retire due to ill health and because of this I had to switch style, luckily for me another club moved into the same location which was conveniently located and I gave it a go. It was Tang Soo Do – A Korean form of Karate.

Apart from a few changes and the language, everything else was compatible, everyone was friendly, and within a few months I was in a car up to Coventry to take my first belt in the new style and taking a firm first step on a path that would change my life.

In this new club endless opportunities were presented, I travelled around the country, often winning the competitions I was entered into, I tested in front of the very best, with glowing reports and even triple grading, my confidence grew and I knew this is where I should be. So when I took my black belt test at 17, I was eager to start my own club.

At 17 this was harder than I imagined, it's hard to gain peoples' trust and respect at such an early age, but I stuck with it. Now, almost 20 years later I'm proud to say I have produced a number of very high quality Black Belts, as well as Regional, National, European and World Championships. I have fought as team captain and coached the UK Fighting team (the only team from the UK to ever win the World Championships) and taught seminars internationally. I coach people to improve their confidence, and break down techniques to make Tang Soo Do accessible to everyone. And when I remember back to that first ever Karate session, blinded by the sun, and intimidated by all the noise, I would never have guessed I would be in the very privileged position that I am in now, surrounded every week by close friends who I have travelled the world with, fought beside, taught from white belt and socialised with countless times. Yes I learnt the necessary self-defence, but Karate/Tang Soo Do also gave me so much more. And I hope and aim to pass these benefits on to every student who walks through the door of my School.

Robert James, Chief Instructor ISK Martial Arts Academy

I first encountered orienteering on an outdoor pursuit's course. A few years later, I took part in the inaugural event of Cornwall Orienteering Club - and came first! What more encouragement did I need to keep on orienteering?

I'd always enjoyed running and the map-reading element of orienteering just gave the running a purpose and provided extra interest. Orienteering is not about PB times for particular distances - it's about interpreting the map and facing up to the challenges that the course planner has set. Which is my best route to the next control? Do I take the direct route through rough terrain or the longer way via easily run paths? Up and over the hill or follow the contours round? And from that come the joys of hitting the control spot-on - and the frustrations of making silly mistakes by misreading the details on the map.

For someone like me who is not fiercely competitive and was never going to be competing at anything like an elite level, the options within orienteering are an added attraction. Most events provide a range of courses of varying length and navigational difficulty so if I'm not feeling particularly fit I can choose a shorter course.

Orienteering has developed since my first event (now over 30 years ago). There are sprint events and urban events in Cornwall, we have sand dune areas and moorland as well as forests. And after each event, we can all compare notes on our route choices and mistakes. Because whatever the terrain and whatever the course we're always aiming for the holy grail of orienteering - the perfect run.

Steve Beech - Cornwall Orienteering Club

A lot of people ask me why I go fishing. After 27 years, I really should have the most compelling answer, but I don't. And believe me, I've thought about it. I've tried to think of that profound one-liner that leaves people thinking, "Wow, I've got to go fishing right now!", but I can see all I achieve is leaving them thinking, "he's another idiot that sits in the rain catching nothing." I actually heard a group of cyclists riding past a lake me and friends were fishing once say to his friends and I guess their sons, "they're probably all there because they've been signed up for anger management classes." At first, I was really angry, (the irony) but I could only laugh. I was a little sad that his son would never get the chance to go fishing and enjoy what I do but hey, not everyone does and not everyone gets the chance.

The truth is, there are so many reasons why I go fishing (or angling) and some are very different to others. When I caught my first fish, a Garfish aged five from Dawlish Seawall in South Devon it certainly wasn't to get away from the stresses of work and a hectic lifestyle. At that age, like every kid, I was naturally curious about everything. My parents didn't fish, my friends didn't go fishing and to be honest no one in the family can really remember how it all started but start it did. That first fish was quite literally life changing. In my eyes, it was the most incredible thing in the world and it was a huge achievement. I was immensely proud, I know because I've seen the very old video of me clutching that fish for hours after I'd caught it parading it around for everyone who cared or didn't care about that stinky creature.

So initially fishing was my connection to the fascinating world of fish. But clearly I loved the act of fishing and that I can only put down to natural instinct. People have told me in a modern world we should have grown out of that. I don't think WE ever can, I hope not! I've had friends say that you discover fishing and it's most likely to happen when you're young, a theory I subscribed to until recently when I watched an interview with one of my heroes, Sir David Attenborough. He was talking to Barack Obama who asked the question, "When did you learn to love the outdoors?" Attenborough replied, "We all naturally love the outdoors, my question is, when did you *stop* loving it?"

That naturally curious instinct is in us all; I was lucky; I got a chance to connect with the natural world and fire that passion before it was lost forever. My life since has always been close to fishing. Fishing has lead me to incredible locations both on my doorstep and around the world. I've met people through fishing and made lifelong friends that if we didn't have that common ground we never would have met. I've witnessed flora and fauna that I know people don't believe when I tell them, but they won't ever see it for themselves because they won't sit still for long enough, unless it's on their sofa. I've experienced the most incredible weather at the edge of water, occasions that have left me worried for my life and moments to literally bask in.

To share just a fraction of this with Sam was an absolute pleasure. I don't honestly think Sam will rush off to a tackle shop and fill the back of the car with rods and reels, but for a very pleasant evening some of that natural instinct and curiosity was brought back. The fishing wasn't easy and although the fish were biting they were hard to hook and land. Not because they were monsters but because they are wild and not easy to fool. But eventually, after some patient waiting Sam's moment came. That small wriggling Roach sat in Sam's hands like the Garfish did in mine 27 years ago and the smile was there for us both. Congratulations Sam, you are an angler and you are always welcome. Long live Sofa Dodgers!

Alex Ledbrooke, Roche Angling Club

Korfball is normally pronounced *whatball?* When you start talking to someone about it.

Especially when you are still at primary school, PE lessons can all be much the same; usually football and usually with those on the school football team taking 99% of possession.

The other 1% is reserved for everyone else retrieving the ball from a shot narrowly missing. Luckily at that time, another sport was being introduced to the schools of Norwich: Korfball.

A sport where a little bit of thinking is required: You need to pass to your teammates or you find yourself quickly neutralised. Taking shots from the halfway line is unlikely to be that rewarding.

It also has the advantage of the goal post being inside the court, so missed shots land still in play. That makes retrieving missed shots a bit more fun.

The PE lessons of korfball were very different to the other sports. I found I could compete against anyone else; we were all starting from zero and I learnt fast; I think our teachers were trying to learn as well. The school needed a team for the Norwich Schools Championships. And I was in it! I can't remember how well we did; I know we didn't win but that didn't matter. I had decided I wanted to play korfball.

A second year of korfball at school quickly passed and I made the move to high school. They didn't play the sport there but advertised on a small poster was a try-out session at Stingers Korfball Club. I didn't worry too much about getting a lift to the session with people I hadn't met before! Soon I was playing in their teams in the local league and going to tournaments over summer weekends.

It wasn't long before I started to get involved in coaching. Friday afternoons at sixth form kept me fit with a 3:15 finish forming the start of long bike ride out into the countryside to help out teaching school children how to play. These children were the same age as me when I started playing; hopefully at least one of them is still playing. The junior coaching turned into senior coaching through university continuing at Stingers.

A move away from Norwich led to a brief spell playing at Basingstoke, and then, as ever the real world got in the way leading to a couple of years "sabbatical." Once I was looking for korfball again, it didn't take long to find Horfield Korfball Club in Bristol. To my surprise, someone turned up one night with some photos of me refereeing them five or six years earlier. (Luckily I hadn't sent any of them off!) The inevitable happened and I found myself involved with their coaching set up and apparently inventing "fitness by stealth".

Another move placed me in Exeter. The South West is seemingly a hotbed of korfball and the transfer got arranged before I found a place to live; a transfer that was delayed by choosing to "play in purple (Horfield)" rather than "watch in green (Exeter)." Now playing for and coaching at the green end of the M5, fitness by stealth became "five minutes of fun."

So twenty years after playing *whatball?* For the first time at school, I'm still playing and still coaching.

Rob, Exeter Korfball Club

Special Olympics Cornwall is part of Special Olympics Great Britain, one of over 180 countries that form the Special Olympics movement, in which 4 million people take part.

The Special Olympics Movement was founded in the USA in 1968 by the late Eunice Kennedy Shriver, sister of President John F Kennedy. Shriver believed that the Olympic ideals of sport could give confidence and new hope to people with intellectual (learning) disabilities as well as to those who cared for them. Chris Maloney MBE founded Special Olympics in Great Britain (then known as Special Olympics UK) in 1978. Chris had been teaching swimming to people with intellectual (learning) disabilities since the early 1960s. In 1976, after reading a book entitled Times to Remember by Rose Kennedy (mother of John F. Kennedy and Eunice Kennedy Shriver), Chris sent a letter about his work to the author. Eunice Shriver enlisted Chris Maloney to develop the Special Olympics programme in the UK and with help from Sir Hugh Fraser and Sir Eldon Griffiths (then Minister for Sport) he paved the way for a legacy of support for Special Olympics across the country. Special Olympics in the UK was one of the first European programmes of the international Special Olympics Movement. Today, Special Olympics GB serves 8,000 athletes and 4000 volunteers in 150 clubs across Great Britain.

In Cornwall, we are committed to achieving the mission statement of the Special Olympics: "To provide year round sports training and competition in a variety of Olympic-type sports for people with learning disabilities, giving them continuing opportunities to develop physical fitness, demonstrate courage, experience joy and participate in a sharing of skills, gifts and friendship with their families, other Special Olympic athletes and the community."

Terry Stanton, one of the SOC committee members, explains how it all started in Cornwall. "It goes back to the Bath Special Olympics GB games, in the summer of 2013. There was an item on the local news about the Bath event and it was interesting to see that there was a South West team, but I didn't see anyone who I recognised from Cornwall, either competing or being interviewed. I made a few enquiries and discovered that there were only a couple of people from Cornwall competing and that they were with Plymouth and District Club. By chance, in the September, I met the Plymouth and District Club Chairman, Alan Stockdale, at a student recruitment evening at Plymouth University. He invited me along to the club, an offer that I took him up on, dragging my wife along; I say dragging, as she really doesn't really follow or like sport. At the club we met up with another husband and wife team, Donna and David Painter, who were on a similar journey that had started in a similar way to mine. We chatted with the athletes and met the indomitable Steve Dodd (Kayaker) who told us he was going to represent GB at the LA World Special Olympics. He did and won two silver medals for kayaking.

David, Donna, Viv and I agreed to start a Cornwall Club. Now we've all been there when it seemed like a good idea at the time, but nothing happens. Not so on this occasion; we contacted Cornwall Sports Partnership to see if they wanted to get involved. Lo and behold they were on the same path as we were, wanting to start a Cornwall Special Olympics Club.

The rest is history; we had a public meeting in January 2015 that was organised by Steve Hillman from CSP, and the first club session was held on Saturday 1st March at Heron Tennis in Newquay. Since then we have grown and grown, offering a range of sport at different locations. We are supported by our wonderful team of volunteers, who turn up each week come rain and shine." I asked Viv why she got involved, as a confirmed non-sporting person. Her answer was "I just love it because everyone enjoys themselves. People are there for the joy of playing the sport, not for the money. Seeing the smiles on people's faces certainly recharges my batteries; I'm sure I'm not the only one who feels that way."

The incentive of winning a medal is important and keenly played for; something we hope will translate into bronze, silver and gold when we take a Cornwall contingent as part of the South West team to the Sheffield 2017 Special Olympics GB Games.

Terry Stanton, Special Olympics Cornwall

The founding manager was Clive Hodge, and as I spent much time supporting my then 14-year-old daughter, Suzzi, at matches and training, I was soon coerced into becoming the club secretary. This is a position I have held ever since, despite the comings and goings of various managers over the years. Although Suzzi spent periods playing for Saltash Ladies and then Marine Academy Plymouth, in higher divisions, she has now returned to playing for Dobwalls and interestingly, for the first time this season is the only player now remaining who played from the very beginning under the founding manager.

As Liskeard Ladies, the team won Cornwall Division 2 East in their first season. They were also crowned overall Division 2 champions when they beat the Division 2 West champions, Hayle, 4-1 in a play-off final. The Liskeard team continued to do well with a runners-up spot in Cornwall Division 1 the following season and then a 3rd spot in the 2005-2006 season. They were also beaten League Cup finalists that season.

In season 2006-2007, with the team challenging strongly for the Cornwall Division 1 title, a change of chairman within the parent club brought with it differing opinions and attitudes. This resulted in a big change when the team relocated to Lantoom Park, and at the beginning of the following season were renamed Dobwalls Ladies FC. Sadly the team fell narrowly short of winning the title in that year of upheaval. Dobwalls Ladies were third in Cornwall Division 1 in 2009-2010 and were the League Cup winners in the same season, beating the Cornwall Division 1 league winners of that season, Falmouth, in an exciting final.

In the 2010-2011 season, Dobwalls Ladies FC finally won Cornwall Division 1. The championship was decided on goal difference over Callington, following a draw away to their rivals in the final game of the season. The team were consequently promoted to the South West Women's League Division 1 West, where they currently compete at a very good level. The squad for the forthcoming season promises to be one of the strongest to date and there are high hopes for a successful campaign.

Despite it being hard work at times, I have really enjoyed sharing in the ups and downs and particularly the successes of the team over the years.

Terry Porter, Dobwalls Ladies Football Club

I started Bujinkai Karate in 1974 under the watchful eye of Chief Instructor John Smith and Instructors, Phil Barratt and Alistair Clark in Newquay.

My reason for starting my Martial Arts training in Karate is simply that was the only style available for children in the area and I was desperate to be able to kick like the guy on the Kung Fu series.

I continued to train in Bujinkai Karate until I became a 1st Kyu (Last Brown before Black Belt). When the club closed, I continued to train in other Martial Arts before I went to college in 1983.

I went to the College of Further Education in Devonport to study Bakery and in Plymouth I found a whole range of different Martial Arts, over the next 2 years I practiced Bujinkai Karate, Judo, Boxing, WTF Tae Kwon Do, Pak Mei Kung Fu and Escrima (Pilipino stick fighting).

After college I didn't restart my Martial Arts until 1990, when I fell in love with the sport karate scene and trained and graded with Richard Hopkins, Kevin Brewerton and Steve Winsper, where I finally opened my own Sport Karate Club in 1995.

In 1992, I broke the World Slab breaking record a record, I've re-broken since. In '92 I broke 80 slabs (10 stacks of 8 slabs) in 8.16secs, the previous record was 80 slabs in 56 seconds, I re-broke that again at the Pencalenick Special School open day in 2006 in 7 seconds, and in 2007 at the Cornwall Sports Awards in 4.84 seconds. I also broke the power breaking record in 1994 at the Granby Halls, Leicester at the Martial Arts event 'Clash of the Titans'. In 2007, I was invited by ITV1 to appear on "Superhuman-Superstrong" where they wanted to test my strength whilst breaking a stack of concrete slabs. It was a fantastic opportunity and programme; you can still watch the programme on YouTube. The outcome was that I broke the stack in 0.2 seconds at a speed of 60mph and the power was in excess of 200kg (they couldn't record the true reading as I broke the power plates that were recording it).

For the next few years, I worked really hard trying to juggle working as a baker with 3am starts and 3pm finishes, then teaching in the evenings, I did this for over 6 years, before realising my dream in 2006 when I became a professional Martial Arts Instructor.

Since 2006, I've produced 69 World Champions, holding the post of England Team Coach for 3 different organisations and have the biggest Sport Martial Arts School in the South West. This didn't happen overnight and is down to being consistent and working very hard. This is the message I try and give to my students; life is tough and to be successful, you have to be prepared to give it everything, even when the odds are stacked against you.

The last 41 years in Martial Arts hasn't been easy, or plain sailing, you'll be criticised, have negative things said about you, it's how you deal with that, that defines you. We are inspired for success, for ourselves and our students.

Martial Arts is recognised as a key element in inspiring young people to achieve great goals, we are proud to say we are doing this daily.

Ed Byrne, Chief Instructor Byrne Black Belt Academy

Growing up, I never liked PE or Sports Day. I dreaded any kind of exercise and had a note for every PE class. I was never overweight in primary school or early years of secondary school, but by year 9, I got bullied by a few school boys for my 'Gothic' dark, long hair and dark eye makeup and what did I do to handle it? I just comfort ate, completely lost my way and by the age of 16, I was nearly 13 stone. At 17 years old, I had to hide behind size 16-18 baggy clothes covering the tops of my arms, my legs and my tummy because I was really unhappy with my body.

One day I decided to buy my first ever exercise DVD.I don't know if you've heard of Nell McAndrew? But she was a glamour model, now marathon runner; she has released many DVDs, one titled 'Maximum Impact.' The reviews were great on Amazon so I made the purchase; and as soon as it arrived, it went into that DVD player, I got my brand new exercise gear on anxiously raring to go; I started the warm-up and 10 minutes later I was beetroot in the face, knackered and ready for bed! I'd never felt pain in my bum cheeks like I did that following morning - there were jumps, skips and SQUATS!! All in a warm-up!

But everyone has to start somewhere and I wasn't going to give up. So the following day I put in the DVD and managed to make it to the cardio section this time. Still, I didn't finish the program, but I preserved and was improving each day and eventually after months of motivating myself to exercise I completed the program and started to feel fitter. I could see changes in my body and I started to really enjoy this exercise malarkey. I purchased DVD after DVD from Nell McAndrew's other programs to Davina, Pump It Up, Charlie Brooks & much much more! By the age of 19, I was down just over 2 stone in weight and sitting happier in a size 12 dress. I continued exercising and purchased a treadmill. I never ran outside, joined a gym or attended fitness classes; I never found the confidence but could keep the weight off by working out in my own front room.

I never thought about a career in Fitness but after taking IT in school, I found an apprenticeship in admin and worked my way up to IT support, handling HR & Operations which I thoroughly enjoyed but 3 years down the line I realised that this was not what I wanted to do for the rest of my life. Each day after work, I would run on that treadmill or put on an exercise DVD to maintain my fitness and improve my body shape and it would be the best part of my day – my friends would ask me to go running with them, I would bring my hand weights and yoga mats, we would do some weight training and ab exercises and from this I knew I wanted to be a personal trainer.

I spoke to my parents about my potential career change, contacted the nearest college and was sent information on various fitness courses. I read up on the Exercise to Music (Fitness Instructor) Course and it was right up my street. Aerobic exercise is what changed my life, so I signed up to this course and every Saturday I attended college (one of the most amazing but challenging thing I had ever done).

Exercise made me a happier, stronger, fitter and most importantly, a more confident person; I am extremely passionate about exercise and knew that I wanted to help others increase their fitness agility and reach their own personal goals in order to gain the same results as I did. So once I completed my course I made the biggest decision to leave my office job, register as self-employed and create Versatile Fitness Choice (VFC). I wanted to offer fun, upbeat, aerobic classes which were not only enjoyable, help improve fitness levels and shrink waistlines but most importantly would suit absolutely anyone no matter their age, gender, shape or size and a year down the line this is exactly what I have done!

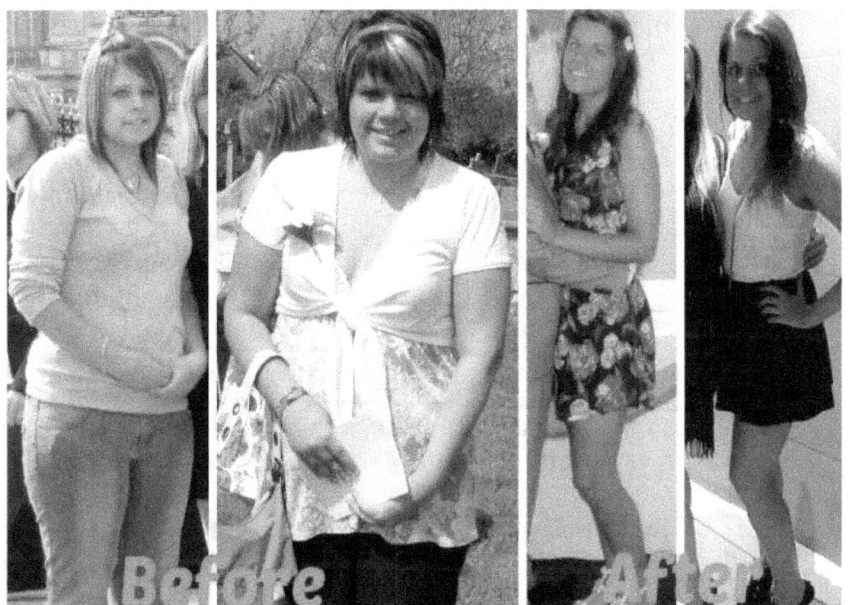

Tara, Versitile Fitness Choice

Many people might think that cheerleading is just about shaking pom poms, but modern cheerleading is so much more than that. Cheerleading is one of the fastest growing sports out there, and is played across the world. Competitive cheerleading sees men and women competing in teams in front of judges performing fast-paced routines with an amazing fusion of gymnastics tumbling, dance, and 'stunting' (lifting and throwing other athletes). It can be nerve racking for new members because it is so new and different, but don't let that stop you. We start at a low level and build up progressions as your confidence builds. It's very addictive and so much fun. As well as physical fitness, strength, agility and flexibility, you build skills needed for everyday life, especially teamwork and trust.

I trained as a professional dancer at Laine Theatre Arts, and performed with many famous faces and celebrities before getting into cheerleading and training with some of the top programmes in the country. After moving from London to Cornwall, I was keen to share my passion for cheerleading, and founded West Coast Cheerleading in 2009. West Coast Cheerleading continues to run cheerleading classes for junior and senior schools across Cornwall, with teams competing in bi-annual County Cheerleading competitions.

In the autumn of 2014, I opened West Coast Academy, a brand new gym in Redruth for cheerleading, gymnastics, dance, parkour and fitness training. With spacious studios, a comfy reception area, specialist sprung floor and plenty of equipment to help athletes achieve their potential, this has been a dream come true for me. The Academy has become a hub for cheerleading in Cornwall, and we are so excited for the future! Our Academy teams are working hard and proudly represent Cornish cheerleading at National and International competitions in the UK, and our next goal is to make links with local businesses and sponsors to help bring them even more amazing opportunities.

Cheerleading is a fun and inclusive sport that has something for everyone. At West Coast Academy, our athletes range from 18 months to 45 years, and our family keeps growing!

Rhea Upsher – Director, West Coast Cheerleading and West Coast Academy

It was September 1999 and the beginning of the rugby season. As parents of three young children we were keen to introduce Tom (number 2), who had just turned 6, to something special for him so that he did not need to compete with sister Lucy, aged 7 years. We pitched up at our local rugby club in Liskeard, East Cornwall and they welcomed Tom with open arms to their u7s/8s side. Not to be outdone, Lucy asked the coach: 'Can girls play rugby?' The coach took one look at her long legs and said: 'Yes, come and join us.' The rest, as they say, is history.

Two years later, our third son, Oliver, also joined the club and they've all played – and are still playing – 16 years later. We have enjoyed watching three rugby world cups, two women's rugby world cups and have, like many families, dedicated our lives to the sport; because rugby is like that. Once you join, you become part of the rugby family. My husband started coaching the week after we joined in 1999 and has coached at Club, County and Regional levels ever since. As a mum, I was soon roped in to managing the teams, washing the kit, raising money, organising rugby tours...

When Oliver was 10, he was physically abused by his rugby coach during training, coming on the back of months of poor coaching techniques. This led to my interest in Safeguarding young people in rugby and I have had a thoroughly fulfilling, if sometimes harrowing time, learning how to do this better and now manage safeguarding in Cornwall. As with many aspects of governance, this has grown in sophistication over the years and now all clubs in Cornwall looking after u18s have at least one safeguarding officer. Volunteering can become quite a full-time job!

But how did we get into ladies rugby? Well, obviously young girls grow up into young ladies and in our case, Lucy having played at County and Regional levels since she was 12, was then spotted aged 14 by the RFUW and invited to take part in the elite u18s Talent Development Group. She captained the England u18s side which won against Wales and was part of the u20s Nations Cup winners in Santa Barbara in 2011. She played for Bristol Ladies (premiership club) as a medical student and, now a junior doctor, has made friends literally all over the world because Rugby is a family whatever level you play.

And what of her parents? Well, despite having an elite athlete in the family, we are absolutely committed to the grass roots game because it is at this level that the journey in the rugby family begins. Over the years we have been able to introduce the game to 100's of girls and young women. Some were natural athletes and excelled at anything they tried out. Others were less confident, sometimes unhappy at school (or even unable to face school) but gained in confidence and fitness when they joined the team. Rugby is par excellence a team sport. It is said to be a game for everyone and it really is. Everyone, whatever shape or size, is welcome because everybody has something to offer. There are different skills needed to be a front row forward to being a scrum half, a second row lock from being a full back under the high ball. But everyone is part of the team and without each and every one of those players, the team would not be complete.

Ann Demaine, Liskeard Leopards Rugby Club

Laura Green, Sarah Choak and Claire Burlison Green, three sisters from Plymouth (twin sisters and their sister-in-law) joined together and created a new dance fitness class, Clubbercise 'the night out work out', which has become an international phenomenon. Their classes are taught in a darkened room with glow sticks and disco lights to a soundtrack of banging club anthems from the 90's to the latest hits. This is their story...

The conversation started in 2012 over drinks at Christmas; they were discussing fitness classes and how music makes such a difference to motivation. They shared their mutual love of dance music and the 'good old' days of night-clubbing. Inspired by the conversation, they decided to create their own dance fitness class with a 'clubby' feel. The first dance routines were created in Laura's lounge. They hired a local Methodist Church Hall in Plympton, Plymouth and bought some disco lights and glow sticks then set about teaching their routines to family and friends. However, word started getting out and others wanted to come along. So the fitness class became 'official' and Clubbercise was born in June 2013.

Claire moved to London in December 2013 and decided to launch training courses so that other instructors could teach their classes. Clubbercise became the fastest growing dance fitness class to hit the UK since Zumba, an amazing achievement! The brand has also helped thousands of people around the world gain access to clean drinking water via their partnership with Oxfam.

The secret of Clubbercise success is that it does not just get you fit; it is also great fun, with bags of energy, simple routines and a great atmosphere. During the one hour class Clubbers can burn around 500 calories. It also encourages those that may shy away from gyms or the usual fitness classes to attend, thanks to the darkened room.

For Laura and Sarah instructing has proved to be so rewarding, seeing their Clubbers smiling from start to finish, helping those get fitter, and simply seeing people enjoying their class and WANTING MORE! The girls are in constant demand to run more classes. During the last few years, they've heard so many inspirational stories of how Clubbercise has changed lives, not just in Plymouth but around the whole of the UK and beyond. They have to pinch themselves every day.

Sarah, Clubbercise

I was always interested in sports from a very early age. At school, I was on the athletics team and the swim team. I played Rugby for my school, cricket for London Schools and county at age 10 and was lucky enough to represent my County (Kent) and my Division (South East England) as a hockey goalkeeper throughout my school years. I was also selected for an international assessment weekend when I was 18.

I always believed that sport was going to be able to sustain me not just as a hobby but also a career. After trying to join the RAF as a PT when I was 18, an op 2 weeks before the fitness test put pay to that and then LIFE got in the way for a long time. Although I carried on playing hockey for a few years after school, I eventually gave it up and started playing rugby for a local club.

This was the only exercise I would get and being a smoker and an asthmatic I found training, especially running, very difficult. Eventually, I decided I wanted to get a bit bigger and fitter (Approx. age 30) so joined the local gym. I started going regularly, although still smoking, drinking and eating lots of unhealthy food. I still couldn't run far but I was starting to get stronger. I would still look at other people in the gym thinking that I would never get the muscle tone and build some of them had, which was a bit demoralizing. The Leisure Centre, unfortunately, had to close a year or so later.

I worked in a town nearby which had a gym on the Industrial estate where I worked called Route 2 Fitness. I decided to give it a go and walked through the door. The owner a man called Rupert Jenkins signed me up and gave me the induction. He wrote me a program after a quick discussion and off I went. Over the weeks, I got to know Ru quite well. He was a Powerlifter and on occasion when I was in there, he would train with me (Give me a beasting!) I have never smiled so much in the gym and hurt so badly after our sessions. The man was very inspirational (and also sarcastic and mickey taking but always in a humorous way). He told me to try some of the classes his wife and another instructor ran in the gym. I did this and although having a lot of insecurities about being in a room of mirrors (yes, I had them too) loved them.

Over a period of time, getting to know both Ru and Jayne I talked with them about how I could get into the industry and they told me how they did it. I did some research, got the backing of my then girlfriend (now my wife) found a course to do and here I am.

There are so many things I feel that I have achieved since becoming a fitness instructor. What I would consider a small achievement for me is often a huge achievement for someone else. It makes my day to have someone who has struggled to enjoy exercise and keeps stopping their bid to get healthier, coming up to me and simply saying thank you for taking the time during a class to make sure they are ok. To me I'm just doing my job but to them I'm helping change their life.

I have had a lady at one of my classes with low self-esteem due to being overweight and took a huge leap to come to a class with her friend. Over the course of 18 months since that first class she shed over 4 stone and has now become a qualified Fitness Instructor, Boxercise Instructor, Kettlercise Instructor and will soon be doing her Personal Training study and Qualification. All because I inspired her much as Rupert and Jayne inspired me.

On the Personal Training side, I trained a woman who needed to lose a significant amount of weight so she could get IVF treatment in the hope of becoming a mum. I trained her for 7 months (only stopping as I moved away). When I moved she stopped talking to me and was hurt because she felt I was abandoning her. About 18 months after, I moved for some reason she popped up in my news feed on Facebook, so I sent a message asking how she was getting on and she sent a picture of her little girl with a heartfelt thank you message for helping her achieve what most people take for granted.

I had one chap who came to speak to me after a class, explaining that his daughter was upset because she had tried her wedding dress on and it was too small and she only had 5 weeks before the final fitting. He asked if I could help so I designed a program to help her lose weight and also tone herself. We finished the sessions the day before the dress fitting and I got a lovely message a couple of days later saying that not only did she now fit but also the dress had to be taken in. She got married a month later and on the following Monday her dad came up to me in the gym, shook my hand and said thanks for helping her look so stunning. He had actual tears in his eyes (So did I after he said it).

All these have made what I do worth the aches and pains, the injuries, the tiredness etc.

I think the biggest fear and issue that people have is not knowing what they have to do. The amount of misleading or false information around about the best form of weight loss or class format is almost at ridiculous proportions. If they have a local leisure centre then go along and see what classes are on offer. The biggest step they will ever take is the first one into a class or Fitness centre. Most people have the fear that they will be the biggest/fattest/unhealthiest/weakest person in the gym or class and they are going to be ridiculed. The main thing I have noticed is that people in the gym or class have the same fears as you do. Most of the time they are so busy worrying about themselves, that they don't have time to look at you.

If you go to a class and don't enjoy it, for whatever reason then try something else. Always have a belief that there is something out there for you because there is. Try everything at least twice as the first time you may dislike whatever you're doing just because you feel insecure.

Mike Charlwood, Priority 1 Fitness

What has Table Tennis given me? In three words – an enormous amount! Exercise, competition, laughter, friendship, work, travel – it has become a large part of my life which I should miss so much if I wasn't involved and I am able to put something back into a sport that has given me so much.

It all started when I went to a meeting back in the early seventies to represent my then club in Hampshire at a league meeting as the secretary was unable to attend. The league needed a new secretary and I was foolish enough to ask what the job entailed? Within seconds the chairman thanked me for my offer and, much to my surprise, I was secretary of the Gosport and Fareham Table Tennis Association. It involved meetings, taking minutes, filling in forms and helping to run the league with its activities such as matches and tournaments. I must admit I enjoy organisational activities, which is a good job really!

As secretary, I represented the league on the County Committee. Here, I met people from all around Hampshire, many of whom I still see at meetings today. As I enjoyed umpiring when I played in league matches, I enquired how to become an umpire. I passed my County Umpires Badge that year and started to go to local and National tournaments, then went on to become a National Umpire and then an International Umpire, giving me a chance to travel the world. My friendships were growing and the camaraderie was immense. One top England player with whom I was talking at the English Closed in Kent one year remarked that we all turned up most weekends, players and umpires alike, and all got on together without knowing what any of us did during the rest of the week. There is no "side" in table tennis. How true! What a great attribute for the game. By then I was also running the Hampshire Inter-Town league as well.

When I moved from Hampshire to Hertfordshire in the late eighties, I played in a local club in the North Herts League and was Assistant Secretary there, being responsible for the minutes as well as general duties within a league. During my time there, I was invited on to my first National committee at first as Entry Form Checker for all English Tournaments and then Secretary of the

Tournaments Committee which eventually lead to my becoming Secretary of the Calendar Working Party as well. This involved me in the organisation of the calendar for all the tournaments that take place each season in England. I still hold both positions to this day and spend quite a few hours doing administration at home and attending meetings quarterly in either Milton Keynes or London. More friends, many of whom I had already met through umpiring, more camaraderie and quite a lot of responsibility. I wouldn't do it if I didn't enjoy it. In 2000, with my husband and two friends, we started the North Herts Satellite Grand Prix tournament, a satellite tournament of the National Grand Prix events, and I became a Tournament Organiser. This has run ever since, although I now live in Cornwall.

We moved to the St Austell area in 2003. I joined the St Austell Table Tennis Club and on my first night was greeted by a player who I had known for years as he used to play in all the junior tournaments and I had umpired for him many times. He was now a senior county player, who lived in Cornwall, but the friendly greeting was a delight and a great surprise - I had been remembered! After a year at the club, the secretary resigned and no one came forward to do the job. When I returned from holiday I was asked if I would consider taking it on and said yes. Without a secretary, in the table tennis world, a club cannot exist, so it was that or no club! I am still in post! I attend meetings, take minutes, help arrange the league teams, keep a register of all players in the club, have got the club registered as a Premier Club with Table Tennis England (the governing body), run club nights, play at club nights, do a bit of coaching, play in the league and go to the County Committee. I am now Cornwall's National Councillor and attend the National Council meetings four times a year at Milton Keynes. A year or so later the League Secretary resigned and I was asked to take that on too. There was a league to organise, a handbook to write, minutes to do and members to keep track of. My table tennis family was still growing, it was fun, I enjoyed doing it and I was still putting something back into the sport that has given me so much. Long may it continue.

Table tennis *is* fun. You can play it in all weathers, after dark and at any age. It's good exercise and keeps you young!

Diana Jermyn, County Table Tennis Centre

My name is Ian Wilson and I am 72 and until last year was still playing hockey. I first started playing hockey at the Duke of York's Royal Military School near Dover in Kent. The boarding school was for boys whose fathers were serving in, or had served in the army. Sport was an important part of life at a boarding school and I was able to play in the school team, although hockey was only played during one term in the winter.

When I qualified as a geologist my travels took me overseas and playing hockey was limited. Living in Brazil for three years was mainly playing cricket in Sao Paulo as there was no hockey team at the time. I settled in Cornwall but was an overseas geologist for English China Clays taking me to many countries. In Cornwall I played for Newquay and Truro and on returning to Cornwall played for Bodmin, now my current club. At the age of 62 I joined the England LX Club (Over 60s) and also played for the West Over 60s and subsequently Over 65s and Over 70s in the Regional Tournament. LX hockey is very good as enables you to keep playing.

I was fortunate enough to play for LX Club in European and World Cup matches in the Tournament Trophy Competitions. I played in the World Cups in Germany (2006), Hong Kong (2008), Cape Town (2010), Oxford (2012) and The Hague (2014). I have also played for LX team in Australia and Argentina and European Cups in Canterbury (UK), Holland, Belgium and Germany. Unfortunately, I had a stroke in 2014 but I am recovering very well. I am getting back to fitness now and hope to play hocked in 2016 again. Hockey has always been an important part of my life and I look forward to playing again. I have been married for 43 years now and I met my wife Kate in 1967 playing mixed-hockey at University of Leeds. So I encourage all to keep playing sport as long as you can.

Ian Wilson, President of Bodmin Hockey Club & Cornwall Hockey Association

Rewind 12 years and I was your typical sport-shy teenager who was terrible at PE and did everything I could to avoid it throughout my time at school, usually somewhat successfully! By some stroke of luck, a fast metabolism and a general liking for being outdoors I managed to reach my final year at college without being morbidly obese. This was despite my love of food, passionate avoidance of anything which resembled sport and having never stepped foot in a gym.

All things considered, at 18-years-old I was in pretty good shape and while I certainly lacked any discernable muscle mass, I was by no means fat and had a good 'blank canvas' on which to develop. Not that this was a concern or priority at the time. Half way through my final year at college, a friend introduced me to his latest new craze. He was the type who was always finding creative new ways to hurt him and Parkour was his new sport of choice. The conversation went something like this:

Grant: "I've started a new sport called freerunning!"

Me: "Is that like going for a jog with no clothes on?"

Grant: "No, it's more like jumping and climbing stuff."

He sent me a link to a website which had photos of people jumping between railings in London landing on the narrowest of surfaces with huge drops below. It seemed mad, insane and borderline suicidal and whilst I could think of many, many reasons why I would never want to do this, somehow there was something undeniably appealing and powerful about the concept which was now firmly rooted in the back of my mind. The idea that it is just you and the city: no rules, no limits, no safety nets. Just your own mind and body and the environment in front of you. The ultimate freedom of expression.

After a brief moment of reflective thought, I casually dismissed this craze as another one of my friend's crazy activities and thought little more of it. However, a week later I happened to have the TV on one evening and caught the introduction to a documentary on Channel 4 which was talking about the origins of parkour and the philosophy behind it. The programme was called Jump London. Channel 4's biggest budget documentary of 2003. I watched the whole thing through and by the end, I was hooked. All my doubts, worries and questions had been answered. It may have taken me 18 years but I had finally found a sport which captured my imagination.

The great thing about parkour is it has very few barriers to entry. It didn't require any expensive purchases of clothing or equipment; in that respect, it was risk-free. With other new sports, I might have been reluctant to make the commitment to a big financial outlay to purchase boards or equipment which would then go unused if I changed my mind a few weeks later but with this I already had everything I needed. I started practicing parkour in early 2014 not long after watching Jump London and for the first 6 months, my progress was slow. I had no one local to train with, nowhere to seek advice, and no previous experience to fall back on. It was very much a case of getting out there and doing it, falling over, picking myself up and trying again whilst attempting to learn from mistakes along the way. Parkour/ Free running would not be where it was today without the internet. Jump London brought the concept to the masses but it would not have been able to reach out and influence so many people without the hundreds of teams and individuals who built websites, created discussion forums and shared their videos and experiences with the world.

In October 2004, I moved to a new city to start a four year university course which gave me the opportunity to meet new people, see new places and crucially get to know the local parkour team who were just as dedicated as I was and had lots of new knowledge and skills to share. In this new environment, with not a lot of money but lots of free time, some new friends and a new city to explore, parkour became my way of life and was pretty much what I lived and breathed whenever I wasn't studying. We would go out and train in the city every day of the week at all times of day and night always looking to push ourselves further and finding out the limits of what we were truly capable of. It was an exciting adventure and being in a team with likeminded people made learning new moves many times faster than when I was training alone.

I think it is fair to say that parkour changed me as a person. Between the start of my journey in 2004 and when I left uni in 2008, I conquered fears and achieved things which I would not have previously thought possible. I took up other sports, took an active interest in nutrition and eating properly and gained huge amounts of confidence which extended into other areas of my life. I had become one of the founding members of the largest parkour / free running team in Berkshire, trained and became friends with some of the top free running athletes in the country as well as starring in two parkour documentaries, "Jump Britain", the ch4 sequel to Jump London and "Parkour: Way of Life" a DVD which sold millions of copies across the world.

After graduating and moving back to Devon, I wanted to take the knowledge and experiences I had gained whilst at uni and share the skills I had learnt with new people who wanted to have a go at parkour/ free running. My vision was to create an indoor space with obstacles and mats where people could train all year round without being affected by the weather and have access to equipment which would allow them to practice techniques which would be too risky or undesirable to try outside first time. In May 2011, the vision was realised and Street Motion was born. Operating from a small dance studio at a secondary school in Exeter, once a week on a Wednesday evening we started the first free running academy in Devon and never looked back since!

Dominic Rott, StreetMotion

I gave birth to my daughter in June 2014 and was keen to start exercising again; I soon realised that the logistics of exercising with a new baby was a lot easier said than done! The cost of childcare added to the cost of an exercise class was so much that it just wasn't feasible and the other option of exercising at home using a DVD was often advised however I know that I am not the only one who lacks motivation when I am on my own. I had heard of Buggyfit whilst doing my degree and although at that time I didn't have children I was interested to find out about it as loved that the classes were not only great at getting Mums active, the classes were held outdoors in parks and public spaces which can be really beneficial for improving a person's mental health.

With this in mind and with nothing on offer in my area I got in touch with Buggyfit and signed up to do the course. You need to have at least a Level 2 Fitness Instructor qualification to take on a Buggyfit franchise and I was also reminded that a sense of humour is a must. Buggyfit has been a brilliant opportunity not only for me to be able to exercise, work and take my daughter along but the feedback I have got from the Mums has also been really positive. I run four sessions a week in different locations, all outside so Mums are reminded to bring their buggy rain covers and wrap the babies up warm. These are some of the comments I have received from the Mums in my class.

"I really wanted to get fit after having my boys but was nervous about starting a class as thought I would be the slowest and most unfit, I was also scared that I would have to run which I just can't do. Contacting Nel she reassured me that the classes were aimed at beginners and there is not any running in her classes so I went along. The classes as great fun and she does make us work and get a bit of a sweat on! I have been with her for 13 weeks now and really cannot believe the difference in my energy and fitness levels from just an hour a week. My posture

has improved as she really drums into us the way in which we should be pushing the buggies properly"

"Buggyfit to me has meant I get an hour a week to do something for myself, the group is really friendly and it is great to swap tips on feeding and coping with a new baby. The class has meant I have regained my fitness levels so feel confident in going back to my previous exercise classes."

"Buggyfit to me has really been a fun way to lose the baby weight and meet other Mum's in the area. I love that the babies laugh at us doing our exercises and some of the older ones try and do the exercises with us whilst sitting in their buggies."

Nel Savage, Buggyfit

I started training the art of capoeira in London 2007, when I first saw the BBC ident of 2 guys on a rooftop gracefully throwing kicks and moving into cartwheels. I knew that was what I wanted to do. I was so lucky to find those actual teachers and who are now my (metres) masters today. Through training I have gone through finding out about myself, my body, pushing through setbacks such as finding moves/sequences difficult. I have wanted to quit training many times, but also have been addicted and never will quit. The social training of capoeira has given me so much, you admire students who have trained longer and want to move like them. Through camaraderie, you become great friends.

I began teaching in Cornwall 6 years ago through my Master who gave me the opportunity. My group's lineage goes back as old as capoeira and I am very proud of this and teach this to my students. Capoeira is so much more to me as I have seen it help so many different people. From getting fit/flexible, losing weight, building confidence and even finding friends. Teaching is the most rewarding thing and I feel privileged to be in the position I am. I have worked with so many beautiful people from children to kids and adults with learning disabilities including severely disabled. To see the glimmer in someone's eyes when they understand what you are teaching, understand how much capoeira gives them or see the passion when I express myself through my art, it gives me a feeling of such joy that I can't even put into words. Through capoeira, I have developed my fitness, flexibility, rhythm and timing. I have learned about the body and anatomy, have learned about the mind and not giving up and pursuing through struggle. I have travelled the world and met so many beautiful people. It has totally moulded me and my life and I owe it a lot. I encourage anyone to find something in their life that they are passionate about. Art for me is expressing yourself. So anything from exercise to music or painting will help you develop so much, and you will literally find yourself enriched with a new energy.

Josh Kana, Apêiara Capoeira Cornwall

In September 2013, I found myself watching The Great North Run in a mental health hospital. Until then I was unaware of the effect of mental illness on oneself and family and friends. I was probably like many people who have never had personal experience; totally ignorant of how debilitating it could be. I listened to wonderful stories and told staff that next year I was going to get fit and run it for MIND.

In previous months, I had messages from Niall who was recruiting players to join Devon and Cornwall's only Gaelic Football team Plymouth Parnells. I was always too busy, then I had my breakdown. When I got out of hospital, I was encouraged to come along to a training session. On getting home from hospital, I was such a nightmare for family and friends, who were so kind but I was really struggling. A few days after, I jumped on a bus and headed to Plymouth to catch a training session with Parnells. That day was to have such a positive effect on aiding my recovery. There was a great bunch of lads who made me feel welcome and over the next few months offered me the encouragement to get active. Gaelic Football is a sport I have always played and this familiarity was priceless. It was great to be part of a team and on that pitch, I felt myself and felt so positive. I started running and getting fitter and I managed to complete The Great North Run as I had promised the following September. For me, this was an incredible achievement in a world of "constant failures' which seem to blight the mind of someone who struggles with depression.

With this, I came off my anti-depressants and found exercise was a natural substitute. They are necessary and invaluable for most people but I personally found they totally numbed my train of thought and dealings with life. Three years later and I still really struggle but I have not done as much exercise in recent months and writing this makes me realise that it is time to get back on track. It is making me realise how important exercise is maintaining a healthier balanced outlook in life. For me, Plymouth Parnells were central to my recovery, my advice is get those trainers on and get active, join a class, a group, a club, a friend... Set small goals. Go for it and enjoy...life is not a Dress Rehearsal!

Shaun McDermott, Plymouth Parnells

I first learnt to sail when I was a young boy at Restronguet Sailing Club, near to where I grew up. We started sailing in dinghy's which is a great way to learn how to read the sea and wind, and then balance the sail and rudder to get the most speed and manoeuvrability from your boat. I have always loved sailing because there is always something to do, like adjusting the sails to get the best use of every breath of wind.

As I grew, I moved up to bigger and more comfortable sailing in yachts with cockpits, for both comfort and safety on longer passages. I now sail a 29ft yacht that has taken me to Ireland, France, Guernsey and the Scillies to date. I really like that you have to go at a pace that is dictated by the wind, tide and your hull. You can watch the world go by, enjoying the view as you go past Newlyn Mousehole, Tater Du and Longships en route to the Scillies or round the Roseland en route to Fowey where the view changes daily, but hasn't changed for centuries. There is a total freedom in that the only limiting factor of how far you can go is the amount of food and water you have on board, because you are in the endless ocean. That is, until the weekend is over and you have to return to work - until next weekend!

Simon Scholes

In 1986, I was asked to go game shooting by a friend and join a small syndicate; I had some experience with shooting pigeon on my father's farm when I was in my teens. I applied for a shotgun certificate and eventually purchased my first Beretta shotgun. The game season is only 4 months of the year, but I was hooked and now I owned my own shotgun, I wanted to carry on shooting, so decided to shoot Clays, and I joined a small Skeet club in Hemel Hampstead, Hertfordshire.

My work was very stressful; I was a general manager of a very busy business hotel in Watford, going clay shooting was the best release of stress.

The more I shot clays the better I became, winning several little local competitions. I joined the Clay Pigeon shooting association (CPSA), I shot my first major Skeet competition, the English open and ended with a score of 96/100. I loved the sport to the point of wanting to change my career from hotel management to owning my clay shooting ground. With most people this would be a dream but I wanted to make it into a reality.

In 1989, the CPSA were doing courses for shooting ground owners to become professional instructors, I informed them that I wanted to purchase a shooting ground and wanted to do this course but was told that I couldn't pass the exam as I wasn't a ground owner, but they would let me do it for experience only. The course was intense and very demanding, but I excelled and the 12 ground owners doing the course said that I was the best pupil and should be the one to pass this very difficult course. The last day a competition was held and the instructors of the course also joined in the shooting. I didn't only beat all 12 candidates but also the 3 instructors who ran the course. I had to coach for one year on different shooting grounds before getting my certificate in 1990.

I purchased Lower Lake shooting ground in June 1991. It's a beautiful shooting ground situated in the heart of the most beautiful country side of Cornwall, and it's also on the border with Devon. The ground has a picturesque view, the topography makes it ideal for simulating high and challenging targets. I developed the valley and introduced high towers. Now it's the most successful shooting school in Cornwall.

Having shot most all my life with an over/under shotgun, I found it difficult to take a side by side (s/s) shotgun from a client and shoot it myself, I decided in 1994 to spend a year practicing and shooting only with a side by side, that year I won the English open and British open skeet with the s/s and shot 150/150 in the British open a record that had never been done before and nor since up to now.

I enjoy all form of shooting, but skeet is my passion. I can compete in skeet at the highest level; I have been a member of the winning England team for the last 3 years.

If you want to achieve a high standard in any sport, you must have good coaching and lots of practice. Good luck.

Bill, Shooting In Cornwall

"I started gig rowing because I had moved to Cornwall and seen rowing out at sea on various coastal walks and thought it looked interesting. A man at work happened to be involved at Padstow Rowing Club, and so I went along to a beginner's session and was soon hooked. The rest, as they say, is history.

My highlights of gig rowing are definitely, but not limited to:

- A great group of friends! We all get on well, because we all row for each other and know we can rely on each other, as we have rowed in some scary sized waves and got back into the harbour safely (if a little wet!).

- The great sense of achievement when we do really well in a race. We are all really competitive and push really hard, whatever the weather conditions.

- A gig event is a wonderful day out; as we sit on the beach, eat cake and race against some amazing competition. Rowers bring their husbands/wives/children and enjoy the day together.

- The rowing is so exhausting, but so exhilarating eg. rowing out alongside Fowey harbour front or racing back into the beach at Marazion beside St. Michael's Mount, or racing in the Camel Estuary from Daymer Bay. Each event is beautifully scenic and a fun day out with your friends and family.

- We have the annual World Championships held on the Isles of Scilly, where 140+ gig boats will line up at St. Agnes and race back into St. Mary's harbour. The noise as the starter shouts "go" over the VHF is deafening as every rower, aided by much shouting by their cox, heave the boats into action followed by 20ish minutes of sweat, blood and blisters, before rounding the harbour wall and collapsing in your seat. It is the most amazing way to start the weekend and each one is memorable no matter how many times you have done it. The pubs are filled with rowers from clubs from as far as Bermuda, the USA and Holland come to join us in the post-rowing celebrations every night.

- The teamwork that is required to get a crew together for each training session, with a cox and to row out into the sea; whether a calm beautiful evening or a more wild evening as we crash down over the peaks into the troughs. We all keep rowing as a team and that way we all get through it, together. We enjoy the highs and lows as a crew, if we have a hard day at work, or at home, we get in a boat and we work our hardest with support from the rest of the crew.

- Lastly, it is the only sport where you can sit down and wear wellies whilst getting the most amazing cardio full body workout!"

Elizabeth Scholes

Here is what some of our active players say about floorball:

"I started playing floorball when I was 19, after playing football for 15 years. The fast pace of floorball keeps you not only physically fit but is a great team sport, demanding a high level of sportsmanship and camaraderie. After running a team in Finland for 8 years, when I moved to England I was keen to maintain my passion and have thoroughly enjoyed being part of Bristol FUC and watching it go from strength to strength. Friendship is a big part of our team, making it fun both on and off the ring." -**Jani Osterlund, Finland**

"The first time I came in contact with floorball was when I was at about six years of age, moving to Sweden. I got immediately hooked on it and have played ever since. For many years, I had the chance to play competitively, which has been great and formed many good memories and friendships. After arriving in the UK, I had the pleasure of joining the Bristol FUC, which has been another great experience. The fascination of floorball to me is that it's a combination of simplicity and complexity. Everyone can play with minimum equipment and preparation but you feel immediately that there is so much to learn individually and as a team with your mates. It's a beautiful game!" -**Jussi Halmetoja, Finland-Sweden**

"I enjoy floorball a lot because it combines a team sport with an intense workout. You get physically tired without notice because it is so quick, no time to think. Afterwards, you feel good. I like floorball for the fact that you have to communicate well, and help each other improve and I like to do socials outside the training sessions, to get to know more people or to get to know people better." -**Joost Iwema, Netherlands**

"I come from a field hockey background and in floorball, I am challenged to use the backside of the blade of my stick. I played in the Scottish league before and currently I am playing in the South league with Bristol FUC. I like the floorball because it's fun and fast sport." -**Robert Bragg, England**

"I started to play floorball around 18 years ago back in Finland where the sport is hugely popular. To me, it's a great team sport, which definitely keeps me fit. The social part of it is also important and you can really see that the better you know the guys you play with, the better you perform as a team." –**Jukka Hautamaki, Finland. Jukka, Bristol Floorball & Unihocky Club**

"I started working at Kernow Wake Park in March 2014. I had never wakeboarded in my life! Alex Sly, who owns the park, met me when I worked in Sessions Surf Shop back in 2013 and I remember asking Alex was he sure he wants to hire me as I had never wakeboarded in my life and how could I teach something I couldn't do?
I never thought I'd pick it up. How wrong I was. It wasn't as hard as I thought, I had great coaches and it's so progressive, I always had something to learn. I've been trying to surf for the last 3 years and wakeboarding is just so much more progressive. Since working in a surf shop, working at a wake park and trying to be a part of these extreme sports I've noticed how hard it is for girls to be a part of it. It's a man's world and only recently have both sports started to have girls as a part of it. I remember seeing wakeboarding when I went to Australia but it was quite intimidating with all boys sitting on the dock laughing at each other with loud music and everyone looking rather 'cool'.
This is what Alex didn't want Kernow Wake park to be like and why he hired me; because I was a girl. It makes it less intimidating and we make an effort for families, ladies and everyone to feel comfortable and at ease.

339

1 year later and I don't think I could love anything as much as teaching and wakeboarding.

In September 2014, I won Grass Roots lady's open category; this was a huge achievement for me, I was over the moon. I felt a lot of pressure being a girl and being the girl that worked at the wakepark but I wanted to prove to myself that I could do it and give it a go.

It might be a male dominated sport but ladies night is our busiest night and we sure are trying to give the boys a run for their money! I love it and I'm so happy I didn't shy away from it.

Katy, Kernow WakePark

Chapter 16 - Get Involved

If you would like to try something, here is a list of contacts. If you do give something new a try, I would love to hear about it. Please tweet me @sofadodgeruk, find SofaDodger on Facebook or you can email me at sam@sofadodger.co.uk

- British Nordic Walking
- England Short Mat Bowling Association, Welsh Short Mat Bowling Association, Scottish Short Mat Bowls Federation, Links to Bowling in Northern Ireland
- GB Boxing
- England Cricket Board, Cricket Scotland, Cricket Wales, Northern Cricket Union
- English Petanque
- British Baseball Association
- The British Wheel of Yoga
- Croquet Association
- British Stand Up Paddle Association
- The British Horse Society
- British Fencing
- Powerhoop UK
- Badminton England, Badminton Scotland, Badminton Wales, Ulster Badminton
- GoCanoe
- British Gymnastics
- Tai Chi Union for Great Britain

- England Handball
- British Rowing
- British Aikido Board
- Rounders England
- British American Football Association
- British Athletics
- UK Tang Soo Do
- British Krav Maga Association
- British Orienteering
- GB Archery page
- National Ice Skating Association
- Angling Trust
- England Korfball, The Scottish Korfball Association, Welsh Korfball
- Surf Lifesaving GB
- Pilates Foundation
- Fitsteps
- National Fitness Day
- Special Olympics
- GB Boccia
- British Judo Association
- UK Dodgeball Association
- English Lacrosse
- BarreConcept
- UK Climbing
- UK Karting
- The Football Association
- Roller Sports Foundation

- England Netball Association website, Netball Scotland, Welsh Netball, Netball Northern Ireland
- English Karate Federation, Scottish Karate Federation, Wales Karate Federation, Northern Ireland Karate Board
- Piloxing
- British Cheerleading Association
- Get Into Golf
- England's RFU, Scottish Rugby, Welsh Rugby Union, Ulster Rugby
- TRX
- Lawn Tennis Association
- English Association of Snooker and Billiards, Welsh Snooker and Billiards Association, Scottish Snooker, Northern Ireland Snooker and Billiards Association.
- Gymcube
- Clubbercise
- Kettlercise
- Table Tennis England, Table Tennis Scotland, Table Tennis Wales, Irish Table Tennis Association
- CrossFit
- British Gymnastics
- Volleyball England, The Scottish Volleyball Association, Volleyball Wales, Northern Ireland Volleyball
- British Kickboxing Council
- England Squash & Racquetball Association, Scottish Squash Association, Wales Squash & Racquetball, Ulster squash
- Zumba
- Walking Football United

- British Wrestling
- GB Wheelchair Rugby Website
- Basketball England, Basketball Scotland, Basketball Wales, Basketball Northern Ireland
- England Hockey, Scottish Hockey, Hockey Wales, Ulster Hockey
- British Ski & Snowboard
- Parkour UK
- Buggyfit
- Provincial Council of Britain GAA website
- British Swimming
- Royal Yachting Association
- UK Ultimate
- The British Octopush Association
- British Shooting
- Cornish Pilot Gig Association
- UK Floorball Federation
- British Cycling
- British Water Ski & Wakeboard

Chapter 17 – Thanks

Thank you to all of the clubs, instructors and coaches who helped me with my challenge and they include:

Kelly at Walk Kernow

Blisland Short Mat Bowls Club

Bodmin Amateur Boxing Club

Wadebridge Cricket Club

The Core in Falmouth

Tregony Pentanque Club

Torbay Barons

Cornwall Yoga Centre

Cornwall Croquet Club

VixyStrawberry

Extreme Academy

Nina Rogers & Spot the Horse

Truro Fencing Club

Funfit Dianne

St Austell Bay Badmin Club,

St Austell Canoe Club

The Callywith Centre

Green Man Tai Chi

Newquay Handball Club

Mike at Priority 1 Fitness

Caste Dore Rowing Club

TBAA Aikido Cornwall

Devon & Cornwall Wild Swimming

Cornish Sharks

East Cornwall Harriers

ISK Martial Arts

Kernow Martial Arts

Cornwall Orienteering Club

St Austell Bay Archers

Mad Ferrett

Atlantic Reach

Plymouth Ice Skating Club

Roche Angling Club

Exeter Korfball

Polzeath Surf Life Saving Club

Iconik Dance & Fitness

Tempus Leisure

Cornwall Segway

Special Olympics Cornwall

Camelford Judo Club

Bedford Mighty Eagles

Hatch End Hawks

The Keay Studios

Magjic Wood Climbing

St Eval Karting Circuit

Dobwalls Ladies FC

Plymouth Skating Club

Bodmin Netball Club

Byrne Black Belt Academy

The Retallack Resort

Tara at Versatile Fitness Choice

West Coast Cheerleading

Lanhydrock Golf Club

Liskeard Leopards Ladies Rugby

Bodmin Dragon Tennis

Clubbercise Plymouth

St Austell Table Tennis Club

CrossFit Newquay

Kernow Volleyball

Bodmin Squash Club

Cornish Wrestling

West Country Hawks

Bodmin Dragons Hockey Club

Plymouth Ski Slope & Snowboard Centre

StreetMotion

Nel's Buggyfit

Dorchester Athletics Club

Apêiara Capoeira Cornwall

Plymouth Parnells

St Austell Water Polo Club

Liz & Simon for letting me on board Lady P

Devon Ultimate Frisbee Club

Kingsbirdge Krays

Shooting in Cornwall

Padstow Rowing Club

Bristol Floorball & Unihockey Club

Limitless Mpr

Kernow Wake Park

www.ingramcontent.com/pod-product-compliance
Lightning Source LLC
Chambersburg PA
CBHW071328280526
45787CB00001B/31